W9-BNE-974

College Health

JOHN E. EICHENLAUB, M.D.

College Health

THE MACMILLAN COMPANY – NEW YORK
A DIVISION OF THE CROWELL-COLLIER PUBLISHING COMPANY

First Printing

Library of Congress catalog card number: 62-10638

The Macmillan Company, New York
Brett-Macmillan Ltd., Galt, Ontario

Printed in the United States of America

PREFACE

Health teachers dream vainly of students with an avid thirst for knowledge, and spend a disproportionate share of their energies trying to whip up interest or motivation. Part of this problem seems inevitable. Any required course has two strikes against it. A required course which many students expect to reiterate the hated brush-your-teeth injunctions of the recently-thrown-off parental domination has further handicaps. Moreover, a health course must take up and emphasize facts according to their ultimate importance to the student, not according to his established interests.

However, part of the motivational difficulty in health courses stems, in my opinion, from orientation and presentation of facts in a somewhat didactic rather than an empathic, emotionally acceptable way. Health textbooks traditionally state facts pragmatically, establish their importance through statistics, and express applications as thinly veiled injunctions. Popularized material traditionally sets a helpful tone and creates interest before even approaching intricate facts, relates everything to reader self-interest rather than incomprehensible population entities, and concludes with either how-to-do-it directions or (if any prior convictions or contrary behavior patterns are involved) with an impartial marshaling of facts.

After teaching health to several thousand students and discussing individual health problems at length in countless Health Service hours, I decided that there was a middle ground between the traditional academic approach and the popular writer's method. This book is the result. The problem was first, to decide exactly what should go into the book on educational grounds —what health facts and ideas would prove most helpful to students throughout their entire lives—and second, to apply every acceptable technique from the field of popular writing to make that material more clearly cogent, helpful and interesting. The content is the result of my own ideas and a nationwide survey involving teachers in over 200 institutions. The actual presentation follows the freer rules of you've-got-to-sell-them-again-in-each-paragraph-or-they-won't-read-on popular writing.

I have largely avoided direct statements recommending specific attitudes or behavior, particularly when any large number of students might be presumed to hold contrary views or follow different practices. This seeming omission results from my strong feeling that a textbook has a limited place in total instruction, and largely vitiates its effectiveness when it tries to do too much. Health *courses* involve human interplay and educational participation through which attitudes and behavior can often be effectively molded. Health *textbooks* can provide the background for classroom discourse and suggest educational activities, but cannot achieve the give-and-take relationship needed to influence prejudiced or previously misguided people. The absence of authoritarian statements and preachy pronouncements does not mean that I lack convictions or that I regard faulty attitudes and behavior patterns as beyond range of attack in the classroom. It merely means that a summary of pros and cons to permit classroom debate seems more likely to affect attitudes and behavior than an injunction to quit smoking, eat properly, or wave banners for the economic status quo.

This book generally follows the well-established principle that education should present the ideal course, not compromises. It emphasizes the establishment of relations with a personal physician and stresses the need to consult him with every illness of consequence. The book includes absolutely no home remedies or home treatments of any kind, and recommends consultation with a physician or marriage counselor in the event of sexual or marital difficulties.

Now as to techniques. My first consideration has been *empathic presentation.* In approaching every subject, I have asked myself: "In what way does an individual college student feel concerned about this?" Not: "How is he concerned?" because I would then be tempted to answer in terms of risks and effects which only an expert acknowledges rather than in terms of genuine, motivationally useful interests. I have not asked myself: "How should he be concerned?" because this would put me in the position of basing my approach upon the very health consciousness and community consciousness which seem deficient. I have tried to use the student's own viewpoint and interest as an entering wedge for each set of facts. The approach to old age, for instance, is through problems students are likely to encounter with older relatives and difficulties for which they themselves must prepare, not through statistical consideration of a vast, impersonal aggregate known as "the aged." This book introduces the problem of tuberculosis from the standpoint of seemingly healthy individuals (with whom the students can readily identify) who want to keep down the disease's ravages rather than from the standpoint of the community's program for hospitalizing advanced cases. I sincerely hope that this approach, which takes the reader by the hand in the here and now, leads him to see how these tremendous problems could affect *him* and others. I hope that it will interest him in community action to lessen the burdens of those already afflicted. Certainly, it has a better chance of doing so than the traditional statistical or nonempathic approach, which tacitly assumes the very community interest which it is trying to create as the fulcrum for all motivational leverage.

Another technique which may need explanation is journalistic foreshadowing; that is headings and lead sentences or paragraphs to point up the applicability or usefulness of the ensuing material. Many passages start by "telling them what good it's going to do them to read on." By planting the idea of possible applications in advance, this method makes the main exposition more interesting and useful, while no extra wordage is consumed (since terminal discussion of applications becomes unnecessary).

A further departure is deliberate variation in structure, person, etc. to enhance interest. Although the ease of finding a given fact by its location in a precisely systematized treatment justifies pedantic regularity in a reference book, the author believes that variation in phrasing and structure adds desirable interest in a book which is meant to be read instead of consulted. Therefore, this book uses "the mass audience you," occasional anecdotes or personal references, and several other techniques which have been long accepted in general usage, even though they are somewhat foreign to texts.

Since certain subjects (e.g. heredity, community programs of medical finance) can be presumed to suit only the more deeply interested and able groups, while others (e.g. physiology of reproduction, complexion problems) are too fundamental for advanced groups but very necessary for certain students, the level of difficulty in this book is not completely uniform. I have tried to suit difficulty to the student group which seems likely to utilize each portion of the text rather than allow the innate difficulty of the material presented to govern reading level. This deliberate variation in level conforms with the general use of a textbook as a resource rather than as a literary entity, and should permit its use by groups with widely different background and objectives.

Incidentally, I have tried to use short sentences, a march rather than a jumble of ideas, and the simplest terminology consistent with clarity at *all* levels. One will have to appraise level mainly by the depth of material presented and the nature of the facts rather than by reading level, which seems well within the grasp of all college freshmen.

Since a textbook should allow the teacher to present subjects in any order he desires, and to omit some topics altogether, I have made each passage essentially independent of all others, even at the price of some duplication. This amounts to only a few hundred words throughout the book, however, and seems worthwhile for the sake of the extra teaching latitude it provides.

Perhaps specific comment on deviations from the traditional approach in each chapter of this book might serve to clarify their purpose. In Chapter One, the self-quiz aims at showing the practical value of the course content, and that previous household and high school instruction haven't really done the job in addition to its stated purpose. Chapter Two uses the newly independent student's self-interest to bestir his interest in housing, environmental safety, and food sanitation rather than approach these subjects purely as community problems. Chapters Three, Four, and Five use problems the student has or might develop to secure his interest and try to build his awareness of mental illness and his concern about it both on a personal and community level. Chapters Six and Seven also put primary emphasis on situations and problems the reader might encounter. They attempt to introduce him to the larger aspects of sedative and stimulant addictions in a way which makes these things a personal concern to him. They lay the groundwork for classroom discussion and educational exercises aimed at molding attitudes, influencing behavior, and creating interest in community measures to control abuse, but do not attempt any exhortations. In my experience, positive anti-alcohol or anti-smoking injunctions make most college students classify their promulgator as a blue-nosed prig and ignore everything that is said, while a presentation which allows students to participate in evaluation of the facts often has real impact on their attitudes and behavior.

Chapter Eight will probably prove of interest mainly to fairly well-qualified, science-minded students who want health knowledge rather than pure guidance. For this group, the straight physiological approach seems apt. The prevailing lack of background in the area of heredity makes such an approach almost necessary, anyhow. The remainder of the hormone-reproduction-parenthood material centers on clearly felt reader-problems.

The food choice chapter deserves special comment. Most college students do not plan their own meals. Instruction in nutrition according to the classic Basic Seven or Basic Four plan therefore proves impossible to apply except either retrospectively (in deciding that last week's diet was or was not adequate) or at some distant future date. The student simply cannot make out a properly varied menu and then secure the recommended foodstuffs. He eats what the dormitory, lodging house, or family provides and regards the nutrition lesson as something rather divorced from reality when it is phrased in daily diet terms.

On the other hand, students *can* control some elements of their diet. If one can teach nutrition in terms which help them to choose a snack that fills out their nutritional needs or select a proper diet meal by meal from a cafeteria line, there is at least a chance that they will put those lessons to work. Lessons applied in daily living stick with you, while lessons filed away in a desk drawer for use years hence rarely see the light of day. Thus the "count 4–5–5" plan on pages 168–70, which worked well with the several thousand patients whom I handled while in charge of the University of Minnesota's nutrition clinic for students. This plan takes up eating in one-meal units to aid students in filling out requirements as they go along instead of dealing in terms of daily food values which students usually find unmanageable.

Chapters Eighteen, Nineteen, and Twenty use enlightened self-interest to motivate both learning and behavior in the field of infectious disease. Once again, I hope that insight and concern developed through personal appreciation of a problem will develop into awareness of and concern over the community aspects thereof, and feel confident that classroom discussion and educational exercises can achieve this result. The traditional presentation *assumes* such awareness, and I believe is largely ineffective in generating it for that reason. You might also note another writing device here: the use of a practical rather than didactic *organization.* The classic division of material according to mode of transmission divides it into entities highly useful to the public health administrator, but accomplishes very little for the man in the streets. Division according to degree of urgency emphasizes the value of this material in general and simultaneously makes a practical point through writing structure alone.

The chronic disease chapters use a physiological approach mainly because healthy young collegians cannot readily identify with the chronically ill. Family problems afford opportunity for enlistment of self-interest as a motivator, and community concern with such problems, receives considerable discussion, too.

In discussing safety, the crying need of most students seems to be safety-consciousness and safety motivation. High school courses, community organizations, and perennial campaigns make almost everyone aware of what should be done in such fields as fire safety, traffic safety, and household precautions. The trick is to get them to do it. Statistics simply do not do the job, especially statistics phrased in terms of accidents per hundred thousand population which do not penetrate the student's mental shield against unbearable anxiety. By coming down hard on safety motivation and on a few major areas in which the student's behavior patterns may not yet be established, Chapter Twenty-four seems to me to accomplish more than statistical analysis or an all-pervasive (and thus necessarily superficial) treatment.

The chapter on health emergencies differs from standard first aid in that it recognizes the resources normally available and tells the student how to use them instead of attempting to make him totally self-sufficient, as most first aid and civil defense training does. In this way, a brief chapter provides rather complete guidance upon urgent health problems instead of giving the whole field of first aid a once-over-lightly. For students who want more detailed knowledge of first aid under circumstances requiring prolonged self-sufficiency, the Red Cross manual makes a suitable supplement.

The three chapters on health facilities and economics prepare students for crucially important decisions in the health sphere. The problems involved are very real and very vexing to people outside the health professions, and deserve considerable emphasis. Once again, I have tried to use enlightened self-interest as the opening wedge for instilling genuine concern with community problems in these regards.

A brief explanation of the chapter arrangement might prove of some interst, even though many teachers may choose to take up subjects in a different order. The first four chapters were put up front because they equip entering freshmen for many of the decisions and problems they face during their first few weeks in school, but with no sacrifice in logical order. The book then moves into personal problems and mental or behavior difficulties, into sex and marriage (where mental and physical problems merge), into bodily health, and into resources the student can call upon in maintaining or restoring health.

Since students can find up-to-date, pertinent data through ordinary library channels without difficulty, and since teachers are always well aware of locally available resource materials, this book does not include a bibliography. In the author's experience, lists of further recommended readings tend to limit the students' inquiry into the full resources of a large library, virtually eliminating his use of periodicals and new accessions, and to create feelings of frustration when recommended books are not available in a small library.

Since students often read without having a dictionary at hand, I have provided a glossary, with special emphasis on technical words not specifically elucidated in the text and words with special meaning in the health context. The index includes many cross-references and synonyms to aid readers in pursuit of specific bits of information.

May I express my thanks for the many helpful comments and reviews which various authorities submitted during the preparation of this book. Whatever degree of freedom from error this book has achieved serves as a monument to these people rather than to myself. Over seventy reviews came through my hands, with at least one expert analysis of every chapter. Since critics enlisted by a publisher's staff traditionally make their comments anonymously, I do not know most of these people's names. I do know the extent of their contribution and want to express my grateful appreciation for it.

Perhaps you will still find elements in this book with which to disagree. If so, please write to me, and join the vast team whose comments have contributed so greatly to this book's usefulness.

TABLE OF CONTENTS

CHAPTER 1

Why Study Health?

WOULD YOU LIKE TO ENJOY MAXIMUM STRENGTH AND ENERGY, FREEDOM FROM illness, and length of life? Would you like to develop stable emotions, a mature, contented viewpoint, and increased mental efficiency? Would you like to achieve respect and acceptance in your community, rewardingly close friendships, the joys of love?

Ideal health is a key to each of these goals. With it you can fully exploit your physical, mental, and social capacities, and bring yourself as close as possible to your many objectives.

What you learn from a course in personal health can make a real difference, too. Admittedly, the courses in health which you have taken so far may have had little effect: your present health is mainly the product of heredity, environmental factors beyond your own range of influence, and practices formed or influenced more by family and community pressures than by logical choice. From college age on, however, your own decisions and practices make a bigger and bigger difference. If you choose to apply the facts about health which this course offers, you can substantially improve your effectiveness in every sphere—mental, physical, and social. You can accomplish more, feel greater satisfaction, and avoid considerable discomfort, disability and unnecessary mortal risk. You can put generations of scientific progress to work in your daily life.

Of course, you can also study this material without getting any benefit from it whatever. You can learn vital facts as pure academic flotsam, explain it, recite it, but never let it affect the way you think or act. Health knowledge *applied* can aid your health in college and throughout the years of your remaining life. It can increase your personal and vocational effectiveness from the moment you acquire it until you die. But nobody can *make* you put it to work for you. Nobody can *make* you change your approach or behavior instead of merely pass your tests.

Science Already Helps Your Health

From mankind's emergence until the nineteenth century, economic and social factors influenced health much more than deliberate application of scientific knowledge. Today, however, science clearly has a profound and dramatic effect on health. And science has made a real difference. For example:

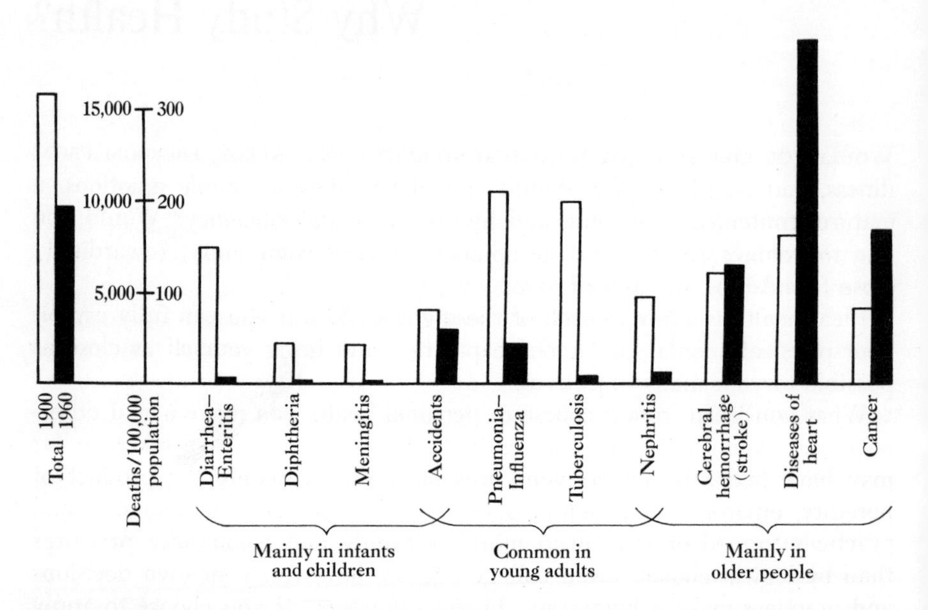

Figure 1. The dramatic reduction in total death rate (left pair of bars) from 1900 (hollow bar) to 1960 (solid bar) is only part of the story. When the top ten causes of death at the turn of the century are arranged by age group commonly afflicted, you can see that tremendous progress has been made against those which strike younger people. The increase in deaths from disorders of the aged is due solely to the increased number of people who reach this age group.

••• Today's college student has a much better outlook for long life and freedom from serious disease than his turn-of-the-century counterpart. The accompanying figure shows the extent of this improvement as reflected in mortality statistics. Note that the number of deaths from every disorder striking mainly among children and young adults has substantially decreased. Some such diseases, like enteritis and diphtheria, have almost disappeared. In a sense, the increase in stroke, heart disease, and cancer reflects health progress, too. These hazards of later years have not actually increased within the affected age group. Stroke, heart disease, and cancer have become more common because more people now live to the age when these conditions frequently strike.

••• School physical examinations reveal substantially fewer physical defects than a generation ago.

••• Students entering college today measure almost two inches taller than those a generation ago, probably mainly because of better nutrition and health care.

Present Knowledge

In the field of health, there is a tremendous lag between knowledge and application. Right now, about one-third of all disability and death occurring before normal retirement age could be prevented through measures already known but not applied. Some of these measures require sacrifice or effort, such as weight reduction, periodic health examination, and a home safety campaign. But many would actually make life easier and more pleasant: better chosen social and recreational pursuits, more variety in food selection, improved light, heat, and ventilation. You can put the most important known health measures to work *right now* for yourself and your family. You need not wait for further research discoveries to cut cancer's death toll by at least one-third: The American Cancer Society says that reasonable alertness and prompt use of measures known today could do that job for you. You need not wait until your community extends its mental hygiene program to every citizen: New outlets and supports are available today. You need not wait for wonderful new tests to reveal the bare beginnings of disease: Methods your doctor already knows can add literally years to your expected life.

Future Discoveries

In all probability, science soon will make substantial progress in the fight against the common remaining fatal or serious diseases. Almost all of these diseases result from the damage of daily living burdens accumulated through the years. They are not like typhoid fever, which scientists can prevent by cleaning up water supplies, nor like pneumonia, which doctors cure after it has struck. Almost certainly, they can be controlled only through changes in daily living habits. Assume for instance that scientists devise dietary rules which effectively ward off hardening of the arteries. You will then be able to avoid crucial bodily changes—changes more likely to kill you than all other diseases and injuries combined—but only if you put the scientists' advice to work in your daily life. No one else will be able to do the job for you, or cure you with these techniques after difficulties have already appeared. You will benefit only if you let science guide your eating habits through the years, even when you feel entirely well.

Your Own Position

A self-scored survey of your own health practices may help to bring these points home. Make two different answer sheets, each with spaces numbered from 1 to 10. Basing your selections entirely on what you actually have done, not what you believe you should do, record answers to these questions on your first sheet:

1 During the last month, the longest you have gone without a bath was: (*a*) 10 days (*b*) 7 days (*c*) 4 days (*d*) 3 days or less.

2 You brush your teeth: (*a*) irregularly (*b*) once a day (*c*) twice a day (*d*) each and every time you eat.

3 In the past 18 months, you have been to your dentist for complete dental attention: (*a*) not at all (*b*) once, within six months (*c*) once, more than six months ago (*d*) on two separate occasions, at roughly six-month intervals.

4 When you read or study, you: (*a*) never sit upright (*b*) rarely sit upright (*c*) usually sit upright, but slouch sometimes for relaxing variety (*d*) always sit upright.

5 The shortest night's sleep you had during the past month was: (*a*) 4 hours or less (*b*) 5 hours (*c*) 6 hours (*d*) 7 hours or more.

6 During the past year, your weight has never been: (*a*) 20 pounds or more above or below the recommended range (see p. 173 if you do not know what your weight should be.) (*b*) 15 to 20 pounds above or below the recommended range (*c*) 10 to 15 pounds above or below the recommended range (*b*) more than 10 pounds above or below the recommended range.

7 On a piece of scratch paper, write down everything you have had to eat in the past 24 hours. Rate your diet as "excellent" if you have consumed at least two servings of meat or eggs, at least one pint of milk, at least three servings of different vegetables, at least two servings of fruit, and at least two servings of food made from whole grain, such as whole wheat bread or breakfast food. Rate your diet "good" if you have fallen one serving short in any division, "fair" if you are short two servings, and "poor" if you are short three servings (extra servings in other divisions cannot be used as substitutes). Your dietary rating is: (*a*) poor (*b*) fair (*c*) good (*d*) excellent.

8 In the last 100 miles which you have traveled by automobile, either as driver or passenger, the vehicle in which you traveled has come to a dead stop for stop signs, obeyed speed laws and followed safe driving practices: (*a*) very seldom (*b*) half the time (*c*) most of the time (*d*) all of the time.

9 You have: (*a*) no personal physician or family doctor (*b*) a personal physician or family doctor whom you have not consulted for five years or more (*c*) a personal physician or family doctor whom you have not consulted for two to five years (*d*) a personal physician or family doctor whom you have consulted within the past two years.

10 The present extent of your health insurance coverage is: (*a*) none (*b*) $8 per day or less for hospital expenses; no medical or surgical (*c*) hospital expense covering at least 80 per cent of usual daily charges; no medical or surgical (*d*) at least 80 per cent of hospital, medical and surgical costs.

When you have finished answering these questions on the basis of what you actually do, take your other answer sheet and go through the same questions once again, but answer in terms of what you believe should be done according to ideal health and safety practice. Most health experts would say that the (*d*) answers are correct. On your second answer sheet, you probably agree with them at least eight out of the ten times. Your actual health practices most likely are somewhat different, though. If you were honest with yourself, you probably have fewer (*d*) answers on your first sheet—possibly only two or three. A marked difference between these scores indicates that you have learned many health facts in a way which makes them stick in your mind, but which does not encourage you to put them into practice. If you learn in the same way now, you will miss most of this course's possible benefits.

Using This Book

If a health fact is to help you live more efficiently and happily, you must apply it now and deliberately keep it at work until it becomes a habit. Moreover, health facts that are working for you automatically make more sense and are easier to learn. Many students report that deliberately finding and adopting applications of health facts makes learning easier and more effective. Here is one approach:

••• At the end of each assignment or class, review the major points and ask: "Is there an issue here I face right now? Or expect to encounter soon?"

••• If "yes," ask: "Should the facts I've just learned change my viewpoint about this issue? If so, how?"

••• Whether your previous ideas were right or wrong, ask next: "Am I doing everything I should about this? Is there some practical, worthwhile way to put these facts to work for me?"

••• If "yes," write down the action you propose to take.

••• Now comes the hard part: pin the memorandum to your calendar dated one week ahead. If you do exactly as you planned during that first week, move the memo next two more weeks ahead. If you arrive at the two-week mark without a breach, move it ahead a month, and if you make it through to that date, move your memo ahead three months. Whenever a check-up date finds you remiss, go back to the start of the progression. Within six months or so, you should have acquired a new health habit.

The more you put health facts to work in your daily life, the more interest you will take in your health studies. You will enjoy your reading and class-work more, learn more, and get more value out of what you learn if you continually apply your new understanding. So constantly seek for applications as you learn, keep your calendar bristling with health memos or use whatever techniques you find effective for revising your health habits, and make this course as worthwhile as possible for yourself!

CHAPTER 2

Selecting Suitable Surroundings

ENVIRONMENT IS A VITAL BUILDING-BLOCK OF HEALTH: IT AFFECTS EVERY FUNCtion of mind and body. Because it is the building-block most easily modified or changed and because you, as a college student, probably have considerable control over key environmental factors for the first time in your life, "selecting suitable surroundings" is a topic of vital concern. The way you exercise that control will affect your health and success throughout life, not just during college years.

ESSENTIAL FACILITIES FOR YOUR ROOM

In choosing accommodations, there are several things to look for:

Sufficient space for sleep and study. Minimum recommended standards [1] provide width of at least seven feet and floor area of at least seventy square feet per occupant, not counting any portion of the room with less than five feet clearance from floor to ceiling.

Brightness and pleasantness. Decent paint or paper; window area at least one-eighth of the floor area.

Cleanliness. Floors and floor coverings in good repair; room thoroughly cleaned at least weekly; at least two clean sheets provided per week.

[1] Standards recommended in this section are taken from a paper presented to the Section on Environmental Health and Safety, American College Health Association, Thirty-sixth Annual Meeting, Los Angeles, California, March 26–29, 1958, by Richard G. Bond, M.S., M.P.H., and Lee D. Stauffer, M.P.H., entitled "Recommended Minimum Health and Safety Standards for Off-campus Student Housing."

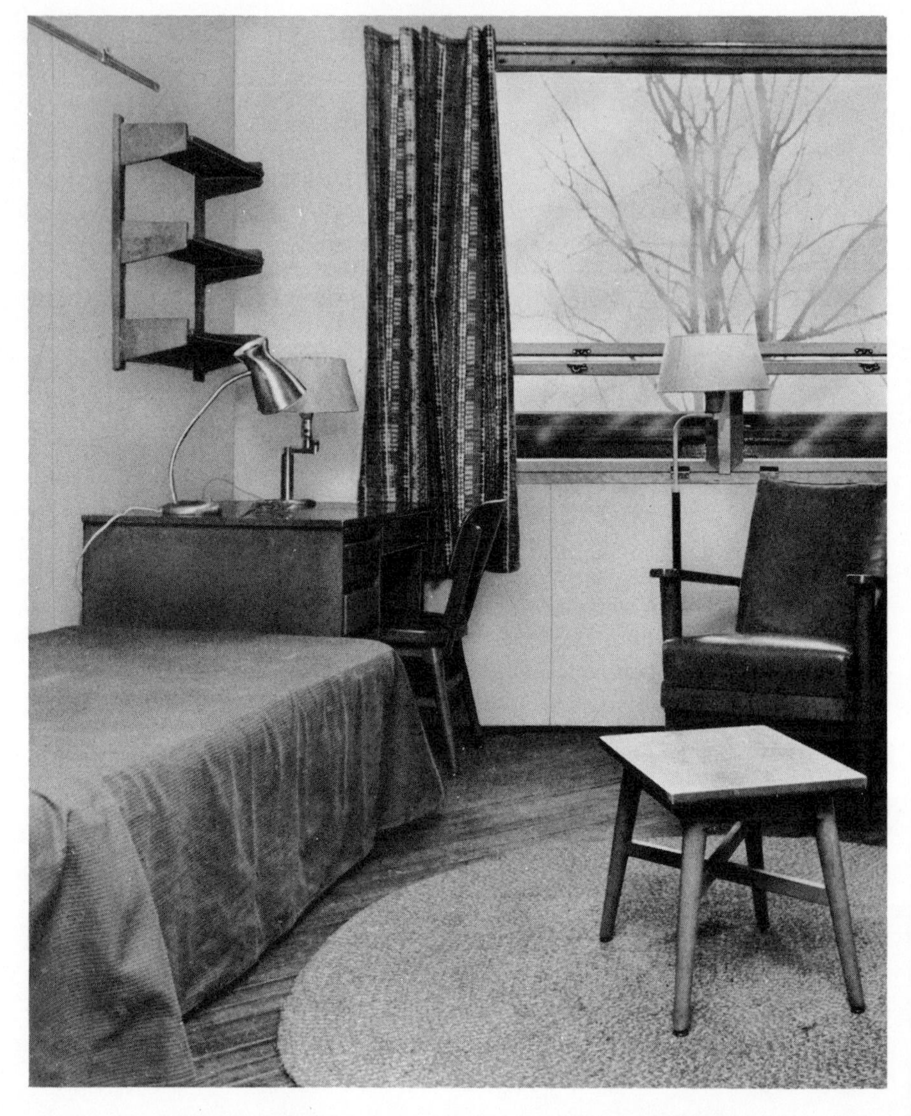

Figure 2. A pleasant place to live—and work. *Gary K. Cowell.*

Heat. Adjustable to meet students' desires; adequate to keep the temperature up to 70° F. at knee height.

Fire safety. Fuses no larger than 15 amperes unless the house has special wiring; at least two ways of getting out of the building, with sturdy stairways located in different portions of the building and unobstructed by furniture or by sometimes-locked doors; no cooking permitted in third-floor units.

Stairways. Well lit, sturdy, with securely fastened tread coverings and sturdy handrail; not steeper than 36 degrees.

Bathroom facilities. At least one tub or shower, lavatory, and toilet for each eight persons; metal or nonbreakable faucet handles (severe hand cuts frequently result when porcelain faucet handles break under pressure); easily cleanable walls and floor.

Furniture. Sturdy bed with a firm, even mattress; desk with a top at least 22″ × 36″; a sturdy study chair; fireproof wastebasket; closet space at least 24″ × 36″; a chest of drawers; a double electrical socket; and adequate lamps (some students provide their own).

Important Extras

Most students find other features desirable. These include:

Proximity. Rooms within easy walking distance of the college grounds save commuting costs and time and give important social benefits from frequently shared activity and ready access to campus meeting places.

Privacy or work-comes-first rules. Your room is workshop as well as home. Work calls for intense concentration. A place to yourself (or one shared only with other considerate students) is very helpful, especially if its location and solid construction help mute the harsh tones of the neighbor's TV. House rules that give sleep and study full priority make a big difference, too, whether living at home or in a many-student unit.

Recreational and social facilities. A place other than a bedroom in which you can entertain facilitates social development, especially with the opposite sex. The dormitory ping-pong table or the fraternity parlor are ideal for relaxing between study sessions, besides bringing together many potential friends.

A student community. Living together makes the close, personal associations of college even more satisfying, helpful, and productive. Sharing interests and experience leads to many friendships and to increased social skill.

Municipal housing codes require adequate wiring, heating, plumbing, and sanitary facilities in any multiple dwelling. If unsafe, inadequate, or unsanitary conditions exist, write or telephone the municipal housing authorities or ask your college housing bureau or Dean of Students to report such conditions. Most housing inspectors are sufficiently tactful to protect the sources

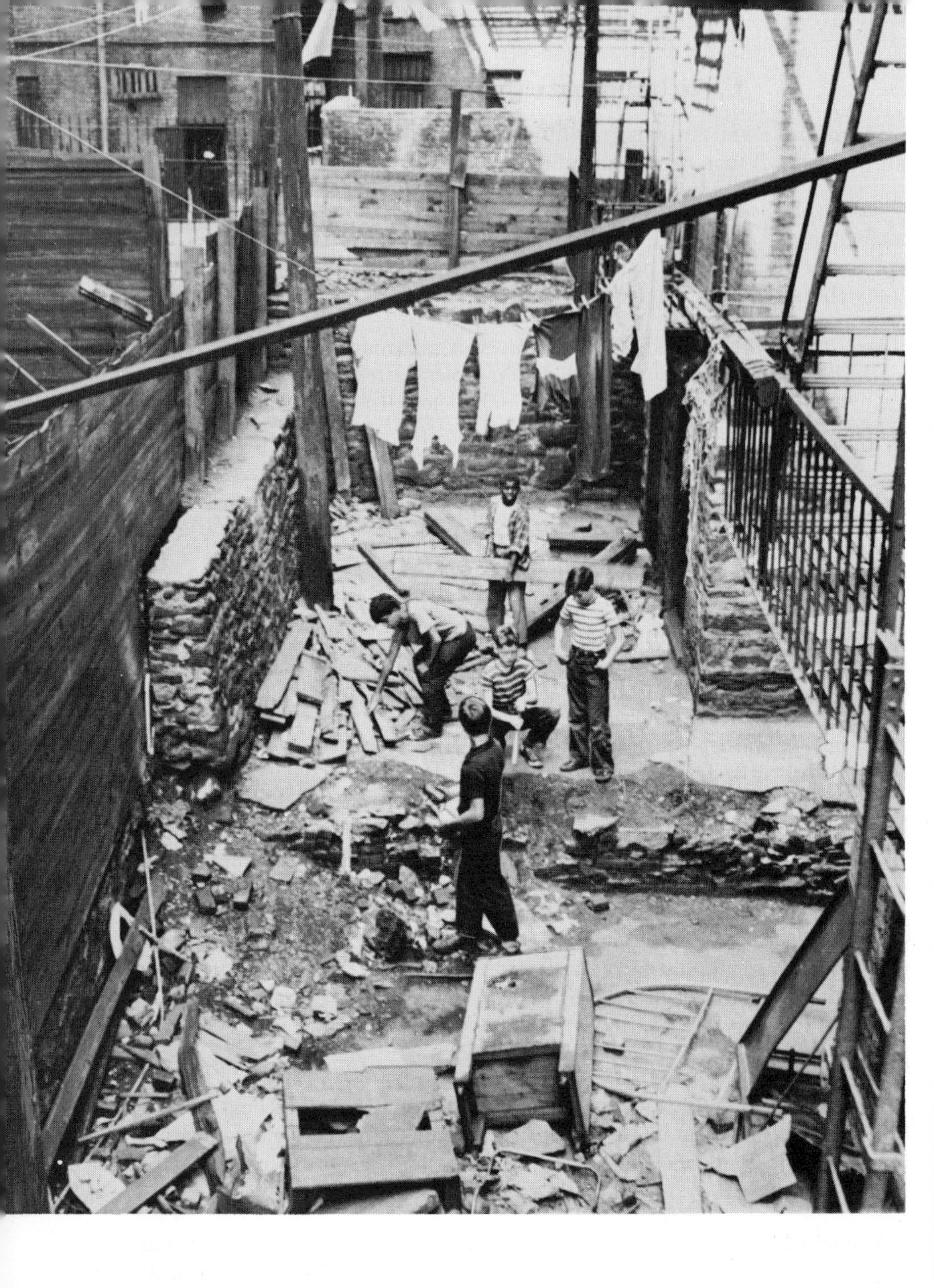

Figure 3. Slum scene. *Wide World Photos, Inc.*

of their information and try to enlist cooperation rather than bully landlords.

A word about slums

While thinking about housing, you might consider the effects of direly inadequate quarters. Slums and tenements harm *you*, because they increase physical, mental, and social difficulties to the detriment of taxpayers and

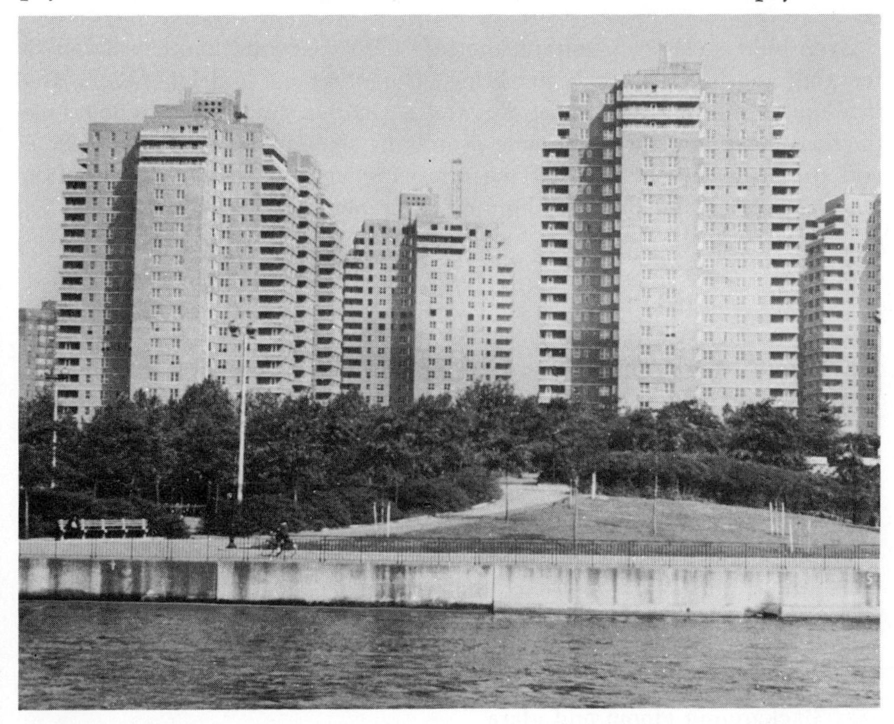

Figure 4. Low cost housing: the ILGWU Cooperative Village, N.Y.C. *Wide World Photos, Inc.*

neighbors, as well as of inhabitants. As many as 4,000 occupy a single block in New York's most crowded tenements. Many must live in slums because disease has sapped their energies and impaired their efficiency or because they are socially maladjusted. Initial seeding with tuberculosis and other communicable disease is therefore heavy in slums, and crowded conditions make for rapid spread. Mental illness, juvenile delinquency, and criminality breed in the tenement districts and impose their burdens upon both their victims and the community as a whole.

Most communities have found that slum-bred illness and maladjustment costs the taxpayers many times as much as subsidized or low-cost public housing. If a community can take people out of squalor, provide decent, healthful surroundings for them and at the same time actually save tax money through decreased expenditures for tuberculosis, mental hospitals, prisons, and welfare workers, what does it have to lose?

Adequate Lighting

Even mild levels of eyestrain interfere with concentration, cause you to feel dull and fuzzy-headed, and bring on nervousness and fatigue. Grossly inadequate lighting may cause headaches, nausea, and other troublesome physical complaints. Troublesome symptoms sometimes can be eliminated and study efficiency increased by improving lighting arrangements, often without investing in any extra lighting equipment at all.

How good lighting helps

You must use the small central portion of your eye's light-sensitive layer whenever you read or do close work. The cone-shaped cells packed into this area are less sensitive to low light levels than the rod-shaped cells which predominate in other areas. Therefore, levels of light perfectly adequate for walking without stumbling or slicing and eating a piece of steak are not sufficient for efficient study. Two 100 watt bulbs or two 20 watt fluorescent tubes in properly shaded and diffused lamps fifteen inches above desk top give proper light. Less efficient or more distant light sources must be of correspondingly greater strength.

Background gloom and glare

Our eyes adjust to the average amount of light they are gathering from the entire field of vision. If the field of vision includes a brightly lit page framed in a dense background of gloom, the eyes adjust to a compromise light level. The brightly lit page overstimulates the eye's light-sensitive layer, causing eyestrain. Every time you look up from the page or back down again, your pupillary muscles and light-sensitive cells make radical adjustments. These adjustments cause further eye fatigue.

Faulty background lighting usually can be corrected with little or no extra expense. One method: face your deck toward a light-colored wall, and use pin-up or floor lamps at a height which lights the wall above the desk as well as your work. In the usual study position, the bottom of the shade should be at least 15 inches above desk level. If the wall is dark, put up a 36″ × 42″ tack board.[2] Be sure that at least 10 per cent of your light is indirect, to eliminate dark shadows.

Glare creates a similar problem. The eye opening and its light-sensitive parts are adjusted for the general light level. Glare overstimulates one patch of light-sensitive cells, causing eyestrain. Some sources of glare are easy to eliminate: glass-covered pictures can be moved or reframed without glass.

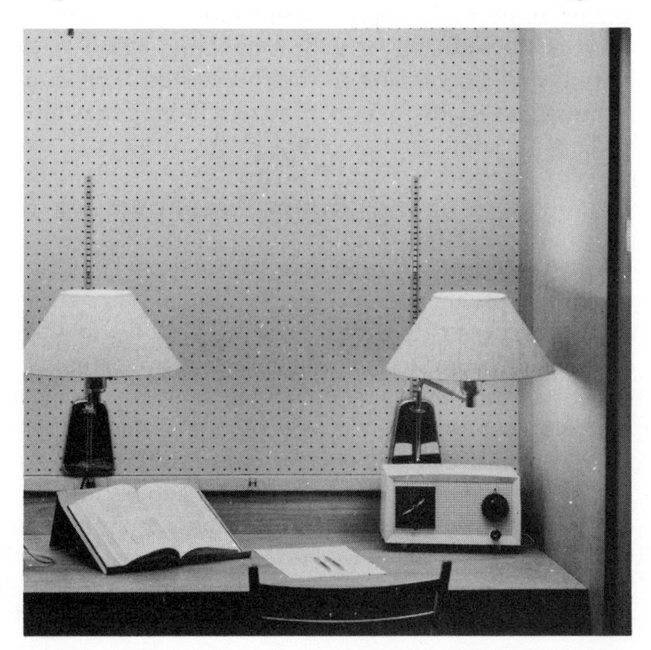

Figure 5. Lots of light from inexpensive lamps by thoughtful arrangement. *Courtesy Illuminating Engineering Society.*

Furniture can be arranged so that light comes over the shoulder or from diffuse, high sources to minimize glare. A dull finished desk can be used, or the desk can be covered with a blotter or cloth. Light-colored window shades, drapes or curtains, and different lampshades may help. Stick to dull-surface paints and satiny lacquers instead of using varnish when redecorating.

Healthful Heating

Heating engineers have found that chilly sensations, goose bumps, and other discomforts people usually blame on inadequate heat are often due to lack of humidity. When this is true, raising the temperature without adding

[2] "Studies of Lighting and Seeing for the Student at Home," Mary E. Webber, *Illuminating Engineering,* Vol. XLIV, No. 5, May 1949.

substantial amounts of extra moisture actually increases the effective dryness of the air by increasing its capacity for moisture. Further sensitivity to drafts and skin discomfort then bring about another push of the thermostat. Very soon, the temperature is over 80°, the air bone dry, and skin comfort, nasal comfort, and resistance to colds (see pp. 219–20) are impaired.

The range of humidity at which you remain comfortable is broadest in the temperature range of 68 to 72° F. Nasal comfort and resistance to colds are greatest at the same temperatures. If you are not comfortable in a room heated to 68 to 72 degrees temperature, increasing humidity with shallow pans on the radiators or with a bubbling steam kettle usually proves more rewarding than running to the thermostat, both in immediate comfort and in preserved health. Warmer indoor clothing may also be needed, of course.

Room Arrangement

Many students can profitably rearrange their furniture, books, and equipment. As a preliminary, list the room's main uses—study, dressing, sleep, and so on—and designate a room area for each. Try to rearrange the room so that each task can be accomplished with a minimum of movement. A further check by listing things for which you must now make an extended reach, get up from your study chair, or walk across the room may suggest additional improvements. One student, for instance, found that he could avoid several study interruptions every evening by keeping his dictionary between bookends on his desk, where he could reach it from both his easy chair and desk chair. Another speeded his morning toilet considerably by putting his dresser and chair near the closet door. Petty things in themselves, but very worthwhile in terms of time saved over the period of several college years.

HOW TO RATE YOUR EATING PLACE

Meals comprise the biggest item in the average collegian's budget. Although most students make arrangements mainly to please their palates, the answers to these three questions also deserve consideration: (1) Is enough food of the right varieties provided? (2) Is food always free of dangerous concentration of germs? (3) Is a pleasant, unhurried atmosphere provided?

(1) Everyone needs nourishing foods of several sorts every single day for ideal strength and resistance. Food choices have a great deal to do with how well the body's nutritional needs are met, but you can only choose from the foods served. Menus should provide:

a. Two large or three medium servings of protein-yielding meat, fish, eggs, or cheese daily.
b. At least two servings of fruit or juice.
c. At least three servings of vegetables.
d. Breakfast food, whole wheat bread or other foods made from whole grain.
e. At least one pint of milk.

If your eating place commonly fails to provide one or more of these items, you may be able to overcome this defect by snacking scientifically. Fruits and dairy products nourish you more than doughnuts and pop; cheese and eggs provide protein; salads and soups provide needed vegetables; sandwiches on whole wheat or rye bread meet deficiencies in whole grain.

(2) Cooking for large groups provides extra opportunities for diarrhea-causing germs to get into food and involves many periods when food is heated to the warm-but-not-hot temperatures at which such germs multiply rapidly. Most cases of so-called stomach flu—mild diarrhea or vomiting which lasts for only a day or so—probably result from such food infection and could be avoided by patronizing only eateries where sound food-handling technique is scrupulously followed. Although you must depend on the local or state health department, college authorities, or restaurant rating guidebook staff for detailed kitchen inspections, these three points may prove revealing:

Food should be either hot or cold. Lukewarm food allows germs to multiply at a prodigious rate. Above 120 to 130° F. and below 50° F. germ multiplication practically ceases. Meat-containing sandwich fillings must be watched with special care—careless cooks often keep them at room temperature because proper chilling makes them hard to spread.

Food should be set out as it is served. If a drugstore counter is set up for the luncheon crowd at 10:30 A.M. and is still serving out of the original food pots when the rush is over at 2:00 P.M., the last few customers will often later become ill. As a rule of thumb, no more food should be set out than will normally be served in an hour.

Dishes should be reasonably free of grease. Some perfectly proper dish-sanitizing methods leave water spots or a film of fine, whitish dust, but no form of dish sanitization works when layers of thick grease or lipstick shield germs from steam or moisture.[3]

When forced to eat in a restaurant or lunch counter where sanitary prac-

[3] So-called dish sterilizers work on the principle that moist heat kills disease-causing germs quickly. It takes two hours of intense heat to kill germs protected from moisture. Therefore, even a hospital autoclave will not kill germs immersed in grease. Unfortunately, this fact is not generally recognized.

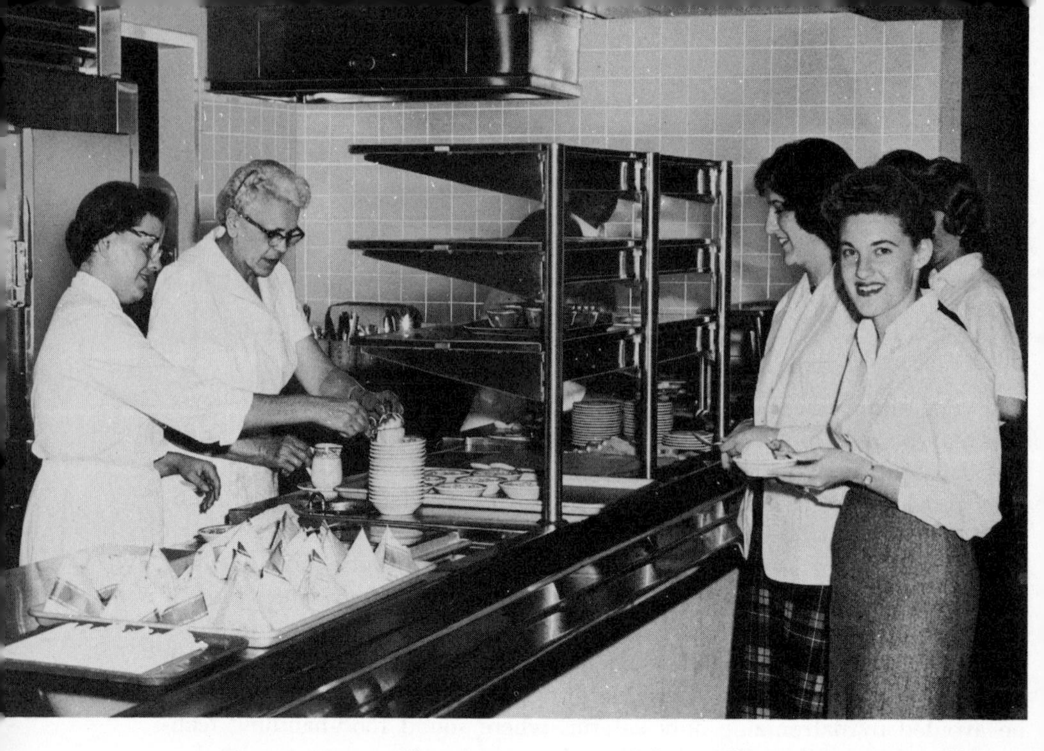

Figure 6. Hot or cold, proper temperature makes a difference. *Gary K. Cowell.*

tices may not be ideal, you can protect yourself from unpleasant consequences by choosing safely packaged or spoil-proof items. Nobody can ruin a freshly opened can of soup, for instance. An unfilled pastry, a piece of fresh fruit, or a peanut butter or cheese sandwich also should be safe. Avoid highly spoilable items like meat or egg salad or cream-filled pastries, unless you have total faith in the chef.

(3) Pleasant mealtime surroundings contribute to better digestion and to satisfying personal exchange. Consider these points:

Less harried meals sit better. Many college students are plagued by complaints which quieter, less harried mealtime would prevent. A pertinent parallel: workers in one industrial plant used to eat in an undecorated, dingy back room with the rumble of machinery droning in their ears. Between fifty and sixty workers came to the medical department for help with indigestion every afternoon. Then management provided a pleasant, quiet, well-decorated cafeteria. Result: less than ten appeals for relief from stomach distress each day, plus over-all improvement in worker morale.

Mealtime is the principal social hour. Mealtime can provide many opportunities for social development and interplay. Key points which make mealtimes socially helpful:

a. A relatively constant, not-too-large group. Unless you eat with the same people fairly frequently, mealtime social exchange will usually be limited to superficial chatter.

b. A group with whom you fit in.
c. Sufficiently convenient location to relieve time-pressure.
d. An atmosphere of quiet.

COMMUNITY SUPERVISION

Although health department inspection can not be depended upon to keep restaurant food, canned goods, and perishables entirely safe (mainly because of budgetary limitations), such supervision certainly helps. Public health employees supervise many aspects of safe food preparation you could not possibly check yourself. They: (1) perform bacteriologic tests on the dishes used in restaurants; (2) visit dairy farms to check milking methods, make sure that the milk stays cool while being trucked in, and examine temperature records from the vats in which it is pasteurized; (3) visit slaughterhouses to be sure that meat comes from healthy animals; (4) supervise food canning and preparation.

Figure 7. Food inspector at work. *Wide World Photos, Inc.*

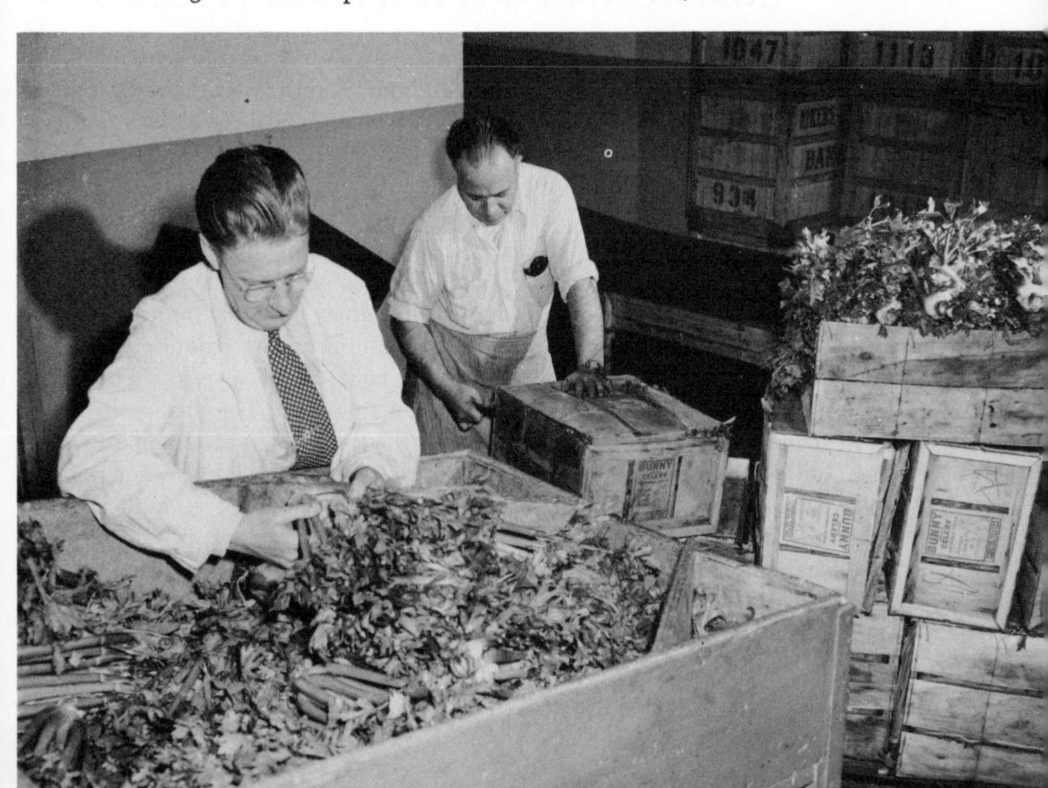

CHAPTER 3

Fellowship, Friendship, and Affection

EVERYONE WANTS TO BE RESPECTED, LIKED, AND LOVED, SATISFYING RELATIONSHIPS contribute greatly to the enjoyment of life's rewards and stability during its upheavals. Although closeness gives others the power to hurt as well as to help you, its benefits far outweigh its dangers. Any effort devoted to broadening and deepening associations without impairing your essential individuality usually proves very much worthwhile.

COMMUNITY-TYPE ASSOCIATIONS

The feeling that you belong to a family or group is a basic emotional support. Back in the days when clans or neighbors had to band together in interdependent groups, the emotional value of being an accepted member was obvious. The community or clan provided security, respect, and recreation; outsiders received something between the cold shoulder and physical assault. Identical emotional values and social opportunities still reward people who "belong," but they belong to an amalgamation of various units and categories with which they feel identified (gentleman, sportsman, scholar) or which they deliberately join (lodges, fraternities, churches) rather than to a clan or geographically distinguished community. The emotionally significant community for each individual is a complex of several groups each overlapping the other in certain spheres of influence. The groups in which you strive to belong do not conform with the boundaries of any one town or neighborhood, nor to each other. For instance, a jazz-loving physician might strive toward moral behavior acceptable to all mankind, seek to conduct himself in his profession according to the tenets of fellow physicians, and still share musical taste only with the very limited group of musicians whom he accepts as "cool." His "community" is compounded of these and other groups, each overlapping in certain spheres of influence and independent in certain others.

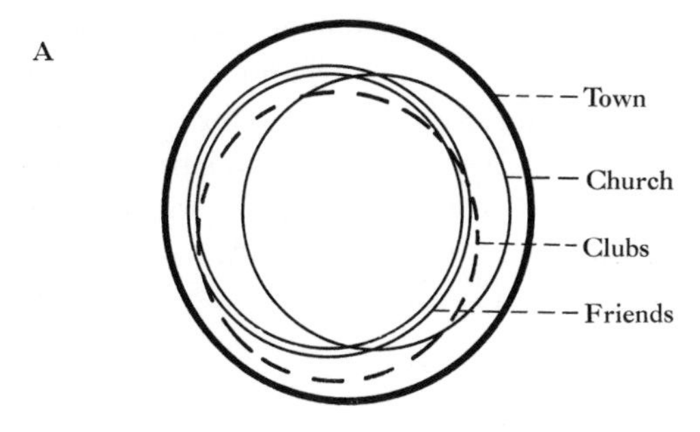

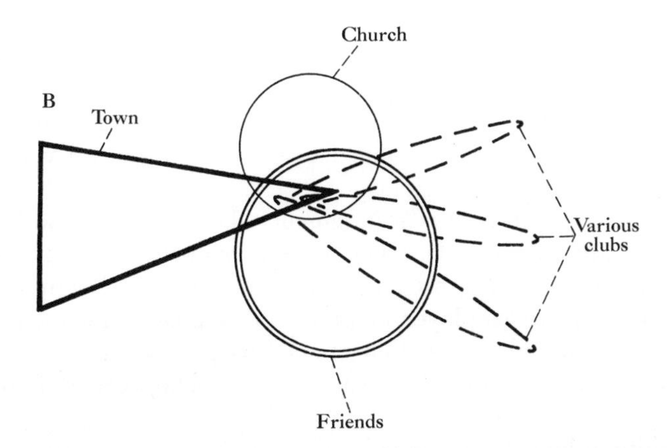

Figure 8. In the boundaried community (A), all your associations overlap. With modern travel and communications your various interests involve you with different groups having little overlap (B) but the over-all feeling that you "belong" remains important.

How the Rewards of Community Acceptance Come to You

Rank, position, or manifest rewards

Election to office in college, fraternal, or other group certainly signifies acceptance and respect. Ratings conferred by authority, such as college grades, military rank, or position in a business organization, usually reflect the judgment of the people whose opinion matters to you.[1] The trust placed in professional men by their clients implies similar respect. Material rewards give an easily determined, but rough index of rank within a vocational group. One lawyer's $40,000 a year salary does not prove him a *better* man than another lawyer who earns $20,000 a year or than a minister who makes only $7,000. However, almost everyone would regard an experienced lawyer who earns less than $4,000 as *unsuccessful* and one who earns $40,000 as *successful.* The tacit assumption is that demand for one's services indicates professional (and sometimes social) worth and also leads to a certain income, not that money itself enhances a man's value.

Supersignificant evaluations

Under certain circumstances, we almost automatically think of ourselves as on display for community judgment. Public speaking provides one good example: you could talk to each member of the audience individually without feeling the anxiety which plagues you when you stand in front of them *en masse.* A hostess' extra housecleaning effort before she entertains is another instance. Each guest probably has seen her house in its customary state quite frequently; yet she feels obliged to battle for approval with mop and waxer before they arrive as a group.

At times, a single individual's judgment takes on similar weight. When you think of a person by title, office, or employment rather than by name, appearance, or personality, his judgment assumes special significance. The parson, a prospective employer, a professor, a policeman—their judgment of you has the same impact as that of the group they represent when they function in official capacities. They carry the symbolic scepter of community-vested authority.

Community judgment by a group or a functionary enhances the value of approval as well as the weight of his criticism. You feel substantial pride when you receive an audience's applause, or when a person in authority praises you. Such manifest community recognition builds your self-respect and confidence quite strongly. Most people find it a distinctly worthwhile reward.

Comparison with an absorbed system of values

You subconsciously rate your own morals, manners, and achievements against the standards of the people whose opinion matters to you, and derive

[1] Not always, because the authorities wielding control may not accurately represent the groups whose respect you desire. For example, bright seventh- or eighth-grade students frequently make deliberate errors on test papers because they would rather be accepted by fellow students who disdain "little Einsteins" than win their teachers' approval.

either self-respect or guilt feelings from this comparison. The resulting rewards and punishments are among the most potent influences in our society. Since your system of values derives itself quite directly from your interpretation of family, church, school and other community-type associations, the groups with which you link yourself become subtle but powerful molding forces in your life.

College as a Community

Your college is a community, set apart to a degree, with its own standards of behavior and achievement, interdependent population, and system of rewards. Some of a college education's most important benefits stem from your interaction with the college community. A more complete understanding of this interaction will help you improve your adaptation to college, and also facilitate transfer of that adaptation to later community life.

College authority

College authorities fulfill many roles assigned in the outside world to bosses, policemen, and chaperones. They have one overwhelming grace: since their only reason for existence is your ultimate welfare, they are unquestionably benevolent. After sincere reflection and study, they set up regulations specifically to benefit the majority of students.

Take the grading system, for instance. College authorities do not, as most students think, use it solely for critical appraisal. The benefits you will derive from knowledge itself usually seem vague and distant; grades provide a more immediate goal and a reward for accomplishment similar in some ways to salary. Grades are of value in guidance and selection; they help you determine what you can do well and which type of career to seek. Grades are essential for maintaining your school's standards. A college degree must signify a certain level of competence before potential employers, for example, will respect it and hire you.

Throughout life we must meet standards of competence within our chosen fields and of conformity to recognized laws and mores. You might find it interesting to compare what is required of an employee in a business firm, a self-employed professional, and a college student with regard to competence, manners, and morals. What are the consequences of one failure or moral breach in college—and later? How do college authorities compare with other bosses in liberality and benevolence?

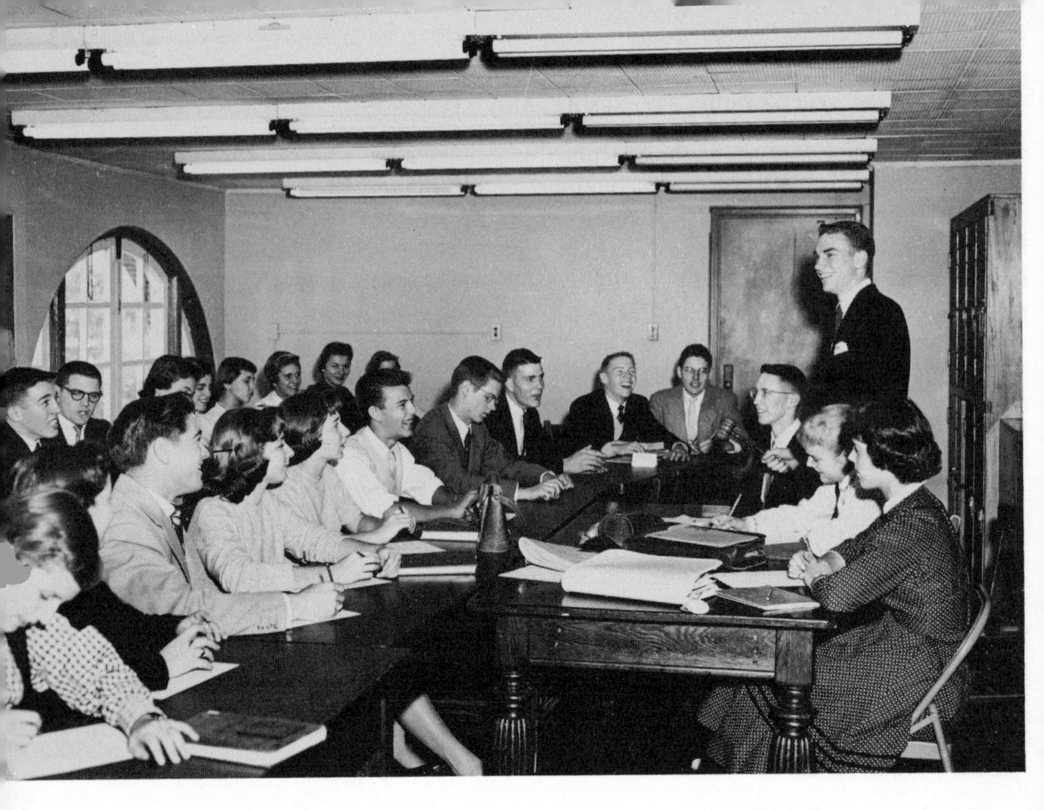

Figure 9. Meeting called to order, social interplay not really halted. *Ewing Galloway.*

Campus organizations and activities

Collegians can satisfy important needs—their need to belong, develop friendships, serve worthy purposes, and improve certain abilities—by affiliating with campus groups and organizations. *Academic, religious, and special interest groups* broaden social contacts and develop leadership potential as well as serve their designated ends, even though such groups may not foster particularly intimate interpersonal associations. You can attend meetings in most such groups on a trial basis without making any commitment and devote as much time to them as you believe they deserve. *Varsity or intramural athletic teams* provide the shared experiences and endeavor from which many close friendships spring. Joining a *fraternity, sorority, or social club* can be one of the most important steps you will ever take for either good or evil as far as social development is concerned. Although the decision to join or not to join is based on a very brief period of superficial acquaintanceship (with both parties very much on their good behavior), there are two saving graces: likes tend to attract likes, and the odds are on your side—most fraternities are devoted to wholesome good fellowship combined with academic success rather than to irresponsible revelry. The deliberate promotion of personal closeness in a fraternity, sorority or social club certainly helps many members toward associations of lifelong value (both as lasting friendships and as models for the future).

Both within interest groups, teams or clubs and in the other groups of college students who are thrown together a good bit, unorganized but coherent social groupings occur. These groupings provide incubation for many of college's closest friendship. They usualy jell within six to twelve months and admit new members only cautiously thereafter. Students who come to college fairly well settled in their interest patterns, residence plans and so forth—or students who decide these issues promptly—usually form friendships more readily than those who make frequent changes.

Campus attitudes toward money

As long as you can meet your fees and expenses, money makes much less difference to your life in college than it will in future years. Your acceptance by the college authorities establishes your basic worth for your associates. Both you and your fellow students know that neither the money you bring from home nor the money you earn during your educational period proves your capabilities. Many other criteria—academic, social, athletic, or other extracurricular achievements, for instance—make more difference to your stature with your fellow-students than your financial worth. Many doors which will close after your college years still remain open. You may want to take advantage of the resulting opportunities for getting to know and understand people from various groups and strata.

Conformity and your social horizons

Compile a list of people whose opinions of you are important to your self-respect. You will probably find that several social groups are represented. You can make these people continue to accept you only if you conform, at least to some degree, to their standards. Nonconformity and rebellion, which may at first glance offer wider horizons, often close many doors to you, thus limiting your circle of potential acquaintance. You can maintain your individuality and retain a broad range of independent thought and action and still meet the minimum criteria of acceptability imposed by the many elements of society within which you might like to move.

Your After-College Community

When you choose neighborhoods, organizations, and associates, you set almost inescapable standards for yourself. Neighbors and potential associates require certain achievements and behavior as the price of continuing acceptance and respect. Although these requirements need not conflict with expressing your own individuality, within broad limits they impose economic and social burdens.

Most college graduates have great faith in their future, and are in a great hurry to have a good home in a good neighborhood. Quite often they overextend themselves by moving into areas out of their current financial depth—areas in which the ladies serve high-priced refreshments at every get-together, in which the children go downtown to luncheon and the movies as a standard sort of outing, and in which the men's ordinary first overture is to invite you for a game of golf (you provide clubs, pay the caddy, and buy refreshments, of course).

Neighborhood-set living standards run the vast majority of young executives and professional people into the red during their first ten years of work. A few of them deliberately choose to live over their heads as a calculated gamble, on the theory that mixing with people higher on the economic ladder will breed further opportunities for success. The larger portion find themselves constantly pinching pennies on every detail of living without understanding how their original choice of housing and social set pushed them out of their depth. An appreciation of this fact can help you toward a much less troubled, anxiety-free apprentice phase in our worldly society.

After-college materialism

After college, your initial screening of people you wish to cultivate from those you do not (and their corresponding appraisal of you) almost always includes materialistic grounds; money influences almost everything you can determine about another person at a glance. Even if you decry materialistic snobbery, you still choose your friends mainly from the people who can afford to do the things you also do, in places which you frequent—points largely governed by available funds. Thus after college you will find that money restricts your range of acquaintance both up and down the economic ladder much more strictly than it does while on the campus.

Most students tend to view the materialistic strivings of middle age from one of two extreme positions. Either they think in terms of the materialistic ladder, with earnings and accumulations as a monolithic measurement of worth, or they apply the relatively nonmaterialistic standards of the college community in their thinking about the outside world.

Both of these positions impose unnecessary psycho-social stresses and distortions.

The materialistic ladder notion takes too little account of differences in success standards applied to different occupations and neighborhoods. Not only do some vocations—notably teaching and preaching—get most of their recognition in nonmonetary form, but criteria of success, expectations of hospitality and many other socioeconomic points are determined in a vocational and neighborhood frame of reference. For instance, you would be perfectly willing to accept the idea that an elementary school teacher who lived in a walk-up flat was successful, but what would you think of a stock broker who lived that way? You would feel graciously treated if the teacher offered you tea and cookies at a party, but how would such refreshments at the broker's impress you?

These widely prevalent attitudes substantially affect the ease with which you can achieve a balanced domestic budget, social acceptance, a feeling of community recognition, and self respect in the lower-paying vocations, and make the relative economic position of the various career choices open to you much less of a factor than the materialistic ladder notion seems to indicate.

On the other hand, a totally nonmaterialistic view also provokes unnecessary strains. Money does for older people what continued acceptance at college does for you: it proves basic worth, provides common activities, and lets them frequent the same haunts with people of somewhat similar attainments to their own. Whether right or wrong, materialistic standards govern most social interplay in America and affect not only your own social

Figure 10. Fun for all within modest means. *Ewing Galloway.*

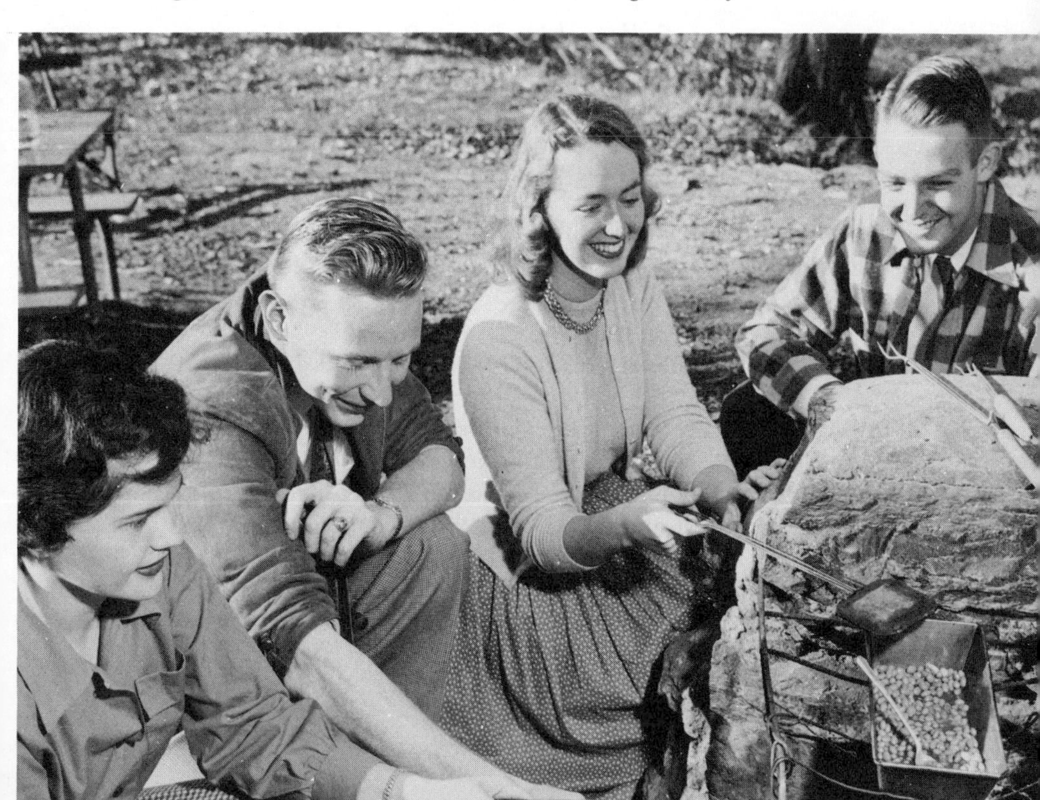

horizons but those of your family as well. Disregard for money during a starry-eyed youth leads many capable men and ladies into either lifelong discontent or bitter disillusionment.

DISTINCTLY PERSONAL ASSOCIATIONS

Personal association goes beyond the acquaintance stage when you become sufficiently involved with the other person to share his feelings and emotions. *Emotional* involvement forges lasting relationships. The more emotional experiences you share without conflict or friction, the further your relationships ordinarily go. The depth of emotional life you enjoy and the degree to which you communicate natural, unforced emotion (without embarrassing the other fellow) affects the speed with which friendships and loves develop.

During your college years you do many things in the company of many people with whom you have a great deal in common. Friendships and still closer relationships form very freely in this atmosphere of conjoint activity and interest.

Fellowship-Type Relationships

At the fellowship level, you build better relationships mainly by doing things together, so that you have a chance to participate in emotional interplay of several kinds. Pleasures usually prove easier to share than discomfiture, but even shared trials cement your personal ties. Friendly competition is helpful and companionable. Conversation permits vicarious sharing of each other's prior experiences and thoughts.

Combating barriers of reserve, dignity, and detachment

Shared emotion promotes friendship. You therefore impel people toward friendship with you in proportion to your own openhearted lack of reserve with them. Emotion cannot be forced, being an involuntary response, but it can be either restrained or freely expressed. The more freely you express your feelings (except those which might cause embarrassment) the more opportunity you give for close relationships to develop.

You want deep attachments to be mutual, of course. You can draw the other fellow into a degree of openheartedness, too, by harmonious response to whatever feelings he reveals.

A good listener inspires friendship—but a good listener not only listens to words but also perceives and responds to emotional overtones and personal, emotional needs. A good listener remains always aware of tone of voice, facial expression (especially around the mouth, which reveals a person's true feelings more readily than the poetically vaunted eyes), body posture and unconscious gestures. From this awareness, he always senses his associate's emotional state and responds to it keenly—not by thinking out the situation, but by interplay at an emotional, distinctly non-analytic level.

Of course, you always should spare the other fellow's feelings. The closer you are to someone, the more easily you can hurt him. Call a stranger in the street a nasty name: he simply shrugs and moves on unconcerned. Use the same appellation with a friend, and you give him real pain. Likewise with omissions and affronts: the closer a person feels to you, the more hurt he is at being left off your guest list or ignored out on the street. You hurt budding friendships when you make an acquaintance the butt of your jokes, the target of your repartee or the victim of minor discourtesies. Good friends may endure these things, but they stick in spite of such sallies, not because of them.

The time factor

It takes time to forge close friendships: time in the company of your friends and time within ready range of communication. Don't become impatient if a few months pass before you develop close college friendships.

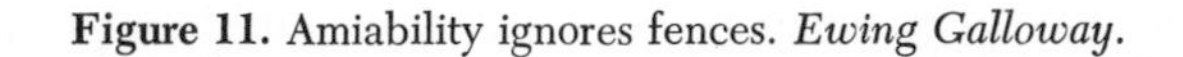

Figure 11. Amiability ignores fences. *Ewing Galloway.*

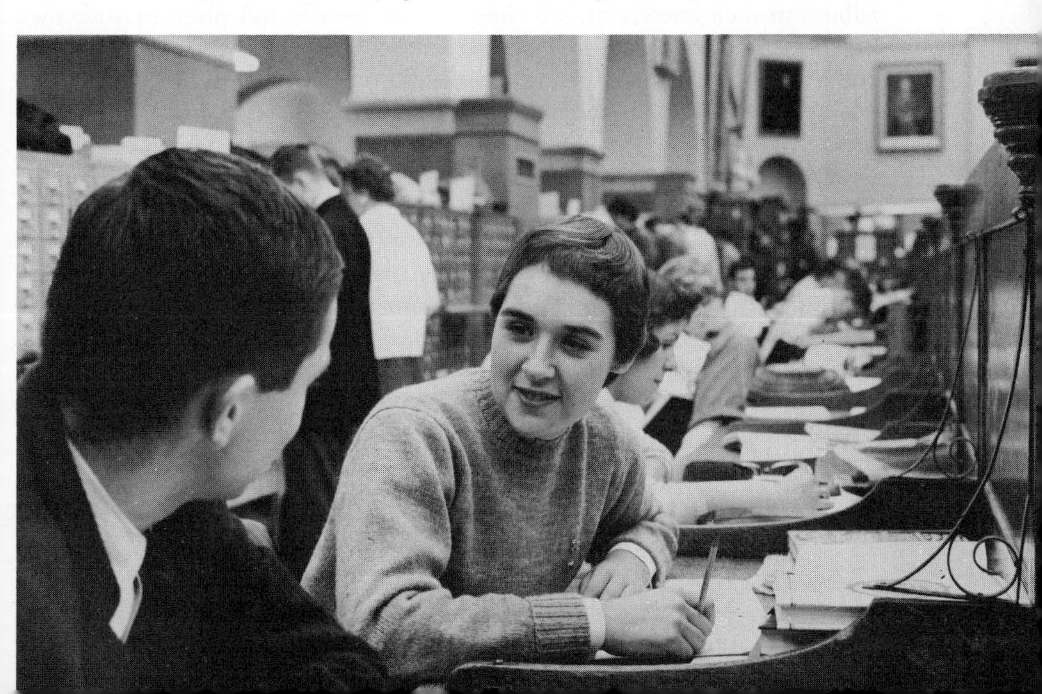

On the other hand, your long-range plans must always take into account the fact that friendships become progressively harder to form as the years go by. Most friendships are forged before age twenty-five, when school and sporting interests throw you much into each other's company and when family responsibilities and interests do not yet compete with or displace budding friendships. If you relocate after you are twenty-five or thirty, you will find the social patterns in the new community thoroughly jelled and your position hedged about by mutual reserve. If friendships are important to you, and if you form them slowly, stability of residence offers very real social advantages. The effect of moves on your own and your family's social relations deserves considerable weight in choosing your career and your method of pursuing it.

Identification

The most complete form of personal involvement with someone else is identification, in which the other person's experiences and feelings have the same impact on your emotions and your self-esteem as your own. The father who bursts with pride as Junior romps for a touchdown, the lover who gets more pleasure from his fiance's enjoyment of a gift than he could have derived by buying something for himself, and the collegian who feels personally ashamed when his close friend is caught cheating in an examination clearly illustrate this reaction. They do not merely soak up contagious feelings from the other person: they react as if they were totally involved, with lasting impact on their pride and self-respect.

Identification offers many obvious advantages. It makes family service a joy, not a sacrifice: whatever you do to give your children pleasure or contribute to their success stirs feelings of satisfaction and pride in your own breast. It allows intensifying spirals of emotion: as lovers go about their courting, each person's feelings bestir the other's passion to new heights, which in turn bestir the other's feelings further. Moreover, identification overcomes barriers of time and space: a mother still feels pride in her daughter's successes even if she hears about them a week later, and by mail.

Common origins, current objectives, or future prospects help promote identification. Family relationship and marriage score on all three counts. Shared activities or living experiences also help: this is one reason for the large number of fast friendships which start in college. The feeling that you sink or swim together also promotes identification, giving team play and group endeavor an important place in welding close human ties.

Roles and relationships

Few human relationships function perpetually on the same plane. When a father criticizes his son's poor table manners, he acts as a community member imposing a standard of acceptability. Later, the two might toss a football back and forth in friendly fellowship. Still later, an intimate discussion of future ambitions and desires might weld them into the intensive mutual concern of identification.

You must evaluate a relationship by the depth it reaches at times of need or opportunity, not by the level at which it is working at the moment. Yet you must govern your actions toward another person according to the roles you occupy at the moment, not your over-all relationship. The bride who pushes down her husband's morning newspaper to kiss him passionately is apt to bestir annoyance rather than affection, especially if the bus to work is almost due to leave. A father who berates his son for staying out quite late has to expect hostility and anger, or even hatred, in response, no matter how much the boy really loves him. There is no reason to feel guilty about such reactions or to regard them as defects in normal affection: love continues just as strong beneath the transient indifference or upheaval.

Roles supersede relationships still more frequently in determining proper

Figure 12. Amuse Baby, Mother also laughs. *Columbia News Office.*

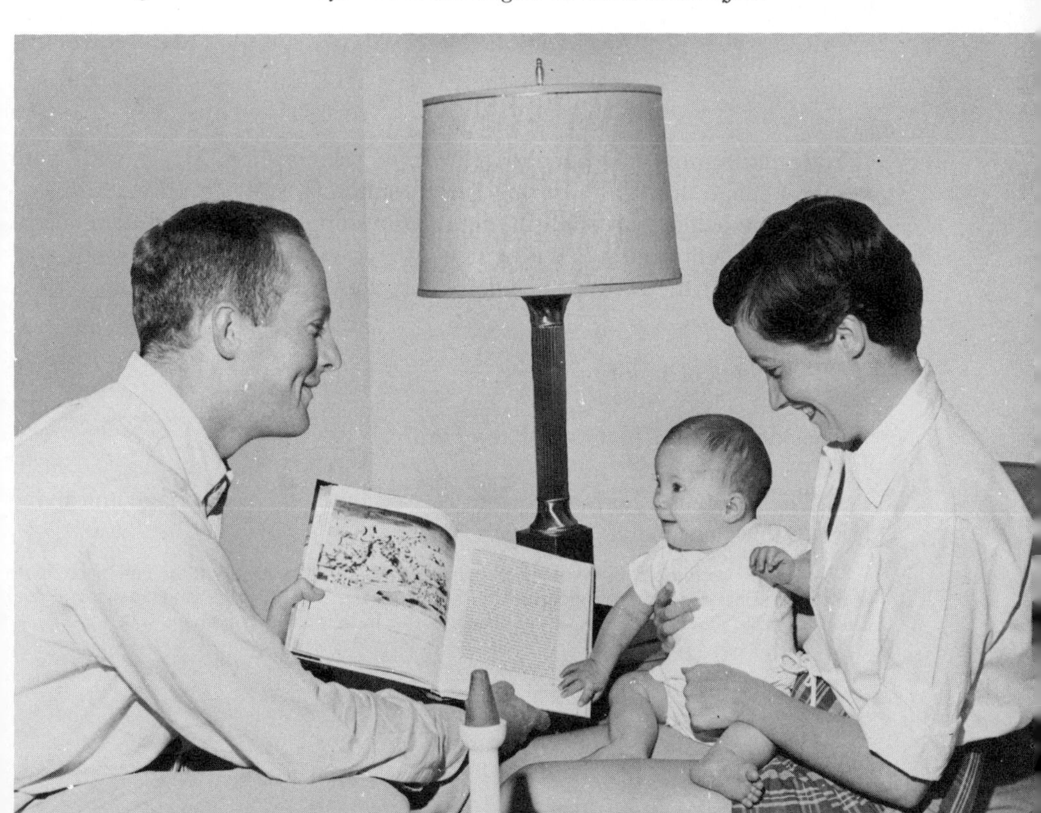

behavior where relative strangers are concerned. A teacher must act quite differently toward a pupil during class than in personal counseling, and differently again when acting as football coach. He must remain constantly conscious of what role he is operating in if his behavior is to be appropriate.

Strengthening identification-type relationships

A love-type relationship or close friendship generally increases in depth when it is functioning in a role which permits identification. When you participate directly or indirectly in another person's emotion-charged experiences you intensify your identification with him.[2] You can provide many opportunities for such experience through picnics, noncompetitive sports, and other noncompetitive activities. Functioning as a team or partnership also helps. Sharing emotionally burdensome duties and decisions welds many couples, families, and friendships. Sharing your reactions to experience through later conversation also helps.

Keenly competitive activities set one person against the other in quest of stature, and thus interfere with identification. Likewise with repartee and debate: they may make people respect your wit and keenness, but they win very little love. You can weld closeness more effectively with conversation which concentrates on shared experiences and acquaintances or on experiences related in such a way that the other person enjoys or reacts emotionally to them.

Family Ties

Your most important identification-type relationships, those with your family, change drastically during early adulthood. College provides an opportunity to achieve an adult-family relationship gracefully and completely. This crucial adjustment is easier if you have explored the two major concepts involved: the concept of family and the concept of dependency.

The idea of family

Consider these definitions of the family:

1. The family is a body of persons related by blood or marriage and living in the same household.

[2] A similar mechanism is involved in adoration of athletes and actors. You participate in athletic contests or drama vicariously. The resulting identification may make you feel a considerable emotional quasi-attachment to the individuals concerned.

2. The family is an institution binding kindred individuals together in a web of mutual concern and responsibility, which transcends distance, time, and even the death of senior members.

These two definitions embrace markedly different concepts. The first conceives of family life as a kind of domestic partnership, presumably involving lines of authority and means of dividing the spoils, but involving few attachments after you leave the old homestead. The second, a broader concept which makes each individual a standard-bearer for the proud family name, makes family ties and debts indissoluble, and makes the family itself an immortal institution through which your own germ plasm can survive for generations.

Which concept do you acknowledge? If you are like most people, you acknowledge both. You feel that once you are on your own, your parents have no right to regulate your behavior, and yet you know that your whole family will bear the shame if you disgrace yourself. You feel that your primary obligation will be to your own household after you are married and establish it, yet you cannot shirk responsibility if your parents are in need. Certainly, you expect the bonds of mutual concern and interest to remain after you cease to occupy the same home with other family members.

To clarify your own idea of family attachment, you might ask yourself these questions:

1. What would you do if your father were arrested and convicted of embezzlement?

2. How much debt would you be willing to assume to keep your mother in a private hospital if a long illness exhausted her resources and her only alternative was to go on charity? What about an uncle? A cousin?

3. How much debt would you be willing to assume to help your own children through college?

How does the picture of your family attachments reflected in your answers to these questions compare with the separate-households-equal-separate-families notion implicit in the phrase "out on your own"? These are your lasting family attachments, with which you must live out your adult life. How can you fit them into your future plans? How can you reconcile them with your partner's somewhat different ideas when you marry?

Dependency

No man is an island. A web of human relationships is necessary support. In infancy, that support is a one-way street: you depend wholly on your parents or their surrogates for food, warmth, and other care, and give nothing in return. You learn the security of placing your welfare in the hands of others, and they learn the satisfaction of meeting a loved one's needs. This basic pattern—dependency on your part and gratifying acceptance of responsibility by your parents—continues for many years. It serves as the secure foundation for your personality while independent behavior patterns form, and rises to the surface when those patterns fail to achieve results.

Dependency in childhood and youth continues to be *actual:* your parents take over key decisions and responsibilities. In adulthood, dependency ideally becomes *unconfiningly emotional:* your parents and their surrogates stand behind you and are palpably concerned when you have difficulties, but do not preempt your prerogatives or assume your obligations.

The shift from actual to unconfining emotional dependency is often difficult. Early adulthood almost inevitably involves rejection of actual dependency. You no longer want your parents to make crucial decisions for you. You no longer want them to take over every responsibility which involves difficulties. But your parents find it hard to let you make what they feel sure are mistakes, or leave you to struggle against difficulties they can remove. So you usually break the actual dependency of childhood with rebellion, undergo a period of hard feelings, then finally bring the adult-type, emotional pattern into play.

College can help you through this change in several ways. If you live away from home, you have substantial control over which issues you discuss with your parents and what role you assign to them. However, you cannot mold a relationship by putting it on ice. Letters and conversations about your daily problems and how you are handling them, without requests for advice or help, carve out a new role for your parents in your life. No letters or failure to mention your problems and activities accomplishes nothing.

College offers qualified professional help with many key decisions, allowing you to assume responsibilities for which you would not otherwise be entirely ready. Perhaps your experience does not qualify you to judge the adequacy and safety of certain quarters or the sanitary preparation at meals, but if your college has an active housing bureau or other supervisory facility you can avoid turning to mother. Your experience may not be sufficient for selecting a career, but your college probably provides qualified counselors who will help you make a sound decision for yourself.

Finally, college gives you a chance to make mistakes. You can start taking a business course and switch into education with very little lost time or money, while an ill-advised business venture would set you back considerably. You can get in a jam that would lead to dismissal in the outside world and still probably get another chance. You can do sloppy, slipshod work below your capacity for a few months or years, and still have an opportunity to pull up to where you belong after you find yourself. Colleges are not in business to mollycoddle you, but they are sufficiently concerned with your welfare to provide some degree of lenience. While you are trying your wings, it's nice to know that you are flying over a safety net.

Whether in college or out, you will ultimately have to make almost all of your own decisions and assume almost all of your own responsibilities. You can reach that position without giving up the tacit support of those upon whom you need to depend (at least emotionally) in crises. To do so, however, you need to make a deliberate switch from actual to controlled emotional dependency: to ask and accept concerned interest instead of material or intellectual help, and to do your planning before or after rather than during your family conferences. College is a wonderful place to make this change.

Figure 13. Choosing a career. *Cornell University News Bureau.*

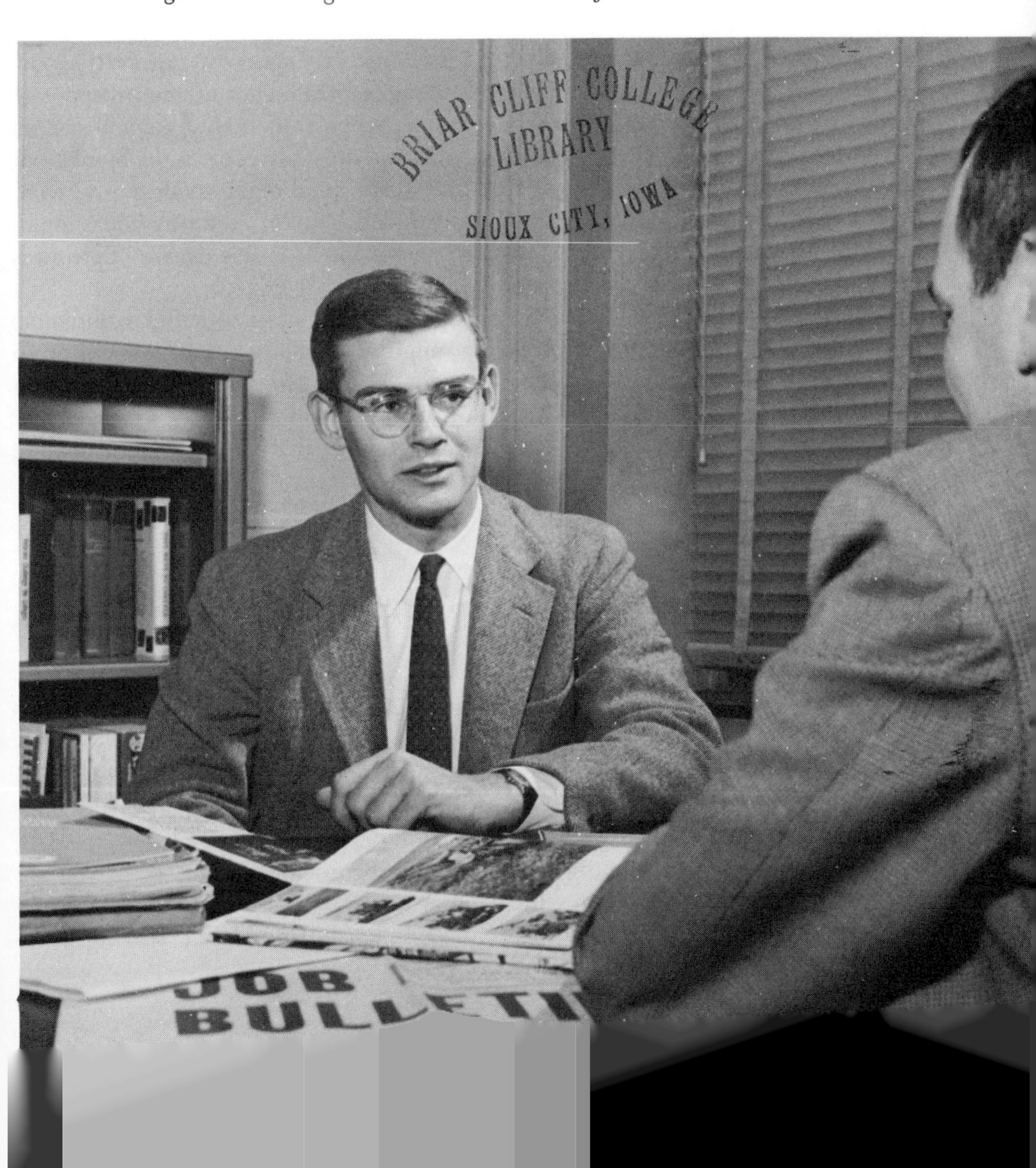

CHAPTER 4

How To Meet Personal Problems

PERSONAL PROBLEMS CAUSE EVERYONE TROUBLE AT TIMES. YOU GET INTO A LOW mood or feel tense and anxious, you develop headaches at the prospect of an evening with your books which vanish when somebody asks you out on a date, you get so keyed up for an examination that your mind blanks out on some of the answers you should know. You plod along inefficiently, wondering why you can't get as much out of an hour of study as you should, until you realize that you've lost your conviction that this course of study is the right one for *you.*

When you are confronted by an upsetting situation or suffer complaints of seemingly emotional origin, a few minutes of deliberate effort will often help you formulate your problem and deal with it effectively. Generally, you can handle problems for yourself and handle them efficiently. Occasionally you need help. This chapter should aid you in identifying problems, dealing with them personally, and getting help when necessary.

ENTERPRISE IN PROBLEM-SOLVING

It is a real relief to get past the sharp psychologic conflict created by most problems. Conflict between incompatible desires or between your desires and your conscience makes you quite uncomfortable. You want to get over an illness, but you do not want to endure the operation required for cure. You want to stay on campus for a sociable weekend, but your conscience urges a visit back home. As long as the issue remains undecided, you suffer some continuing conscious or subconscious strain.

The same variety of stressful conflict accompanies less immediate problems, even those which you have not consciously formulated. Solving problems reduces psychologic strain, even if those problems do not seem pressing.

Problem-solving Technique

An orderly approach to formulating and solving problems brings your intellect efficiently to bear upon personal difficulties and incapacities. When you recognize the existence of an immediate problem, certain definite steps often help bring about a prompt and adequate solution. Actual written formulation of problems and step-by-step written solution helps you become conscious of your own reasoning processes and ultimately improves your capacity to deal rationally with problems even when written exposition is impractical. Why not try focusing your intellect on some problem which is plaguing you now, using a pencil and paper to carry through each of the following steps?

1. *State the problem clearly.* The mere act of formulating a problem in concise words promotes its resolution. Most full-fledged worrywarts suffer mainly from failure to take this crucial first step. So long as you leave your problems vague and poorly formulated, you cannot think them through to a solution.

2. *Reformulate your problem in constructive terms.* You can attack problems constructively only if you put them in the present tense, and orient them toward action. If a problem seems to lie in the past, you have to choose significant aspects in the present before you can do anything about it. Take these problem pairs, for instance:

Retrospective: "My girl and I broke up last night."
Constructive: "Should I patch things up or look for greener pastures?"
Retrospective: "I flunked my midquarter exam."
Constructive: "What can I do to pull myself up in this course?"
Retrospective: "If only I hadn't made such insulting remarks to poor Mary last night!"
Constructive: "Would an apology or some other step help, or would it be better to let the matter lie?"
Retrospective: "He's dead. Poor Harry is dead."
Constructive: "This grief is getting me down. What can I do to pick up the pieces?"

What if constructive formulation is impossible? If the problem situation obviously cannot be altered? Facing a problem in fully crystallized form helps you resign yourself to its continued existence, and to make the most of life despite the persisting difficulty.

3. *List all possible courses of action, including combined attacks.* Probably more mistakes are made by failing to consider all alternatives than by making the wrong choice. You ask yourself: "Should I marry this person now or not?" without considering the possibility of continued courtship. You try to decide whether you want to try for an M.D. degree without investigating other health careers your special aptitudes might make both easier and more satisfying for you. Or you choose between business administration and teaching without considering whether the advantages you see in both might not be available in a field such as public school administration.

4. *Marshal facts for and against each course of action.* All pertinent facts, including your own uncontrollable feelings and prejudices, deserve some weight in your thinking. If you hate harsh winters, for instance, this feeling should be considered in choosing between job offers from Minnesota and California.

5. *Get expert advice if necessary.* Important decisions may involve facts readily available only from experts. An objective view sometimes proves helpful, too, especially where your own capacities are concerned. Your legal rights, your fitness for marriage, your academic capabilities in a certain field, and many other crucial facts can often be appraised at reasonable cost by an expert.

6. *Make a definite decision.* After gathering all the facts and giving them due consideration, your first decision is usually the best. Where results can be accurately measured, as in examination questions, reconsidering your answers leads to more changes toward error than toward rectitude. The misery of perpetual worry as well as the probability that you will do more harm than good attends continual reconsideration of already-made decisions. The best course probably is to set a definite time period for considering the possibilities, then make a definite decision, to be reopened only in the event that new facts emerge.

UNSOLVED AND OBSCURE PROBLEMS

Unsolved problems create vague but troublesome uncertainties: although you may not have faced up to them, you subconsciously know that they exist and that they demand changes in your viewpoint or way of life. You hesitate to build plans or dreams on an insecure, shifting foundation. The result is usually a combination of listlessness, indifference, and fatigue. More obvious effects of stress, such as uncomfortable nervous tension or psychologically induced physical disorders, may also result.

Certain very common disorders and complaints among college students stem from the emotional stress of unsolved personal problems. The direct effects of stress are compounded by its effects on the autonomic nervous system, breathing control centers and so on. A direct or indirect emotional basis is much more likely than physical disorder to cause the following complaints at college age:

1. Excess tension, manifested by nervousness, easy fatigue, headache unrelated to colds, excess perspiration, and insomnia.
2. Emotionally induced overbreathing with deep, sighing respiration, which leads to chemical changes in the blood producing dizzy spells or light-headedness, and tingling hands and feet.
3. Functional disturbances of the intestinal tract, such as upset stomach, indigestion, gas pains, constipation, or periodic attacks of diarrhea.
4. Acute anxiety, causing pounding or racing heart, difficult breathing, tightness in chest, and cold sweats with weakness or tremor.

Figure 14. One way to boost morale. *Cornell University News Bureau.*

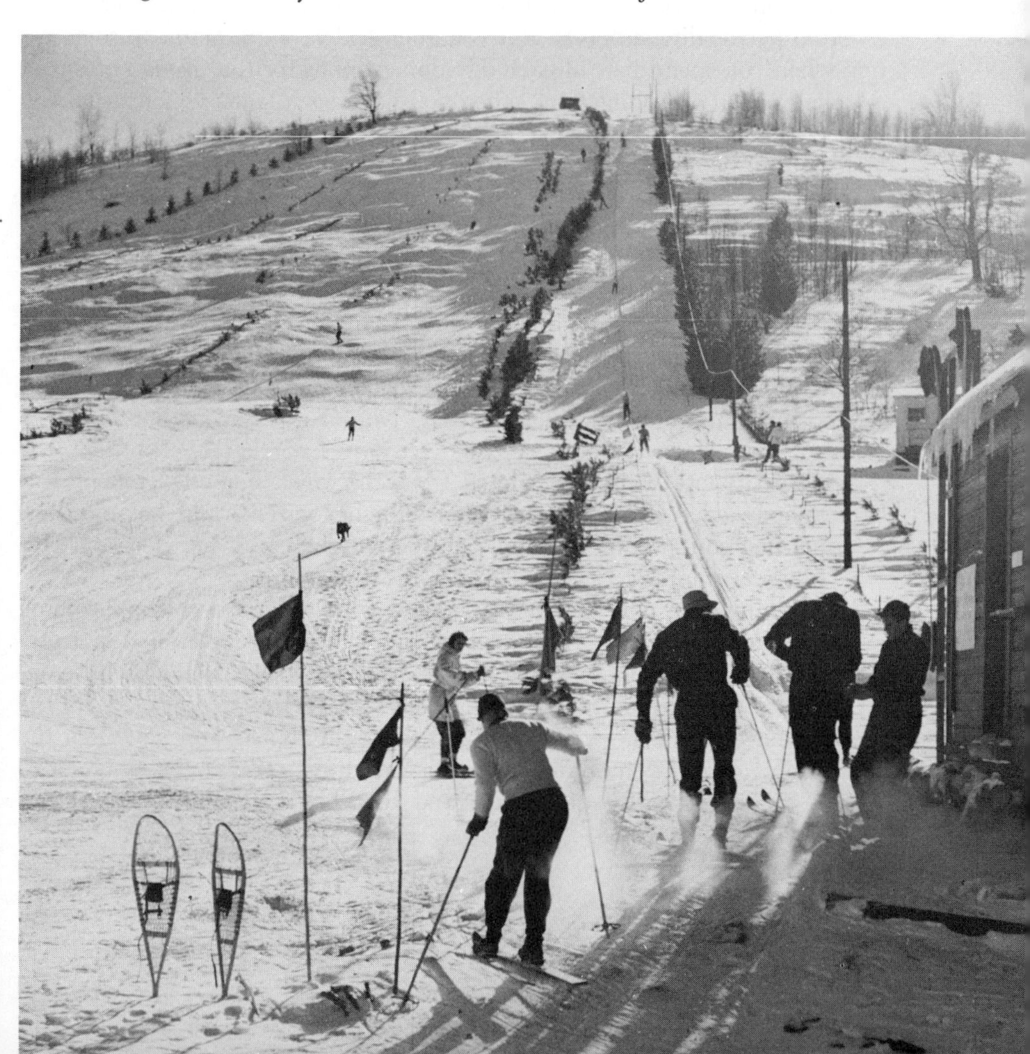

Most of these complaints call for a medical checkup, partly to discover possible underlying physical disease and partly to keep undue concern about the presence of such disease from adding further emotional strain. If no physical cause is found, three further steps are possible.

1. *Provide extra leisure, and use it for general psychological relief and support.* Your mind works very efficiently in promoting your psychological comfort. Given free rein, it impels you toward behavior which meets your inner needs quite well—often better than what you would have selected in a deliberate effort to combat stress. For this reason, leisure time often serves to restore emotional balance. You tend to use leisure time for hobbies or sports which give you just the kind of outlets you need, or for personal association providing just the kind of emotional support you need, or for reading, religious observances and other activities through which emotional balance can frequently be restored. Leisure time spent in pure loafing may or may not help: quite a few people with emotionally induced complaints get worse instead of better when they are at loose ends, since scheduled activity and the proof of worth involved in work or achievement are often essential personality supports. But you almost always get better to some extent when you spend part of each day doing things for fun instead of out of a feeling of duty or obligation. When you have complaints which make you suspect the need for boosted morale, a little more time each day following your natural bents may prove quite helpful indeed.

2. *Set your own house in order.* When troubled by psychogenic complaints, people who have been complacently muddling through should review their own living patterns and goals critically. Although you should not dig for quirks and complexes without professional guidance—morbid, retrospective self-searching almost always does more harm than good—you may be able to identify problem areas and take constructive action to set them right without profound, unguided self-analysis. To give a few examples:

a. A girl whose complaints dated from the week her engagement was announced reviewed her decision with her parents and her minister, gaining considerable assurance in the correctness of her decision. Her physical symptoms disappeared.
b. A young man who had been plagued with fatigue ever since coming to college decided to review his plans for the future. Enrolled in a premedical course mainly due to his family's wishes, he had little intrinsic motivation to study. Considerable self-searching led to the conclusion that he was actually in the right course, and gave him the feeling of self-determination for the first time.
c. A victim of indigestion discovered that his complaints were aggra-

vated by continual disagreements with his roommate. A new rooming arrangement proved much more satisfactory.

3. *Seek help and guidance.* If complaints interfere with your efficiency or comfort to any considerable degree, a trained psychiatrist, psychologist, or psychiatric social worker can probably give you considerable help.

A great deal of behavior and emotion is determined by associated events without truly logical connection. For example, a small child was riding in the open back seat of a convertible on a road paralleling a railroad track. As a train approached behind the car, somebody said: "Look, there's a train!" The child turned to look. At that moment, the train gave a frightening blast with its whistle, the automobile stopped suddenly to avoid collision with a truck, and the child tumbled screaming into the car's footwell. For months afterward, the youngster whimpered at even the distant sound of a train whistle and ran from the room when even a toy electric train was operating. Scarcely logical behavior when the train had nothing to do with his being hurt, but typical of emotional association!

Such obscure associations may cause considerable difficulties, and can usually be brought to light only with the intellectual guidance and the emotional support of a trained counselor.

ACKNOWLEDGED COLLEGE-AGE PROBLEMS

Certain problems arise so commonly during your college years that you probably either face them right now or will face them in the near future. The need for self-set vocational goals, problems related to courtship, and difficult financial decisions fall in this group.

Vocational Goals

When most students enter college, they still derive their impetus from a desire to please or fit in with other people. They study mainly because it is expected of them. The switch from this other-directed motivational pattern to the pursuit of self-chosen goals usually occurs sometime between college entrance and the end of the sophomore year, although it may come earlier or much later (and sometimes not at all). When it occurs, you gain new drive and intensity, and derive considerable gratification from your progress toward your various objectives and goals. To encourage formation of inner-directed goals, you might ask yourself these questions:

1. Do you have a valid goal now? You may have an entirely valid vocational goal already. Three points will help you feel greater confidence in your choice:

a. Normal progress to date or other evidence that your capacities fit your ambition.

b. Resources (including cash, family assistance, marketable skills, and ready credit) to meet your needs without cutting in disastrously on study time.

c. An interest which originated in genuine affinity for the subject rather than in a desire to avoid difficult courses, conform to the wishes of others, or emulate a respected relative.

2. Can you conceive of the living conditions and work day of a person successful in each of the careers you have seriously considered for yourself? To choose among careers on the basis of the life you will lead in them, you must know what that life will be like. The practice of medicine, for instance, involves the closest interpersonal relationship short of marriage, a pleasant degree of community respect, and frequent intellectual challenge, but it also involves a very long work week, continual emergency calls, and an uphill battle with the books in trying to keep up to date. Until you can outline a doctor's hour-by-hour schedule for both work and play, you cannot really decide that medicine is the right career for you.

3. If you do not have a valid vocational goal, could you set one today? Remembering that a definite decision today can still be altered if new facts emerge, can you use the problem-solving technique set forth above to arrive at a valid vocational goal? If not, can you settle on one field even if you have not determined what role you are capable of playing in it?

4. Would testing or counseling help? Although nobody can make up your mind for you, vocational counseling often helps you to make a sound decision. Objective tests of your capacities help you set realistic academic goals. Interest tests have two values: they help direct your attention toward the most suitable fields, and they group vocational choices in a way which brings to your attention many suitable careers you would not otherwise have considered. Counselors help in decision-making technique and can often provide facts not readily available to you from other sources.

Courtship Problems

Courtship has two major functions: to encourage the deep emotional attachment upon which a sound married life must be built, and to permit the discovery, trial (within limits), and selection of prospective mates. In pursuing the first objective, sexual attraction and practice create many problems. The second objective calls for decisions on how long and intensive a courtship should precede marriage and what issues should be settled before the final vows are solemnized.

Sex and courtship

Physical attraction unquestionably plays a part in the formation of close personal relationships. Propriety establishes different limits at each stage of courtship in every culture and permits emotional experience within those limits as a welding interpersonal force. The problems that arise out of sex play and indulgence stem mainly from conflict between the forces impelling you toward improper indulgence and the standards you have acquired by birth, training, or association.

Perhaps you can resolve or prevent some of this conflict by asking yourself these questions:

Figure 15. When you share an emotionally significant experience—especially a wholesome and pleasant one—you increase mutual attachment. *Ewing Galloway.*

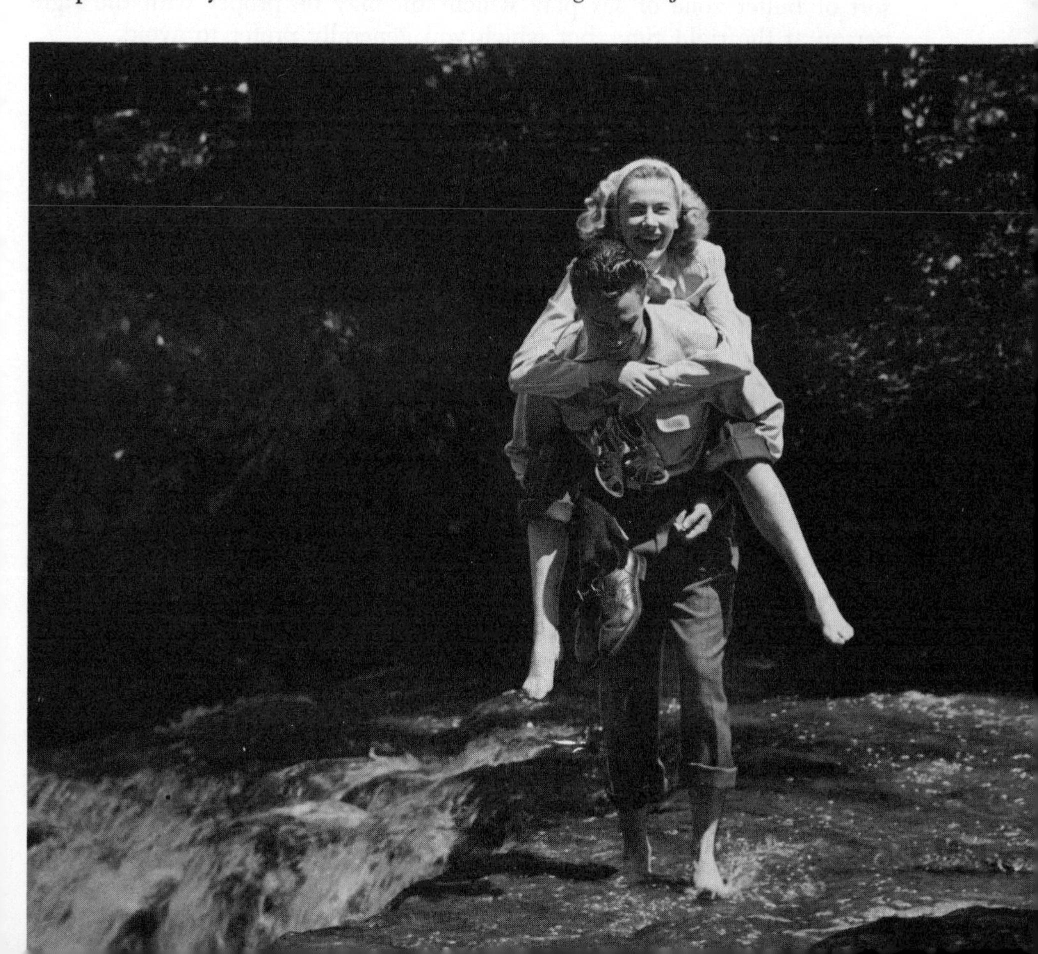

What is improper indulgence? Sex can be a welding sacrament which continually revitalizes marriage, or be a pleasant sport to which marriage gives license but no added significance and from which marriage gains only momentary values. The basic difference is whether the participants think of sex play and indulgence as expression of their feelings toward one another or as purely carnal pleasures to be sought for their own sake or given in exchange for specific rewards. The value of sex as affection-building communion through the many years of marriage weighs heavily in comparison with the transient pleasures of casual sexual contact.

You gain something important for your own future marriage, besides conforming to religious and social demands, by limiting premarital sexual relations. What level of sex play belongs in the marital preserve depends largely on your cultural background and personal views. Defining this preserve precisely *right now* may save you the distressing need for making crucial decisions under highly stress-ridden circumstances.

How much of a buffer zone do you need? Sexual excitement which has been carried beyond a certain point and left unconsummated leaves uncomfortable and distracting congestion in its wake. Very intense sex play may, therefore, yield less net enjoyment during courtship than somewhat more moderate indulgence. Understanding this fact may help you establish a sort of buffer zone of sex play which still may be proper with the right person at the right time, but which you generally prefer to avoid.

Courtship as prelude to marriage

Faced with the overwhelming biological pressures of youth, it is hard for college students to consider their relations with any member of the opposite sex to be a mutual employment interview for a lifetime contract. Yet continual reappraisal of candidates is the only way to avoid the difficult problems arising out of deep emotional attachment for someone you recognize as an unsuitable mate. You might find it worthwhile to write down right now the absolutely minimum criteria your future spouse must meet: religious, social, personal, and so on. Perhaps these standards will change considerably through the years, but at least they will guide you somewhat. Another simple aid is to keep a diary or an active correspondence with a parent or close friend about your social life. When you try to write something meaningful about a suitor, you automatically appraise some of his qualities.

Once you have pretty well settled on a certain prospective spouse, continued reappraisal serves another purpose: it helps you to get some of the burden of adjustment to each other out of the way before marriage. Differences in feeling toward family ties, differences in viewpoint about the roles of the sexes in marriage, differences in desire for children, and a number of other issues deserve discussion.

Financial Decisions

Most financial problems in college revolve around three questions: Is further penury and struggle worthwhile for the sake of more education? Is the relief from penury gained through part-time work worth the price in reduced efficiency in college? How far should you mortgage your future to resolve present difficulties?

Although facts and figures relating to your particular career help resolve these questions, many intangible factors also merit some consideration in your decision. You cannot decide whether more education is worthwhile by weighing its cost against increase in lifetime earnings after taxes. You must also consider difference in the type of work you will be able to perform, added professional stature, and the benefits in family, social, and community life. You cannot decide whether part-time work is worthwhile solely on the basis of its effect on your ability to make passing grades. Many of the most important benefits of college involve opportunities to pursue interests and acquire knowledge and skills beyond bare requirements, not to mention the social development and noncurriculum benefits of living with a select group of young people, participating in campus affairs, and so on. You cannot set your debt limit according to your borrowing capacity alone. You need a cushion of credit with which to meet emergencies, relative freedom from old debts when you undertake new family responsibilities, and as much relief as possible from the debt-multiplying burden of interest over the years.

In most colleges, you can get substantial help with financial problems by consulting the dean's office, loan and scholarship administrators, or student employment and housing bureaus. Many of these agencies can offer financial aid as well as guidance and help. The resources they tap are not charity: the increased value of your own services to the community more than repays the cost of keeping you in college or maintaining your study efficiency if you have real need. Why not go over your financial position with a counselor at intervals throughout your college career? You will be surprised at how many helpful suggestions he can give.

CHAPTER 5

Your Mind and Illness

HAVE YOU EVER SPENT A RESTLESS NIGHT BEFORE A CRUCIAL TRIP OR INTERVIEW? Do final examinations disturb your appetite or other bodily functions? Have you ever muffed an opportunity through undue embarrassment or other emotional upset?

Such psychologic, physical, and social difficulties can all originate in the mind. Even if your troubles have nonpsychologic origins, your mind determines how much hardship they will cause. One man can meet phlegmatically a type of pain which drives another to distraction, a third becomes a recluse after accidental loss of a leg while number four lives a full, rich life within the confines of a wheelchair.

Your mind coordinates all your physical, emotional, social and intellectual activities. It determines your response to all varieties of stress and strain. If its responses lead to any substantial decrease in your efficiency or comfort, you suffer some degree of mentally generated difficulties. Few people escape such problems altogether.[1] However, you can build and sustain personality strengths with which to meet them. You can learn to recognize and handle your own and your associates' problems.

PERSONALITY STRENGTHS

Your personality should provide two advantages: a stable psychological base and a set of well-developed abilities with which to pursue your various personal and social goals.

[1] The figure usually quoted, "one in ten will suffer mental illness," is based upon need for care in a psychiatric hospital. It does not include the infinitely more common episodes handled in the offices of psychiatrists and other physicians or by other types of counselors, the psychogenic illnesses whose physical component requires office or hospital care, or the vast number of upheavals you survive without expert help.

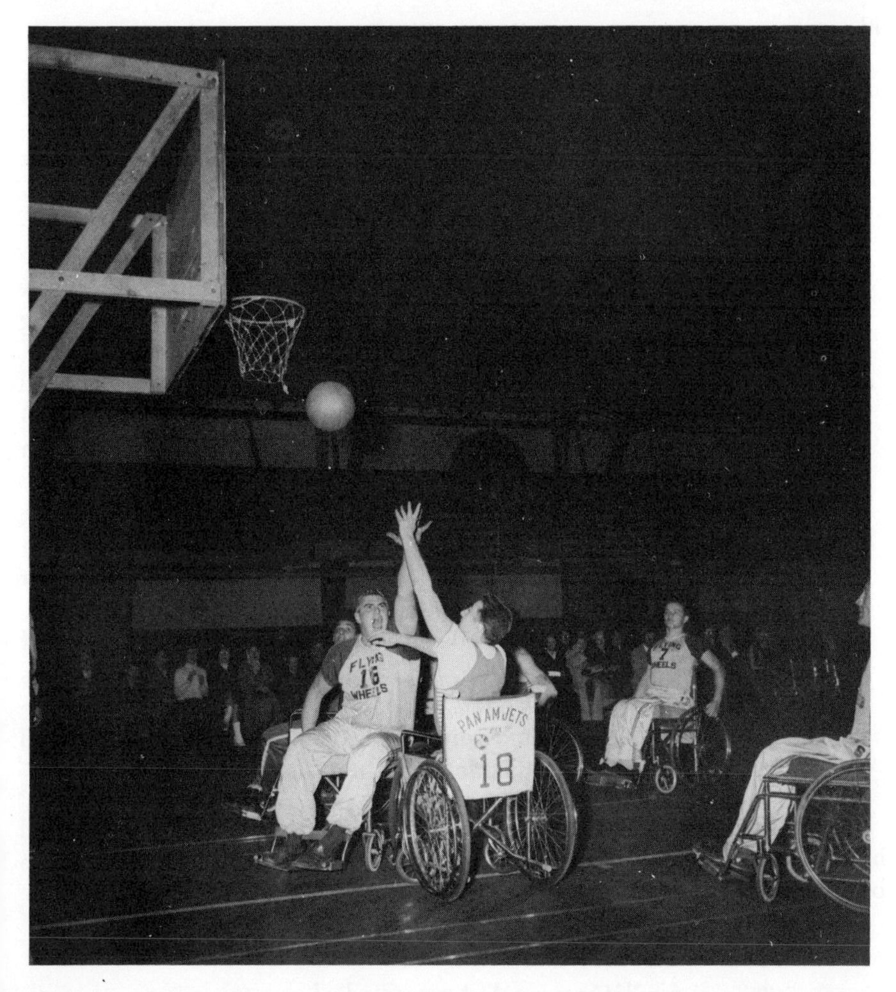

Figure 16. Living happily within physically imposed limitations: the Flying Wheels won 65–53. *Wide World Photos, Inc.*

A Stable Base

Archimedes once said: "Give me a solid fulcrum and I will move the world." In a sense, sound mental health is the fulcrum through which your efforts and abilities become effective. You need a degree of self-confidence, self-assertiveness, self-control, and stability to keep from being swept away from attained objects and to exert any leverage in reaching further goals. Sound mental health embraces all states of personality which permit effective functioning as an individual and reasonable psychologic comfort within the framework of society. As a rough guide to your own level of mental health, you might consider the list of questions below.

Mental health checklist

1 Do you enjoy life in general, experiencing unhappiness only in response to understandable causes?
2 Although you may occasionally be discouraged, are you generally self-confident and hopeful about yourself and your opportunities?
3 Are you able to maintain close and satisfying relationships with a few people, friendly relationships with a number of others, and get along well on the whole with your associates in business and other affairs?
4 Are you able to meet your problems without becoming more disturbed by them than their degree of seriousness would warrant and without customarily running away from them, asking others to bear them for you, or making life difficult for others because of your own burdens?
5 Except where there is reasonable cause, are you unafraid of people, things, and situations?
6 Are you sensibly concerned about your health without being either overly interested in your body functions or repelled by them?
7 Does your conscience help you keep your behavior good for yourself and for others without punishing you too severely for minor offenses nor endlessly for moderate offenses?
8 Do you only infrequently find yourself becoming angry or irritated and are you able to express justifiable anger in a socially acceptable way?

If you answered all questions "yes," you can be sure that your mental health is quite good. One or more negative answers do not necessarily mean bad mental health, of course.

Abilities and Accomplishments

In situations calling for evaluation of your vocational, avocational, social or personal qualities, you depend mainly upon a subconsciously formulated image known as your self-concept. This image tends to be somewhat static, often falling far behind new developments in your personality, physique, and situation. Common examples: The perpetual sophomore alumnus who obviously thinks of himself as "just one of the boys" long years after the boys cease to think that way; the tall man who wears unbecoming vertical stripes because he formed his clothing tastes during pudgy adolescence and still thinks of himself as overly broad; and the established authority who still expresses his opinions quite hesitantly because he has

[2] Adapted by permission from material in *Psychology for Living*, 2nd ed., by Sorenson and Malm. Copyright, 1957. McGraw-Hill Book Co.

never become used to the idea that people value his opinions. A similar, less extreme lag in your own present self-concept might plague you with feelings of physical inferiority because a late adolescence kept your development behind that of your associates for a time, or influence your choice of career by persistent insecurity based upon already solved financial or academic problems.

Besides being behind the times, your self-concept is often distorted by subconscious psychologic pressures. A homely woman may *need* to think of herself as sexually attractive. A student who has failed three courses may *need* to consider himself persecuted because of race or religion. A person who has found it impossible to win friends or develop other personal gratifications may *need* to think of himself as a dedicated businessman or teacher. These mechanisms are natural and effective ways of avoiding the grim facts of inadequacy or failure. In small doses, they may do enough good by making you feel self-confident and secure to justify the harm they do by keeping you from attacking the basic issues. Gross distortions often cause substantial difficulties, however. A reasonably accurate self-concept can help you in many ways. Two simple methods improve your self-appraisal considerably:

1. Check your appraisal of yourself against results. If you have a false picture of yourself as a tough guy, a great lover, a sharp bargainer, or a wit, the temporary pain of adjusting to the truth is generally far less than the recurrent pain of further errors resulting from your misapprehension. Certainly you should not lose confidence or quit whenever you suffer a setback, but an occasional pause to take stock of what you have actually accomplished with each of your apparent talents and skills may prove very helpful in adjusting your goals and your approach.

2. Watch how other people respond to you in different situations and roles. Since many crucial personality skills concern your interplay with other people, awareness of their response to your overtures helps you to recognize and use your own personality assets. You can learn to monitor your own interpersonal relations, at least on selected occasions, without particularly interfering with their spontaneity. You can become conscious of whether your relationship with any person or group is improving or deteriorating. By correlating these responses with the behavior patterns which evoke them, you can decide whether you do better as a sympathetic listener or an active counselor; whether your brand of humor makes people enjoy your company, causes them more embarrassment than pleasure, or simply falls flat; whether your habit of placing your hand on the other person's arm during conversation or the speed with which you start calling new acquaintances by their first name is well received, and so on.

PSYCHOLOGICALLY CAUSED COMPLAINTS

If we chose complete freedom from psychologically caused distress as our norm, all the world would indeed be mad. Almost everyone suffers from occasional physical, emotional, or social distress on psychologic grounds. Certain amounts of anxiety and tension are normal and desirable motivating or character-molding forces. Would you really extend yourself as much in preparing for examinations, for instance, if you had no anxiety about the outcome? Would you respond as alertly during the test if you were completely relaxed instead of tense?

Even mechanisms typical of serious mental disorders are normal, useful, and effective in certain circumstances. You do not necessarily have anything wrong with you if you get a headache just before a date which you do not want to keep, even though the mechanism is exactly the same as that which induces hysterical paralysis or invalidism. You are not ready for the psychiatrist's couch if you throw your golf club into the pond instead of admitting that the poor shot was your own fault, even although the mechanism is the same as that found in serious paranoia.

On the other hand, nobody is immune to psychologically caused complaints which call for corrective action. There is no reason to feel ashamed of having such troubles, or to hesitate in seeking help when difficulties arise, since everyone breaks under sufficient stress. For example, exposure to the continuous stress of combat during World War II caused a certain proportion of soldiers to suffer breakdown each week. If left long enough, virtually every individual from the original group was ultimately sent back from the front because of disabling mental illness. This fate was so inevitable that military authorities finally conceded to it, and adopted a policy of rotating troops to the rear before combat stress could reach overwhelming heights.

Most important psychologically induced complaints take one of five forms: physical complaints or disorders, mood disorders, dissociative disorders, psychasthenias, and behavior disorders.

Physical Complaints and Disorders

As we noted in the last chapter, physical changes such as cold sweats, racing heart, feeling of constriction in the chest and trembling hands are part of the emotional response to stress. Continual weakness and easy fatigue frequently stem from emotional upset. Other changes, such as tingling hands and feet, lightheadedness, and certain muscle spasms, result from breathing patterns imposed by emotion. Similar alterations in body functioning can lead to a variety of serious physical disorders ranging from indigestion and ulcers to high blood pressure and certain heart attacks.

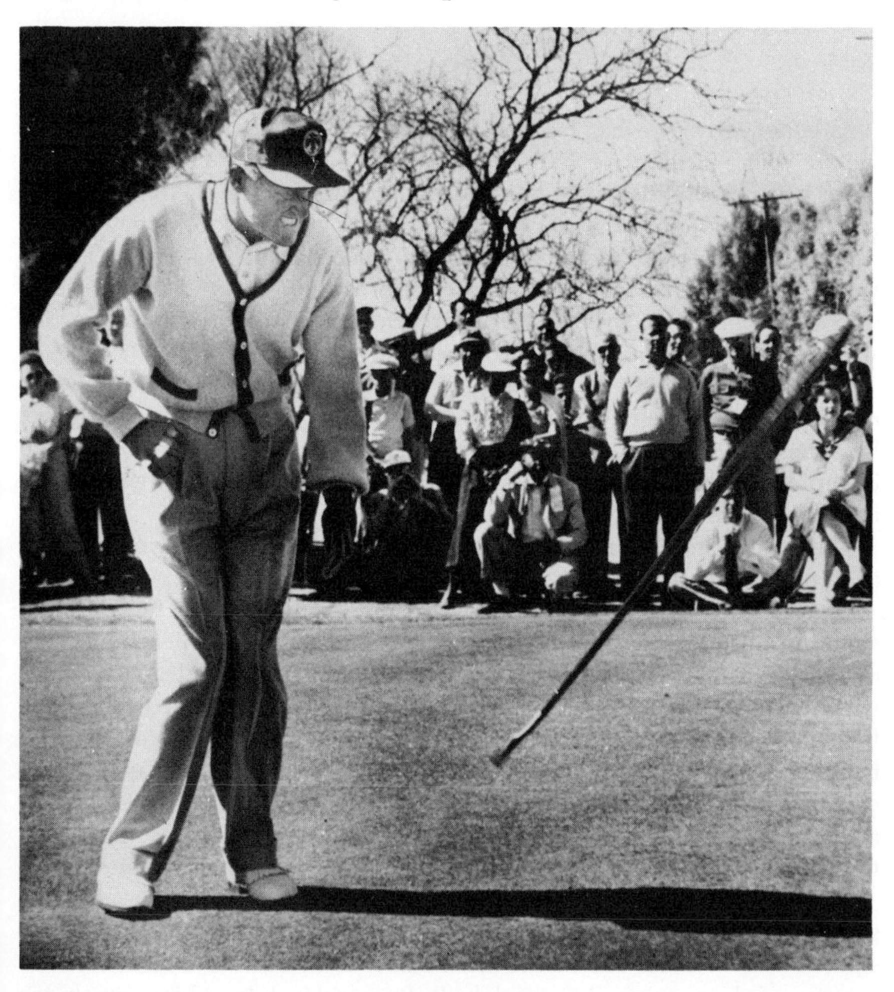

Figure 17. A normal emotional outlet. After flinging away his putter in disgust, Tommy Bolt went on to score a sizzling 65 and win the tournament. *Wide World Photos, Inc.*

Physical complaints also result at times from the mind's efforts to protect itself from conflict or guilt. In our society, a person who is incapable of meeting his responsibilities because of illness is not considered culpable. If you skip an examination because you are afraid of failing it (or failing to fulfil your own and your parents' expectations), you will lose self-respect and the respect of others. If you cannot take an examination because you feel sick to your stomach, nobody (not even yourself) thinks less of you. The miseries of nausea and vomiting are more acceptable than the humiliation of acknowledging fear.

Mood Disorders

Although everyone has his ups and downs, fluctuations in mood which impair your efficiency or happiness certainly deserve attention.

Deep depression lies at one end of the mood spectrum, being characterized by dejection, feelings of unworthiness and guilt, lack of appetite, constipation, loss of sex interest or capacity, and difficulty with sleep. Some victims wring their hands and pace the floor, while others sit in a dejected stupor. Response to conversational approach is slow and distracted. Suicidal attempts, plans, or thoughts are common.

Somewhat less extreme depression causes blue moods, crying in the morning, and a degree of disturbance in sleep, sex, eating, and bowel functions. Suicide is actually more common in moderate depressions than in profound ones, because the victim retains his ability to organize and carry out his plans.

The normal mood range comes next, characterized by relative efficiency and comfort.

When mood swings somewhat upward beyond the normal range, hypomania results. This is the so-called "talking sickness," in which the victim carries on a merry monologue. He often hops from one idea to another without finishing his sentences, although an alert individual can usually follow his meaning. The victim's exhilaration usually overcomes normal moral and social inhibitions. He tells ribald stories in none-too-appropriate circumstances, and abandons most sexual restraint. He is often extremely active, working or playing eighteen to twenty hours every day, but tends to flit from one thing to another much too rapidly for any real achievement.

The most extreme degree of upward mood swing, called mania, goes one step farther to almost perpetual frantic activity. The victim has no use for clothes, rest, or food. His talk is often continuous, but too disconnected to convey much meaning: his mind hops from subject to subject much too quickly to allow him ever to complete a sentence. His behavior serves little useful purpose, usually not even meeting his own bodily needs, so that he requires considerable care.

Dissociative Disorders

Schizophrenia and related disorders involve a dissociation between emotional response and matters with which the victim is currently dealing. To give an extreme example, a hospitalized victim of schizophrenia met the news of his mother's death with thigh-slapping laughter. He had gotten along well with his mother, and would normally have been quite grieved at her passing. His illness was so profound that his expressions of emotion were completely divorced from ordinary response patterns.

This same change characterizes all dissociative disorders. The schizoid personality's emotional responses are flattened. Other people feel shut out by his reserve and he himself feels more like a bystander than a participant in life. A hebephrenic's responses are inappropriate or inept, with silly giggles interrupting his own serious discourse. A paranoid distorts innocent circumstances into cause for hostility, blames imagined enemies for everything that goes wrong and perhaps strives to eliminate his problems by attacking these actually innocent associates. A catatonic's fantasy and its accompanying emotions occupy him to the point of distraction, perhaps even to a degree where he sits in a stupor without meeting his needs for food or basic cleanliness.

Although dissociative reactions interfere greatly with the victim's ability to get what he wants out of real life, they give substantial substitute emotional rewards. The patient frequently becomes so absorbed with his own distorted or unreal perceptions that the return to drab reality seems more a comedown than a cure. For instance, one schizophrenic woman sat in a stupor for years, and on recovery said that she had ignored her doctors and attendants because she thought she was in Heaven, surrounded by the angels, and the doctors were tempters sent to drag her down. No wonder severe, well-established dissociative disorders tend to persist for many years, making early care for this type of disorder crucial!

Psychasthenias

A psychasthenia upsets some specific function of the mind without causing physical complaints or total personality disturbance. Victims of obsessive neurosis are haunted by certain ideas, impulses, or thoughts they recognize as useless and distracting but cannot exclude. A college coed found the statement "You're simply not college material" going around and around in her brain, for instance. A young man at a wedding reception found himself so plagued by the impulse to ask the bride "And when is the baby due?" that he did not dare speak to her, and left the reception precipitously.

Victims of compulsive neurosis have similar fixed and recurrent responses, but in patterns of behavior rather than thought. Patterned behavior contributes to your emotional security by making familiar, reassuring repetition out of many frequently performed activities. So long as such reassuring rituals remain brief and relatively efficient, they are not only harmless but also very useful. You need help only when rituals become burdensome. For instance, one patient regularly required nearly an hour to undress because every article of clothing had to be laid out just so. Any interruption meant that he had to get dressed again and start all over. Another washed his hands with a brush for ten minutes many times each day, ultimately leaving them covered with raw, weeping sores.

A phobia involves intense fear of an actually harmless object or situation. Most phobias are emotional responses which have been transferred from commonly encountered objects to uncommon and socially accepted ones. A woman who exchanges fear of the male sex organ for a concentrated, pathologic fear of some such symbolic equivalent as a snake may find herself in an occasional unreasoning terror, but frees her marriage of a considerable emotional burden. When the object to which fear is transferred is frequently encountered, as in fear of crowds, heights, confined spaces, and the like, psychiatric measures to encourage direct attack upon the basic underlying fear are usually worthwhile.

Behavior Disorders

In a civilized world, everyone's behavior is partly controlled by the demands of communal living. You wear clothes, you eat with a knife and fork, you say what is expected of you more often than what you really think. It takes time to learn the prescribed limits and to train yourself to move comfortably within them. Some people never achieve this goal, or achieve it precariously with frequent breaches in observance. When harmful effects result, a behavior disorder exists. The form of disorder varies, but alcoholism, homosexuality, criminal behavior, and other forms of deviation or rebellion are common examples.

You learn social standards and learn to accept them comfortably at a steady rate from birth. However, society does not expect much of you at first. A three-year old who picks up somebody else's pennies is quite innocent, a thirteen-year old who does the same thing is a budding delinquent, and a twenty-three year old a full-fledged crook. Behavior disorders therefore seem quite prevalent in the teens and twenties, when society's expectations are fully established but conformity still is developing. However, many behavior problems improve without deliberate treatment as the individual responds more and more to social pressures, while most other psychologic difficulties get worse over the years.

PHYSICALLY CAUSED MENTAL DISORDERS AND COMPLAINTS

Physical diseases not specifically affecting the brain may mimic psychologic disorders and complaints. For example, seemingly psychologic difficulties such as nervousness, irritability, pounding or racing heart, and insomnia sometimes stem from overactivity of the thyroid gland with resulting overacceleration of most body processes. Physical diseases not specifically affecting the brain can impose emotional burdens sufficient to cause psychologic disorders, too. Prolonged disability, discomfort, and the need to depend on others for help with even simple tasks may involve enough stress to throw a victim of arthritis into depression, for instance.

Physical diseases which affect the brain frequently cause severe disorders in mental functioning. The main difficulties, in the order of the frequency in which they are likely to strike among your relatives and friends, are as follows.

Delirium

The internal poisonings and disordered bodily functions of a severe illness, or the physiologically similar aftereffects of alcoholic excess, sometimes bring on a state of delirium in which the victim suffers nightmare visions and sensations he regards as entirely real, at the same time losing consciousness of the real world around him. He often takes physical part in the events he is imagining, fighting or running away from the fearful objects he perceives. He frequently injures himself in the process.

A delirious child or an acutely ill adult requires close attention, especially in the early morning hours. Someone should sit up with the victim if there is any way whatever in which he can injure himself (which there always is in the home). Unless the underlying disease has been completely cured, constant attendance at night is more important than extra care during the day for two or three days after apparent recovery from delirium.

Delirium tremens occurs when alcoholic excess leads to poisoning effects plus disordered use of fluids and fuel in the brain. Without treatment a considerable percentage of victims accumulate enough extra fluid in the brain to squeeze it fatally against the inside of the skull. Delirium tremens is a serious disorder. If this illness arises in your family or circle of friends, you can help the victim considerably by making arrangements for prompt, intensive medical care.

Senile Psychosis

The memory loss, confusion, and emotional instability which stem from marked senile change in the brain sometimes constitute mental derangement. Further difficulties arise through the frequent accompanying tendency to distort other people's motives, to blame real or imagined problems on specific individuals, and therefore to develop unreasonable anger or hostility. Many old people ultimately require care in a psychiatric hospital for this reason.

If one of your relatives seems headed toward senile psychosis, two steps often prove worthwhile: remain alert for evidences of deterioration as described in Chapter 23, and (if he has any property) ask the old person's doctor to make and record simple tests of his mental competence occasionally to prevent both dissipation of his resources through mismanagement during the early stages of mental deterioration and legal battles about the validity of his will when he expires.

Alcoholism, Syphilis, Tumors, and Other Causes of Brain Damage

Evidence of memory loss or abrupt change in character in conjunction with headaches or impairment in muscular or nerve-controlled function deserve a doctor's prompt appraisal. Brain damage from disease or injury may be at fault.

Many people wonder why tax-supported institutions give so much care to victims of alcoholic excess and syphilis of the brain while victims of less reprehensible disorders are left to shift largely for themselves. Alcoholics and syphilitics fill enough state-supported mental hospital beds to more than justify intensive preventive and early-care programs for the control of these disorders. In Minnesota, for example, the entire cost of the state's venereal disease control program, which includes free laboratory service, contact investigation, and material for treatment, costs less per year than it costs the state to treat two victims of brain syphilis. Alcoholism accounts for millions of dollars worth of psychiatric care each month, while free clinic care and policing of alcohol purveyors is comparatively inexpensive. Although you may feel little sympathy with drunks and syphilitics, early management of their disorders can save you considerable tax money during your vocational life, and thus deserves your political support.

WHAT TO DO ABOUT MENTAL ILLNESS

If you encounter psychologically induced disabilities or complaints in either yourself, your family, or a close friend, you will wonder what to do about them. The next few pages will tell you what the prospects are for victims of mental illness, what forms of help are available for them, and what you can do to combat mental illness in yourself or your associates.

Prospects

The rate of cure in mental disorders is considerably higher than in most other disease categories. A large percentage of the patients in a mental hospital at any one time seem to be incurable, but this is due mainly to the fact that incurable patients live out their normal life span. One schizophrenic who becomes ill at age twenty-five and remains hospitalized until age sixty-five balances in the hospital census over eighty patients who are cured within six months. Moreover, a large percentage of mental illnesses respond to nonhospital treatment, and many victims of mild or readily curable mental disorders get all the help they need from a general practitioner without even recognizing the psychological basis for their complaints.

Several methods of treatment help to speed recovery from mental illness.

Psychotherapy

Treatment of illness by planned interaction of human personalities or intellects often is highly effective. Many varieties of such treatment are frequently available to victims of psychogenic difficulty.

Reassurance

The fear that serious physical disease underlies complaints and the fear that there will be permanent, severe mental disability add to the burdens of mental illness. If the patient's condition lets him accept reassurance on these points, a doctor's thorough evaluation of his state may itself prove curative.

Support

Personal interest and concern give you a feeling that someone is behind you in your struggles with the problems of daily living, and often proves distinctly helpful.

Guidance or counseling

Failure to realize and make the most of your assets may let mental illness strike when all the raw materials for sound and satisfying daily life are readily at hand. Discussing your situation with a counselor may help you gain a new perspective.

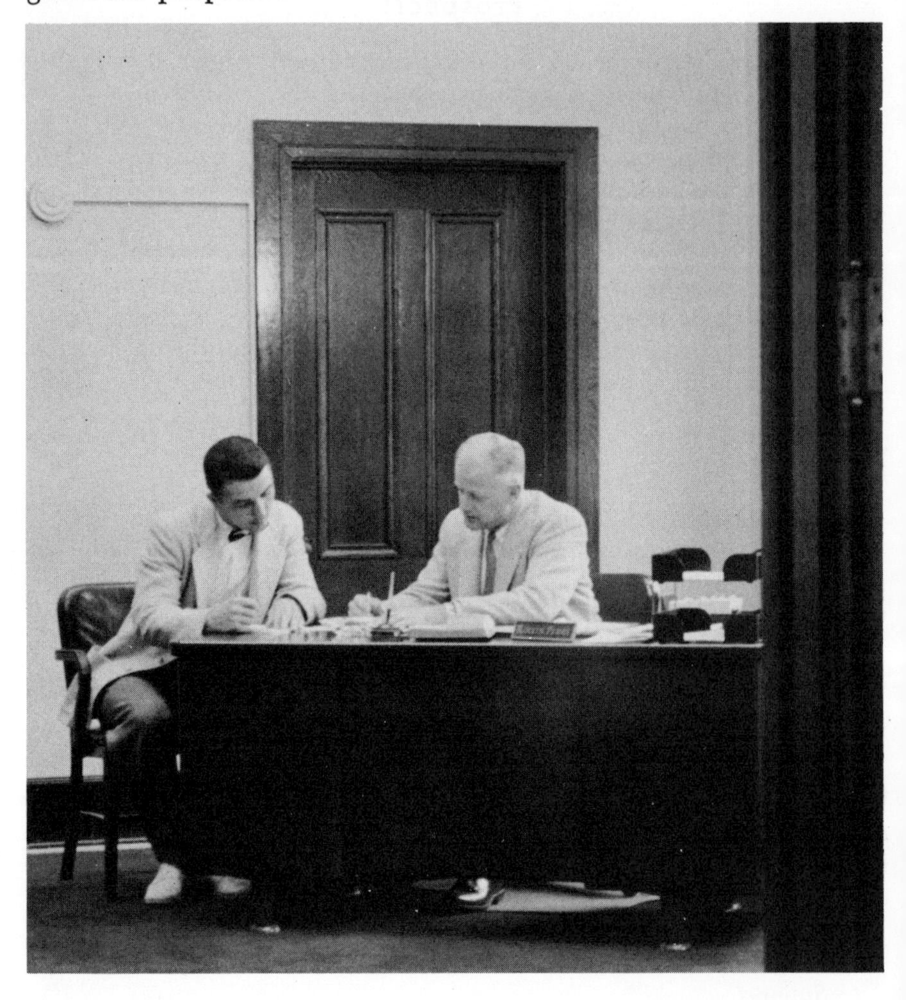

Figure 18. Counselors sometimes help. *Cornell University News Bureau.*

Ventilation

When you talk about past experiences or present problems with a trained therapist, you relive or examine them in a situation ideally suited to intellectual resolution of rankling difficulties. The other person's presence and interest helps you to bear up under burdens of emotional conflict which otherwise would make it difficult or impossible for you to deal with the issues rationally. Deeply rooted psychologic difficulties thus often yield to guided airing of the emotional conflicts and experiences underlying them.

Controlled environment

A psychiatric hospital relieves the patient of most need to make decisions. He does not have to decide when to get up in the morning, when to go to meals, or what to eat. His mental energies are freed for the more important task of self-repair, just as the physical energies of a person with bodily illness are conserved by putting him to bed. At the same time, every psychiatric facility offers noncritical acceptance. Nobody in a psychiatric clinic or hospital greets the unfortunate manifestations of illness with ridicule or unreasoning fear. Even patients with quite evident deviations from "normal" can win friends and achieve respect and acceptance instead of being summarily rejected as freaks. The hospital also permits relative isolation from the patient's usual associations and relationships, some of which either caused or are intimately involved in his breakdown. Most psychiatric hospitals supply a variety of activities for patients, providing a sense of achievement through craft programs, an opportunity for artistic expression with finger paints and so on. Some patients need constant supervision (although comparatively few in this day of effective turmoil-soothing drugs) to keep them from harming themselves or others. The ready availability of medical and psychiatric treatment is also important, especially for patients whose home communities lack such facilities.

Relatives or friends frequently can supply the proper environment for a victim of mental illness. If suicide is a threat, simply having someone around all of the time usually provides protection—mildly depressed people seldom harm themselves except when they are left alone. In other cases, relatives and friends can help by accepting the disease victim in whatever role seems most comfortable for him. In the depression which follows loss of a loved one, a body part, or a function, the normal grieving processes speed recovery much more than injunctions to "buck up," for instance.

Religious ministrations

Religion offers considerable help to many victims of turmoil or depression. Psychiatric attack on mental illness is perfectly compatible with the religious approach.

Drugs and Physical Treatments

Besides attacking problems of the mind through the mind, psychiatrists and other physicians sometimes employ drugs or physical forms of treatment.

Medicines

Several medicines soothe psychological complaints and physical problems with psychological roots. These medicines give comfort during upsets which are temporary in nature, and sometimes permit a better attack on long-range problems by restoring more normal interpersonal relationships.

Shock treatment

Periods of unconsciousness induced by convulsion-causing drugs or electric current have highly beneficial effect in some mental illnesses. Since these treatments not only render the patient completely unconscious but also usually blank out his memory of the preliminaries, no notable physical or mental discomfort is involved.

Physical therapy

Certain special forms of baths and massage sometimes prove soothing or stimulating to victims of mental illness.

Sources of Professional Assistance

You can seek several varieties of expert help with mental disorders or problems. Each has advantages and disadvantages.

Psychiatry

Psychiatrists are graduate M.D.'s with several years of further training in the management of mental disorders. They can prescribe medications, administer shock treatment, and evaluate both physical complaints which have an emotional basis and psychological aspects of physical disease. The firm confidence most people have in physicians, plus the physician's well-established tradition of keeping confidence, help to establish a helpful counseling relationship between patient and psychiatrist.

Most psychiatrists in this country follow one of these disciplines: psychoanalysis, psychobiology, or eclectic. A psychoanalyst applies specific techniques to help you recall and resolve emotion-charged conflicts from your past experience. A psychobiologist works with you to discover and make the most of your personality assets. An eclectic psychiatrist attempts to apply whatever methods he feels will help each individual patient. A psychoanalyst thus follows different theories, but is not necessarily at a higher professional level than other psychiatrists. A limited number of highly selected patients get worthwhile benefits from analysis, while the bulk of psychiatric treatment is conducted in other ways.

Clinical psychology

A clinical psychologist can discover the nature of mental disorders. He can give effective support, counseling, and intensive or ventilative psychotherapy.

Other professional categories

General practitioners and other nonpsychiatrist physicians probably care for the bulk of mental illnesses in this country. Medications, reassurance, support, and counseling are within their scope. These measures frequently suffice for mild or moderately severe conditions.

Social workers, guidance counselors, rabbis, ministers, and priests all get substantial training in recognition and care of mental disorders. While their efforts other than specifically religious ministrations are usually limited to counseling and support, they often get good results. If the measures they can apply do not suffice, they can often help to arrange further care.

How to Arrange Counseling or Care

The services of workers trained in prevention and care of mental illness are available through many agencies.

Specific college facilities

While you are in college, you probably have considerable special counseling help available to you. Many large colleges and universities provide specific mental hygiene clinics staffed by social workers, psychologists, and psychiatrists. Staff members in the student counseling bureau often have considerable psychologic training and are sometimes able to give considerable help for a variety of mild personality difficulties. In institutions too small to provide specialized mental health or counseling services, the Dean of Students' office or certain of the faculty advisers may provide some such guidance or help you to locate further help. The college health service may be another source of aid. Campus religious organizations are usually staffed with workers especially chosen for their sympathetic concern for young adults and their problems.

Private practice

Psychiatrists, other physicians, and clinical psychologists commonly practice their professions independently. Your usual physician can often help you with your problem, or can help you to choose a more specialized adviser and make suitable arrangements.

Psychiatric treatment often involves frequent visits over a considerable period of time. Cost per visit runs at least fifteen to twenty-five dollars for psychiatric care or ten to fifteen for psychologic counseling. Economic barriers thus prevent many patients from using private facilities, especially if their illness interferes with their earning capacity.

Psychiatric wards, hospitals, and clinics

Psychiatric care provided in conjunction with hospital facilities usually embraces the services of a psychiatrist or of a psychiatrist-psychologist-social worker team. Shock treatment and drugs are usually administered quite competently. Many public institutions provide adequate psychotherapy, especially for patients who have recently become ill (among whom psychiatrists expect to accomplish the most per interview hour). These facilities are usually either totally tax supported or are provided on an ability-to-pay basis (patients being assessed full fees, reduced fees, or nothing after a financial investigation).

Mental hygiene clinics

Most mental hygiene clinics give treatment or help with frank illness and with troublesome problems or difficulties instead of the truly preventive care the name implies. If your community maintains such a clinic, you can usually get excellent advice for any psychiatric problem on an ability-to-pay economic basis. Social workers, psychologists, and psychiatrists usually work together in such clinics to provide economical and efficient service.

Family welfare agencies

Since mental illnesses and emotional problems often disturb an individual's ability to fit in well with his family life, most family welfare agencies provide complete counseling service for mental upsets and illnesses. The social worker-psychologist-psychiatrist team approach is most common, and an ability-to-pay basis leaves both the rich and the poor free to use the service.

Juvenile and educational trouble-shooting agencies

Many states and some counties provide special psychiatric, psychologic, and social worker services for juveniles through either the department of education or the department of public welfare. Sometimes these facilities are available to adults whose problems are contributing to the difficulties experienced by juveniles, as when an alcoholic father mistreats his children sufficiently to cause them psychologic disorders. These services are usually rendered on an ability-to-pay basis.

Religious agencies

As trained and experienced workers with considerable knowledge of the victim's background, religious counselors often provide effective psychotherapeutic counseling as well as specific religious guidance. Some churches take their responsibilities in this area so seriously that they provide trained social workers, psychologists, and even psychiatrists for counseling services.

MENTAL HEALTH FROM A COMMUNITY POINT OF VIEW

Mental illnesses requiring hospitalization involve heavy expense in conjunction with prolonged disability, which generally makes their cost too burdensome for the victim to meet with his own resources. Even illnesses which do not require hospitalization frequently call for such long and expensive care that few can afford proper treatment without community help. Mental illness can lead its victims to harm other people as well as themselves, and to neglect or abuse their families in ways which ultimately demand community intervention or aid. The community must also provide means of suspending certain civil rights so that a person whose illness keeps him from recognizing his own need for care can be confined for treatment

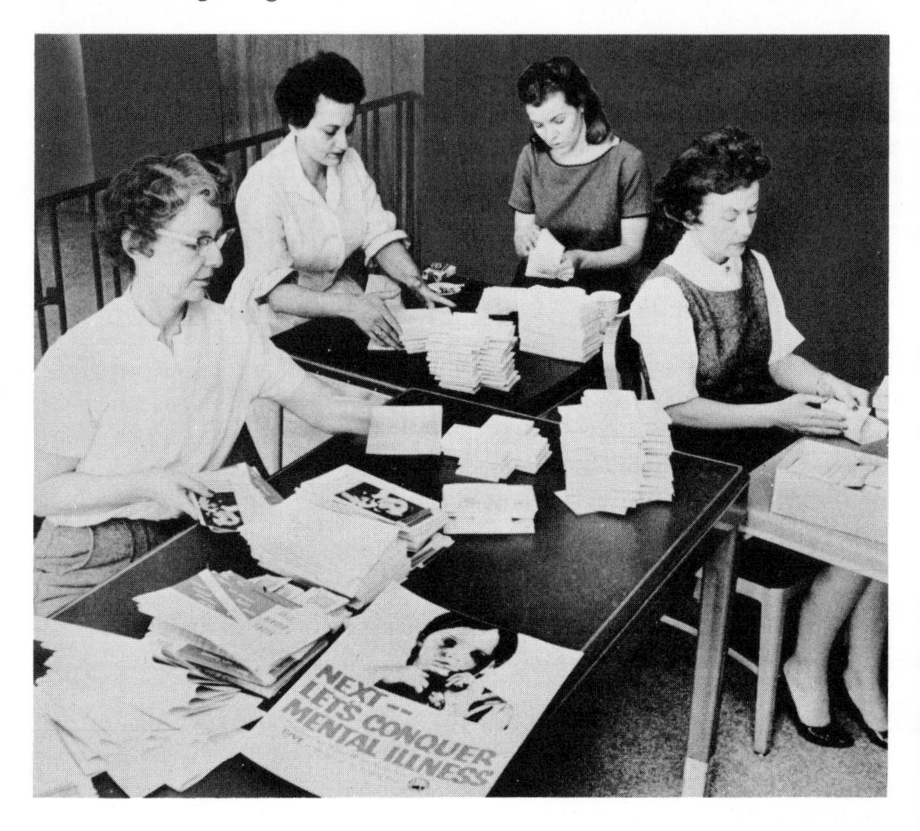

Figure 19. Volunteers at work. *Courtesy Minnesota Association for Mental Health* and the *Rochester Post-Bulletin.*

and so that a person whose illness prevents him from managing his property prudently can be saved from his own temporary ineptitude. It must provide legal safeguards to keep unscrupulous people from abusing these processes of commitment and guardianship.

Some of the difficulties which fall upon your community as a result of mental illness cannot be rectified. Others cost a great deal more to manage if they have proceeded to the point where community intervention is absolutely necessary than if they receive attention earlier in their course. Even long-standing problems may cost less when handled by prompt and intensive treatment than when allowed to smolder along year after year.

With one person in ten requiring hospital care for mental illness during his lifetime, with delinquency and criminality imposing burdens of danger, property damage and expense, and with milder mental illness creating a multitude of milder but still appreciable community-involving difficulties, mental illness is a problem in which you have a definite stake as a taxpayer and as a citizen. Even if mental illness could not strike you or yours (and it can), better treatment facilities, more prevention and an improved research program deserve your support. You can work through many voluntary and official agencies in combatting mental illness with absolute certainty that this goal is worthy.

CHAPTER 6

Alcohol, Tranquilizers, Sedatives, and Narcotics

ALCOHOL RESEMBLES TRANQUILIZERS, SEDATIVES, AND NARCOTICS IN IT PRINCIPAL effect, which is suppression of certain brain functions. All of these materials definitely affect the functioning of your body and mind, and all of them involve hazards and drawbacks. You often have to decide whether you stand to gain enough to outweigh your possible losses from any particular use of any particular agent. If you know how each of these agents operates, you can decide such issues more intelligently.

SHARED EFFECTS

Alcohol, tranquilizers, sedatives, and narcotics all work by suppressing the function of certain parts of your nervous system. The direct effect of such suppression is slowing, diminution or loss of certain sensitivities or reactions.

You can sometimes obtain a desired result by impeding a normal function, but only by risking or surrendering some increment of capability. A degree of release from intellectual or conscience-dictated self-control follows use of alcohol, sedatives, and tranquilizers, for instance. Such release may ease self-consciousness, social restraint, anxiety-inducing perfectionism, and other problems, but involves some risk of numbed conscience, dulled motivation, and muddied intellect. Narcotics produce definite and medically useful insensitivity to pain when administered in the usually prescribed doses, but impair mental efficiency to a measurable (though not disabling) degree in the process. Various depressant drugs often prove useful in inducing sleep, but at the price of somewhat dulled consciousness in the event of an emergency.

Alcohol is not a stimulant

Alcohol works by suppressing mental functions, not by stimulating them, in spite of old-fashioned references to brandy as a "stimulant" still found in many books. Apparent stimulation occurs at times because many mental functions are governed by a complex set of check-and-balance-type controls, partial suppression of which removes normal inhibitions. Perhaps you have seen an ordinarily quiet, humorless young man spurred into lively and witty repartee by a drink or two, for instance. In his normal state, fear of making social errors makes him mull over each remark until the time for making it has long since passed, and he seems rather dull. Alcohol makes him less concerned about the impression he might make, and so relieves constraint. It does not stimulate his brain toward brilliant retorts; it only suppresses the exaggerated self-control which usually keeps him from making them (and in the process also depresses normal self-control and makes him much more prone to social error).

Dependence, Habituation, and Addiction

The main sources of difficulty from use of alcohol, tranquilizers, sedatives, and narcotics are drug dependence, habituation, or addiction. If you acquire a drug *dependence,* you use suppressants to met recurring problems instead of attempting to solve them. With a drug *habit,* you find that you cannot live a normal life without regular dosage unless you first endure an uncomfortable period of readjustment. In full-fledged *addiction,* definite and severe illness punishes any attempt to get along without the drug. Most tranquilizers can cause dependence but not true habituation, while alcohol, sedatives, and narcotics quite frequently cause both dependence, habituation, and addiction.

MEDICINAL USES

Narcotics, sedatives, and tranquilizers help relieve pain, cough, restlessness, insomnia, and undue tension or anxiety. Your doctor may prescribe suppressant drugs when your illness involves such difficulties. The fact that he has medicines effective in fighting psychogenic complaints often makes it worthwhile for you to consult him even though you know your difficulties are too temporary to require lengthy counseling or psychotherapy.

Drugs During Illness

A doctor usually prescribes the smallest dose of a narcotic or sedative which will consistently accomplish his purpose and keeps the total amount prescribed sufficiently small that his patient will not develop habituation or addiction problems. These precautions virtually eliminate the risk of habituation or addiction during a brief illness. You can take as much as you need to stay comfortable if you stay within the prescribed dosage limits and quit within two to three weeks.

In illnesses which may last more than three weeks, ask your doctor whether you should accept mild discomfort in order to avoid habituation or addiction. Medications prescribed for prolonged or recurrent illness account for a substantial number of narcotic addictions and for most addiction to sedatives. While you should take full advantage of the pain relief and soothing effects prescribed preparations can offer, an awareness of hazards will help you work with your doctor to avoid habituation.

Drugs for Situational Stress

Tranquilizers or mild sedatives have a definite place in easing the stress you feel in certain situations. When you feel upset or distraught after the death of a close relative, for instance, your doctor can probably give you definite relief with perfectly safe doses of a sedative or tranquilizer. On the other hand, students frequently ask for such drugs in circumstances better handled without such aid: to combat the tension of an ordinary test or to facilitate calm during an employment interview. You should make a special effort to handle frequently recurring situations and situations which involve character molding, leadership, or personal training without drugs. A few examples of problems better met in other ways:

••• Mary C. asked for sleeping pills because the people in the next room were so noisy that they kept her awake. A complaint to her landlady solved the problem with no risk of addiction.

••• Peter L. wanted help with the jitters he always suffered when he gave a talk in speech class. After some discussion, he realized that calming down with tranquilizers would make classroom experience almost worthless as preparation for later public speaking demands.

••• Jerry N. wanted tranquilizers to help him ride out a crisis in the fraternity of which he was president. Since he presumably would have had difficulties in arousing any feeling of urgency in the brethren as he smiled in unconcerned calm, he finally decided to endure his tensions for the sake of greater effectiveness in leadership.

SOCIAL USE OF ALCOHOL

In many elements of American culture, alcoholic beverages definitely are an expected adjunct to hospitality and conviviality. Even a quiet family dinner may call for a cocktail or two. Here are the main arguments for and against using alcohol as a social lubricant.

Benefits Claimed for Social Drinking

Alcohol numbs one's concern over what others might think of him and thus helps overcome social constraint. Many people find the effect of alcohol on tension and on consciousness of fatigue desirable as an aid to social intercourse and amiable family life. Although alcohol itself does not taste good, centuries of experimentation have evolved many forms of cocktail, wine, liqueur, and so on which some find pleasing to taste or stimulating to appetite. And last, the ability to drink without drunkenness or loss of social grace is one criterion of acceptability in many groups. Different settings apply varying standards which range from the beer bust's demand that you remain conscious to the cocktail party's insistence on profound decorum and tact while your control is under alcoholic assault. However, all have in common a degree of mastery of alcoholic influence over behavior most people acquire only with practice.

Hazards of Social Drinking

Alcohol's capacity to numb your concern over what others think of you and its similar effect on your own conscience sometimes result in improprieties which might have serious consequences. Such alcohol-caused problems range from crude remarks or insults you wouldn't have uttered had you taken one less drink to sexual liberties resulting in an unwanted pregnancy. The slowed reflexes of even moderate drinking create a special problem in this age of fast-moving traffic: two or three cocktails will double your time-lag in emergency response, even though they may not affect your social behavior or ordinary coordination. Any use of alcoholic beverages involves some risk of habituation and addiction, especially use to quell fatigue and tension (which directly involves the hazardous I-need-a-drink-to-get-along philosophy). Finally, the acceptance of drinking as a social norm by people who can handle moderate alcoholic intake permits and encourages others (some of whom cannot handle the drinking situation) to try out various uses of alcohol.

DANGEROUS NONMEDICINAL USES OF NARCOTICS AND SEDATIVES

Many young people sample various drugs to explore a new range of experience: a dream world whose sensuous pleasures they feel can only be appraised by actual trial. This desire to explore is usually supplemented by the forbidden-fruit philosophy of social rebellion or family defiance.

Since drugs usually are available only through illegal channels, experimentation is actually limited to the pusher's routine, which aims at getting as many customers hooked as possible rather than providing a liberal education. Marihuana is the loss leader: it produces real-seeming dreams which are mainly frightening and unpleasant, but occasionally pleasantly erotic and never humdrum. A sense of liberation from time's steady progress, in which hours of experience seem to occur during a minute or two, heightens the sense of escape. However, the drug's unpleasant physical aftermaths quickly drive most experimenters to other drugs. At this point the pusher introduces morphine or heroin, which produce interesting dreams for a few episodes. Thereafter, their use produces very little pleasure unless the dose is continually increased, but if enough doses have been taken to establish addiction the victim feels literally terrible without the drug. He finds himself needing considerable dosage merely to keep comfortable. The cost of a day's dosage runs about twenty dollars on the illegal market. The addict thus has little chance to support his habit honestly, and frequently resorts to crime in an effort to keep his need appeased.

Experimentation with drug action other than through the pusher's web sometimes occurs in conjunction with spiritualism and the like. Sedative-induced trances and drug-aided hypnotism lead fairly frequently to habituation or addiction.

Drug addiction often takes the place of alcoholic indulgence in certain population groups. Alcoholic addicts frequently go from liquor to sedatives and occasionally to narcotics when alcohol is unavailable or when curative methods make alcohol repugnant without helping basic personality difficulties. A surprisingly high percentage of doctors, dentists, and nurses adopt a drug habit under pressures which would lead to alcoholism in other people, partly because drugs are readily available to them and partly because the effects are not as readily recognized by patients, permitting the habit to remain undetected for extra months or years.

ALCOHOLIC, BARBITURATE AND NARCOTIC ADDICTION

Psychological factors predispose the vast majority of victims to alcoholic or other addiction. In a superficial view, it is easy to find examples like the eminent and successful Mr. Jones who had social position, a fine family, and a good job until he took to drink and wound up in the gutter. Upon closer examination, you usually find that Mr. Jones had many chinks in his armor before the demon rum came on the scene. The usual nature of those chinks, the early signs of impending alcoholic or drug trouble, and ways to combat alcoholism and addiction will be considered in the rest of this chapter.

Symptomatic Alcoholism

As a readily available, potent sedative which victims of mental distress can use without even acknowledging that they are sick, alcohol is often the first refuge of victims of depression and other mental illness. An abrupt change in drinking habits over a period of a few weeks or months strongly suggests some such psychological pressure for relief. Accompanying evidence of blue moods or impairment in eating, sleep, bowel function, or sex-pace point strongly toward severe psychological disturbance for which medically prescribed measures will give quick and worthwhile relief.

Alcoholism as Rebellion

Alcohol also offers a spendid weapon of passive rebellion against imposed responsibility. Anyone can become irresponsible without feeling much blame by getting drunk.[1] People who are torn with conflict over self-assertion or hostility *vs.* the demands of vocational, social, and familial responsibilities often take occasional or permanent refuge in alcoholic semistupor. Alcoholism and other addictions thus often result from failure to absorb socially required standards of behavior in a way which permits you to live comfortably within the prescribed limits.

[1] In *The Virginian,* Owen Wister typified this prevailing American attitude by having the hero brag that he had been in jail only once, and that wasn't really his fault because he was drunk when he committed the offense.

Alcoholism and Psychopathy

An unusual tendency to rebel against socially exacted standards of behavior is generally called "psychopathy." In another view, psychopathy is inadequate response to society's program for building comfortable acceptance of the major prevailing standards. Such failure can occur at any of three stages: (1) learning what people expect of you; (2) accepting these demands as the valid price of membership in society; or (3) learning to pursue comfortably your various living goals within the prescribed limits.

Most alcoholism and drug addiction occurs as part of a psychopathic behavior pattern. As will be seen, this fact gives you a potent preventive attack to use upon these problems as an individual, as a potential parent, and as a community member.

The Nature of Alcoholism

Alcoholism is a condition which makes its victims drink in ways harmful to their pursuit of major living objectives. Alcoholism is thus an important problem to each victim as well as to society, because it interferes with living spheres like marriage, vocational success, and acceptance in his proper social circle. Alcoholism is not a matter of quantity: a man can consume only a few bottles of whiskey a year and still be an alcoholic if he drinks in responsibility-shirking bats that leave him unemployed and immersed in domestic strife. Nor is it necessarily a matter of drunkenness: a man who is always steady on his feet, well mannered in society, pleasant to his wife, and capable in his job can still consume enough alcohol day by day to induce memory loss and mental deterioration, or to cause hallucinations and severe derangement if some untoward event cuts off his liquor supply.

An alcoholic generally cannot keep his drinking from being harmful except by avoiding alcohol altogether. Once he has an established pattern which leads to harmful drinking, none of the methods of treatment available today can control the problem well enough to allow social or temperate drinking. Freedom from alcoholic problems in exchange for total abstinence is the most any alcoholic can expect from treatment.

You can achieve as much for yourself by going completely on the wagon if you find your drinking patterns sliding toward the pathological. If you recognize you are headed for trouble before your drinking has caused serious difficulties, you can often quit without professional aid or can achieve a cure through relatively simple, inexpensive varieties of care.

Signs of Impending or Early Alcoholism

How can you tell when you are in danger of becoming an alcoholic? Neither quantity nor frequency of drinking serve as criteria. The way you drink and your reason for taking a drink reveal your status much more definitely.

How incipient alcoholics drink

Concealment or sly supplementation characterizes drinking patterns in early alcoholism. The shift from social drinking to alcoholism often reveals itself in one of these ways:

1. taking a couple of quick swallows while you are mixing drinks for your guests
2. making your drink considerably stronger than theirs
3. taking one or more extra drinks before meeting your companions for the evening
4. drinking alone
5. drinking in the morning

In campus life, the earliest definite sign of developing alcoholism is usually drinking to the point of amnesia. The student who "must have had a wonderful time, because I spent ten bucks and I don't remember a thing" is using alcohol as an escape from social responsibility instead of as an aid to social ease. From this pattern to more profound alcoholic disturbance is an easy course down which most people will definitely slide unless they make a deliberate, pronounced effort at change.

Why incipient alcoholics say they drink

When a person is creeping toward alcoholism, he has somewhat different reasons for taking a drink than the normal social drinker. He drinks to improve his effectiveness, self-confidence, or comfort in various situations. He feels an inner need instead of responding to an external situation. One example is need for a drink to brace yourself or steady yourself before giving a speech, attending a party, or facing some other stressful situation. Another is need for a "hair off the dog that bit you" the morning after alcoholic excess. A solitary nightcap to induce sleep may signify an incipient habituation to alcohol. In fact, any time you feel *need for* a drink, the time has come to consider whether alcohol is on its way to becoming a problem for you.

Help With Prevention or Cure

You can get considerable help in keeping alcohol and narcotics from becoming problems or in managing difficulties which arise among your associates. Here are the main available facilities for prevention and cure.

Public attacks on psychopathy

All the public agencies whose purpose involves molding and regulating human behavior play an important part in encouraging comfortable adaptation to society's demands. This adaptation serves as the best possible protection against alcoholism or addiction. Health and welfare programs distribute important educational material and use many other means of guiding parents in establishing well-accepted discipline. The public schools play an important part in teaching proper response to authority. Law enforcement officials and others concerned with imposing the dictates of society upon individuals have a heavy responsibility to do their work in a way which minimizes resentment. Both the schools and the police and the courts usually have trained counselors available to help with problems which arise either through the individual's failure to observe society's rules or through his psychological distress at having to observe them.

Group work

Most of the difficulties which arise in inducing individuals to conform comfortably to society's demands come out of conflict with individuals in authority: fathers at first, then quasi-parental authorities like teachers, then appointed wielders of the scepter like policemen, foremen, and bosses. Both in achieving comfortable adaptation to society's rules and in overcoming rebelliousness or frank psychopathy, group dynamics detour the individual's roadblocks against authority. A well-integrated member of a boys' or girls' club seldom gets into trouble with the law and builds substantial reserves against later frictions and maladjustments of the sort commonly preceding alcoholism. Team sports and extracurricular activity groups tend to exert similar favorable influence. Groups formed for the specific purpose of combating an evident trend toward psychopathy have proved of great value, too.

Community efforts to control drug and liquor supplies

Control of narcotic addiction through legal regulation of the supply has been very successful. In 1914, when the Harrison Narcotic Act established effective controls and limited use of narcotics to prescribed medicinal administration, there were 215,000 drug addicts in the country. At present, fewer than 50,000 Americans are addicted to drugs, even though the adult population has nearly doubled. Similar but slightly less stringent regulation of sedative drugs through the Durham-Humphrey Law of 1951 has effectively combated the growing problem of barbiturate addiction.

Control of alcoholism through regulation of supplies has proved less successful. Two-thirds of adult Americans drink, most of them being in no substantial danger of becoming alcoholics. Both Federal and state prohibition laws have, therefore, generally failed to develop the degree of public support necessary for satisfactory enforcement. Most communities today concentrate on regulating the sale and use of alcoholic beverages rather than attempting to eliminate them altogether.

Care for alcoholism and addiction

You can get help for psychopathic, alcoholic, or addiction difficulties from any of the mental health resources discussed in the last chapter. In addition, two special aids deserve recognition.

Alcoholics Anonymous is a group of former victims of alcoholism who work with current victims of alcoholism on a voluntary, unpaid basis. A.A. builds its program on the principles that an alcoholic remains an alcoholic for life, with a permanent incapacity to drink normally, and that religion and service to others give him worthwhile goals with which to replace the mere escape provided by alcoholic excess. A.A. works closely with psychiatric and social agencies in rehabilitating victims of alcoholism, and is recognized by most such agencies as a highly worthwhile aid.

The Federal government maintains facilities for treating narcotic addicts at Lexington, Kentucky and Forth Worth, Texas. Although there is no easy way to get away from a serious drug addiction, the medicines and measures provided make it possible for some addicts to manage complete cure. Others are able to reduce their dosage to a level they can afford without criminal activity. Eligible patients get transportation and care free of charge, making their arrangements through any licensed physician.

CHAPTER 7

Stimulants *vs.* Restorative Rest

In a logic-governed college classroom, neither authoritarian condemnation of such customs as excessive coffee drinking and smoking nor the acceptance of these practices because many people follow them has any place. These customs undoubtedly affect health, and the facts about their health effects certainly deserve your attention. You must decide for yourself what influence these facts should have on your behavior.

CAFFEINE AND THEOPHYLLINE

You probably think of a cup of coffee as a pleasant drink rather than as a stimulant drug, yet it contains the same stimulant, caffeine, which effectuates the most widely sold, nonprescription, sleep-postponing tablet. Cola drinks also contain this ingredient, while tea contains theophylline, an equivalent compound. Both caffeine and theophylline have definite actions on the central nervous system, the heart and blood vessels, the kidneys, and the digestive system. You can take full advantage of their helpful effects without being inconvenienced by their harmful ones only by thoroughly understanding their actions.

A cup of strong coffee contains about 100 mg. of caffeine, the same amount contained in each dose of the most commonly used sleep-deferring drugstore remedy. A six-ounce bottle of cola beverage contains about 50 mg. of caffeine, twelve-ounce varieties about 100 mg. Since any harmful effects attributable to coffee stem from its caffeine content, cola drinks can thus be considered equivalent to half-strength coffee.

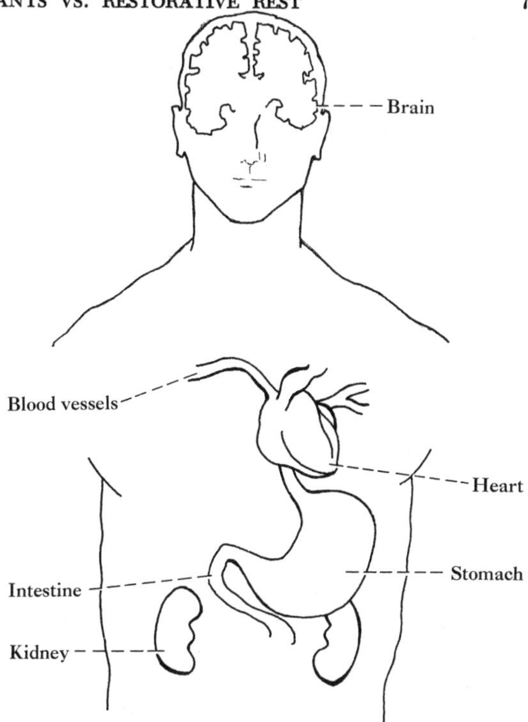

Figure 20. Although generally safe, even one cup of coffee or tea affects the functioning of all the body organs shown in this diagram.

Effects of Moderate Amounts

Moderate quantities of caffeine or theophylline help you fight off sleep and the feeling of fatigue, improve your mood, and produce a feeling of greater mental efficiency. This feeling is not entirely justified. These stimulants actually impair over-all mental efficiency slightly: they decrease accuracy and precision more than they speed thinking processes and reflexes.

Caffeine and theophylline measurably speed pulse and increase blood pressure, effects usually harmless to a person with a normal heart and blood vessels, but which may require consideration when these organs are diseased. Caffeine and theophylline also increase the volume of urine, which neither helps nor harms normal people.

The effects of caffeine or theophylline on the digestive system are somewhat unpredictable but frequently involve disturbance in appetite, abdominal discomforts, constipation, or diarrhea. These effects seem to result from continued exposure to moderate amounts of caffeine (300 to 500 mg. per day) or theophylline rather than to abrupt consumption of larger doses. Appetite effects seem especially marked in children, thus confirming Grandmother's conviction that coffee can cause poor eating and could conceivably interfere with growth.

Effects of Large Amounts

When the average person takes about 1,000 mg. of caffeine, he suffers distinctly uncomfortable effects. Nervousness, jitteriness, giddy spells, insomnia, shaking hands and muscular twitching, racing and pounding heart, nausea, abdominal discomfort, and crushing, heart-type pain may occur.

Psychological factors certainly play some part in the effects of caffeine, especially that upon the nervous system. Students who swear that coffee has no effect on them stay awake all night on a couple of the sleep-forestalling tablets which have identical stimulant action. Experimental subjects find that a bedtime cup of coffee (from which virtually all the caffeine has been removed without their knowledge) keeps them wide awake, while warm milk (spiked with 300 mg. of caffeine) proves very soothing. The fact that such a powerful psychological force as suggestion can enhance or overcome the effect of caffeine really does not mean that caffeine has no action, however. It only means that you may need considerable experience and self-observation to sort out the effects caffeine actually has on your system.

Your tendency to develop tolerance for caffeine makes it even harder to determine how much caffeine you can take without immediate or long-term unpleasant effects. Most people quickly become inured to many or all of the effects of caffeine. They require larger and larger amounts to produce any psychological lift, and they do not get jitters or insomnia from previously troublesome amounts of strong coffee. Although many of these people have some palpitations or indigestion which can be traced to caffeine, these difficulties are comparatively mild.

Tolerance to caffeine often carries with it a degree of dependency, however. When the accustomed morning coffee is not available to lift one's mood and act upon various blood vessels in the brain, irritability and throbbing headache strike. Caffeine-withdrawal symptoms do not last long and seldom prove truly disabling, but they usually punish those individuals whom tolerance frees from other harmful caffeine-caused effects.

AMPHETAMINE AND EPHEDRINE

Your doctor may well prescribe amphetamine or ephedrine if you need medicine to lift your mood in a spell of mild depression or to suppress your appetite during weight reduction. The action of these drugs is very similar to that of caffeine, only about 50 times as intense per unit of weight. The usual 10 mg. tablet thus gives effects five times as great as a cup of coffee, and people who no longer get much stimulation from coffee because of fully developed tolerance still get full effect from amphetamine or ephedrine. Normal doses lift mood, dispel fatigue, and quicken processes of thought and action.

Amphetamine as a Study Aid

A few students depend upon amphetamine-aided cramming sessions instead of spaced out study before examinations. While stimulants can keep efficiency above the level to which fatigue would reduce it during an all-night session, few doctors (if any) will prescribe amphetamine or ephedrine for this purpose because of their possibly harmful effects. Moreover, the cramming system has definite disadvantages in comparison with a spaced-out study schedule and undrugged efficiency during the examination:

1. Stimulants actually decrease study efficiency in a normal situation. Although stimulants maintain or even increase efficiency in motor and semi-skilled activities, they increase distractibility and decrease thinking accuracy. A sense of achievement and success often results from their mood effects, but actual results do not justify it.
2. Stimulants decrease efficiency during a test. Once a student starts taking stimulants, he has only two choices: quit before the examination and let accumulated fatigue catch up with him at the crucial moment, or keep himself alert with another dose of stimulant. If he elects the latter, he generally feels that he has done exceedingly well, again because of mood effects. His actual performance will be somewhat impaired in tests involving both time and accuracy and drastically impaired in tests where time is not a factor.
3. Stimulants make you generate a fatigue debt which draws high interest. A man who must keep himself going for 48 hours with stimulants (e.g., the captain of a ship during a hurricane) generally needs to spend three to five days loafing before he feels completely well again. Attempts to keep going for 72 hours or more frequently result in delirium or circulatory disturbances and almost always lead to a muddle-headed, foggy state which requires bed-bound care for several days.

Amphetamine for Appetite Control

Doctors often prescribe amphetamine products as part of a weight-reduction program. The amount required for appetite suppression is moderate and the effect usually good. However, amphetamine-aided weight reduction gives little help in establishing new eating patterns. Overweight tends to recur quickly after you quit the drug. Succeeding episodes require higher and higher dosage for effectiveness. Ultimately, effective appetite control almost always requires dosage sufficiently high to affect the blood pressure and pulse rate.

Weight control is a lifelong job, not a result achieved forever through one definitive campaign. Your chance of long-range success is very much greater if you can achieve reduction without the aid of amphetamine. Weight reduction gives little help in establishing new eating patterns. Overweight tends
tion through drugs leaves the dietary revision necessary for weight control unaccomplished while weight reduction through diet simultaneously achieves that goal. Most people who tend toward overweight need a great deal of help from a physician or some other interested party during the dietary revision phase. Since the amphetamine program defers this period until after the weight reduction is achieved, they seldom ask for or receive the assistance they need in establishing a weight maintenance program.

TOBACCO

The conviction that the other fellow is plagued by prejudice ruins most discussions of the health effects of smoking. Defenders of the weed tend to regard all their opponents as moralistic extremists whose basic motive is to encourage or impose self-denial, and write them off as fanatics. Tobacco adversaries cite as prejudicing factors the skillful dissembling of Madison Avenue advertising agents, the social pressure toward acceptance of smoking, and a number of other factors which predispose you to find the custom innocuous even though they have no bearing on the issue of whether smoking has harmful effects.

Perhaps you would find it interesting to debate in class the role of preconceived judgment on each side of the Great Smoking Controversy. The debate should not founder for lack of material.

How Smoking Affects Body Functions

The small amount of nicotine that gets into your body through the delicate membranes of the lung increases mental and physical activity somewhat, but at some cost in both mental and physical capabilities. Actual tests show decreased efficiency in both intellective and muscular functions after absorption of tobacco smoke. Absorbed nicotine also increases the flow of stomach acids and activity of the intestine's muscular wall, increases pulse and blood pressure, and decreases circulation to the heart muscle. These effects are sufficient to aggravate digestive and circulatory disorders, but do not usually cause complaints in normal people.

Everybody knows that an unpleasant degree of nicotine poisoning frequently punishes novices at smoking. Nausea, vomiting, pallor, and dizziness characterize such full-blown nicotine effects. After you become inured to tobacco, the complete picture of nicotine poisoning no longer occurs. However, a surprisingly large number of smokers have occasional attacks of nausea, palpitations, weakness, or light-headedness due to nicotine action. These attacks do not inevitably follow overindulgence. They seem rather to follow a periodic pattern every two or three weeks, to conform to the menstrual period, or to occur in periods of emotional stress. Since complaints do not regularly follow heavy smoking, victims of this variety of nicotine poisoning often continue to smoke for years without realizing the relationship of tobacco to their complaints.

Smoking also affects the irritability of nerve endings within nose, throat, and lungs. Smoker's cough results, as well as certain changes in breathing rhythm which contribute to the difficulty of discontinuing tobacco. Heavy smoking ultimately dulls flavor perception to a considerable degree. This dulling often reaches the point of vitiating tobacco flavor itself: most heavy smokers cannot tell whether their cigarette is lit or not if they are blindfolded and if the room is sufficiently smoke-filled to nullify their sense of smell.

Psychological and Psychosocial Factors

The key action in tobacco smoking is suction with the mouth. Most psychologists relate the comfort and gratification attained through this act to its emotional parallel, feeding at the mother's breast in infancy. According to this notion, the soothing associations of mother love and primitive gratification link themselves with smoking to create satisfying emotional effects.

Perhaps less speculative (if more superficial) is the widely prevalent and socially reinforced association of smoking with adulthood and with debonair sophistication. During your childhood years, you were almost certainly told that you were too young to smoke, implying that smoking is a badge of maturity. Books and plays continually use a person's way of smoking to portray his character and emotions, making the smoking behavior an important part of adult self-expression. When you want to assert yourself as adult and express adult desires and capabilities, the symbolism of smoking often seems apt.

Last but not least, smoking is one of the few forms of fidgeting which our society accepts without deprecation. When you are ill at ease, you have a natural desire to fiddle with something. You want to scratch your ear, pick at your clothes, drum your fingers, or pace the floor. Unfortunately, the people around you would readily recognize these evidences of restlessness and lose some respect for your aplomb. You would feel dissatisfied with your own self-control if you fidgeted in these ways. Yet our cultural ground-rules allow you to take out a cigarette, tamp it on the nearest table, light it, fool around with it, get up to hunt for an ash tray, and trace endless figures in the ashes without criticism. Such actions have the same psychological benefit as fidgeting but with a difference. Everyone views smoking as normal adult behavior, not adolescent restlessness.

Tobacco and Circulatory or Digestive Disease

Nonsmokers at thirty years of age have half again as much chance of living to age age seventy as heavy smokers.[1] Almost 2¼ times as many heavy-smoking males as nonsmoking males in the same age group die each year. This means that heavy smokers die off at a rate only equaled by nonsmokers after they are seven or eight years older.[2]

Most of this difference is due to extra coronary heart disease, not to lung cancer. While it is true that hard-driven people are more prone to smoke heavily and also more prone to coronary attacks, recent studies have shown that people who smoked a pack a day or more and then quit for a year or more halved their chance of dying during any one succeeding year. Further evidence that cigarettes deserve some of the blame:

••• While smoking a cigarette and for up to thirty minutes thereafter, a substantial proportion of people have definite electrocardiographic changes of the type usually associated with impairment of blood flow through the coronary arteries.

••• People with narrowed coronary arteries often experience pain and other complaints when smoking, pointing to extra narrowing through nicotine-induced spasm of their already-impaired coronary arteries.

Since most severe coronary attacks result from a clot forming in a coronary artery during a period of decreased flow, since cigarettes appear to cause such decreased flow, and since people whose personality patterns and situations formerly made heavy smokers of them can escape the expected coronary risk by quitting tobacco, the conclusion that at least part of the extra

[1] 45,919 *vs.* 30,393 per 100,000 according to the late Professor Raymond Pearl of Johns Hopkins University.

[2] *To Smoke or Not To Smoke:* © 1957, American Cancer Society, Inc.

coronary disease in heavy smokers stems from effects of tobacco seems unavoidable.

Several diseases in the causation of which tobacco may or may not have a part are definitely aggravated by continued smoking once they are present. Coronary heart disease fits into this group. So does peptic ulcer. Arterial disorders such as Buerger's disease become worse with smoking. Ordinarily arteriosclerosis remains unaffected, because it stiffens the artery walls sufficiently to preclude nicotine-induced spasm.

Smoker's Cough

Tobacco-smoke-provoked cough and drainage from the nasal cavity back into the throat result partly from chemical grating on nerve endings in the breathing passage and partly from increased activity of the mucous glands which normally produce a protective coat for the lining of the upper breathing passages. Both effects aggravate respiratory infections such as colds, bronchitis, and pneumonia. The presence of smoker's cough frequently calls for x-ray and other studies which would not otherwise be necessary. Some victims of tuberculosis or other serious lung disease do not get attention when they first start to cough because they attribute their complaints to smoking. In the main, however, smoker's cough leads only to annoyance, not to serious difficulties.

Tobacco and Lung Cancer

More than 60 times as many heavy smokers as nonsmokers in any one age group get cancer of the lung. This correlation seems too great for mere coincidence. Pathologic studies showing a continuous gradation of change from normal bronchial lining to cancer with increased tobacco exposure also supports the existence of a cause and effect relationship between smoking and lung cancer.

If you smoke two packs of cigarettes a day, your chance of dying of lung cancer runs about one in ten. Nonsmokers have only one chance in 270 of getting this disease [3]—a very real difference.

Filter Tips

The American public's main response to the cigarette-cancer correlation has been a switch to filter tips. However, filter tips have never been shown to

[3] These figures seem to conflict with the sixty-fold increase cited mainly because more of the heavy smokers die of coronary disease and other causes before they reach the age group in which cancer is common.

decrease cancer-spurring irritation in the least. The cancer-causing substances so far identified in smoke pass freely through any usable filter. Moreover, most smokers burn filter tipped cigarettes down to within a puff or so of the filter itself. Since smoke from the last inch or so of a cigarette contains ten times as much tar as smoke from the first portion, the net result of smoking a filter tipped cigarette to a short butt instead of smoking a plain tipped cigarette to a medium butt may actually be to increase rather than decrease the amount of tar reaching your lungs.

Alternative Smokes

Pipe and cigar smoking compare very favorably to cigarette smoking in their effects upon life span and lung cancer incidence. Heavy cigar and pipe smokers have only about 2½ times as many lung cancers as nonsmokers, or about 1/20 as many as heavy cigarette smokers. Undue circulatory disease risks are similarly reduced.

Pipe and cigar smoking definitely cause an occasional cancer of the lip or tongue, usually at the site where the smoke stream hits. This type of malignancy is much less common than lung cancer, however. Its surface location allows detection on time for cure at least half the time, or at least ten times as often as lung cancer. All in all, cigar or pipe smoking probably involves only about 1/10 as much shortening of life span as cigarette smoking.

REST FOR TRUE EFFICIENCY

Although artificial stimulants bolster you temporarily against fatigue and depression, only physical and mental rest truly resolve these problems and simultaneously improve your mental capabilities, your bodily efficiency, and your resistance to disease. A few special considerations may aid your decision as to how much rest you need and how you can get it with a minimum of lost time.

Fatigue and Efficiency

Two types of fatigue have important effects upon efficiency. The ordinary, readily recognizable fatigue which sets in at the end of a hard day or an arduous study session usually passes off after a night's sleep or even a brief rest break. A more subtle and sustained variety of fatigue comes on after three weeks or so of continuous but endurable overexertion, markedly impairs efficiency, but seldom is particularly evident to either the victim or his associates.

Smoldering fatigue

The state of smoldering fatigue shows up dramatically whenever you measure the output of people under extreme work loads. Assume a plant which produces 100 units of goods when its workers put in an eight-hour day. During brief rush periods, production goes up proportionately with overtime: in a twelve-hour day the men produce almost 150 units. During

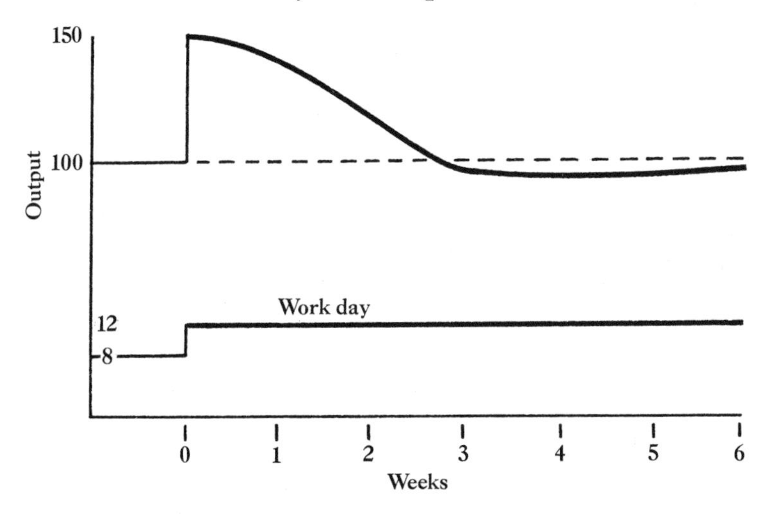

Figure 21. Effect of smoldering fatigue on productivity.

wartime, however, dozens of plants all over England and the United States tried to achieve sustained increase in production by prolonging the work week. Smoldering fatigue produced an almost identical effect in all: after one week on twelve-hour days, a 100-unit plant produced 145 to 148 units, by two weeks the output was about 130, in three weeks it was back to about 100 (in spite of 50 per cent more work hours) and it finally settled at about 90. Sustained effort beyond a certain point not only produced decrease in efficiency per hour, but actually produced net loss in total accomplishment as well.

Fatigue levels for college work

Most college students can stand work levels well above eight hours a day. Their work is varied, they have chosen it on the basis of interest, they enjoy intrinsic motivation, and they are relatively free of household and community responsibilities. The fact that college students are selected for ability and drive also presumably heightens their work capacity. But every student has a work load limit beyond which he cannot maintain efficiency.

After a few months' experience, most successful college students find their limits of efficient sustained endeavor and plan their work to suit this pattern. Every student has limits beyond which more work actually produces less return. A good study program must remain within this limit, and must spread back enough work from peak periods (like exam time) to prevent the inefficiencies of smoldering fatigue.

A collegian's total work load

Classwork and study are not your only burdens during college. Even an easy outside job constitutes work. Many of the social obligations of college also involve burdens, especially for youny ladies who cannot fit dating demands in with their other responsibilities as easily as can initiative-maintaining males. Students who fix their own meals or clean their own apartments have to score extra hours for household chores.

Your own work capacity

Although immediate fatigue, poor morale and nutritional fatigue show up in very evident weariness and inefficiency, smoldering fatigue often reveals itself much more subtly.

Probably the best single check for smoldering fatigue is the covered-clock time test. While you are still fresh at the beginning of a quarter or semester, work every other problem on one page of your last year's math book, memorize twelve lines of an unfamiliar poem, or perform some other easily defined task. Look at the clock at the beginning and end of the task, but not between. Note the exact time required, and put the materials aside. A couple of months later, after prolonged and uninterrupted school attendance, try the equivalent task. If the time required is markedly longer, you probably have too heavy a total load.

If you feel markedly stale and inefficient late in each school session, such precise tests probably are unnecessary. You unquestionably have some degree of smoldering fatigue, and should probably revise your academic or living schedule.

Rest or recreation?

Short-term fatigue commonly results from changes in mood and morale you can sometimes fight off better with recreation than with rest. Smoldering fatigue, however, responds to rest and to rest alone. The extra exertion and excitement of most recreations often makes such fatigue worse instead of better. If rescheduling to spread back work loads is not practical, perhaps some of your recreations, chores, and general responsibilities can be rearranged. Otherwise, reduced work load may be the only way to achieve efficiency.

Special Rest Techniques

Certain techniques actually make brief breaks during the day three or four times as efficient as extra resting time at night, besides making nocturnal rest more effective. If schedule pressures make it difficult for you to get as much sleep as you need or if your sleep requirement runs much over eight hours a day, you will probably find these techniques especially valuable.

Figure 22. Getting ready for next week's long grind. *C. Hadley Smith.*

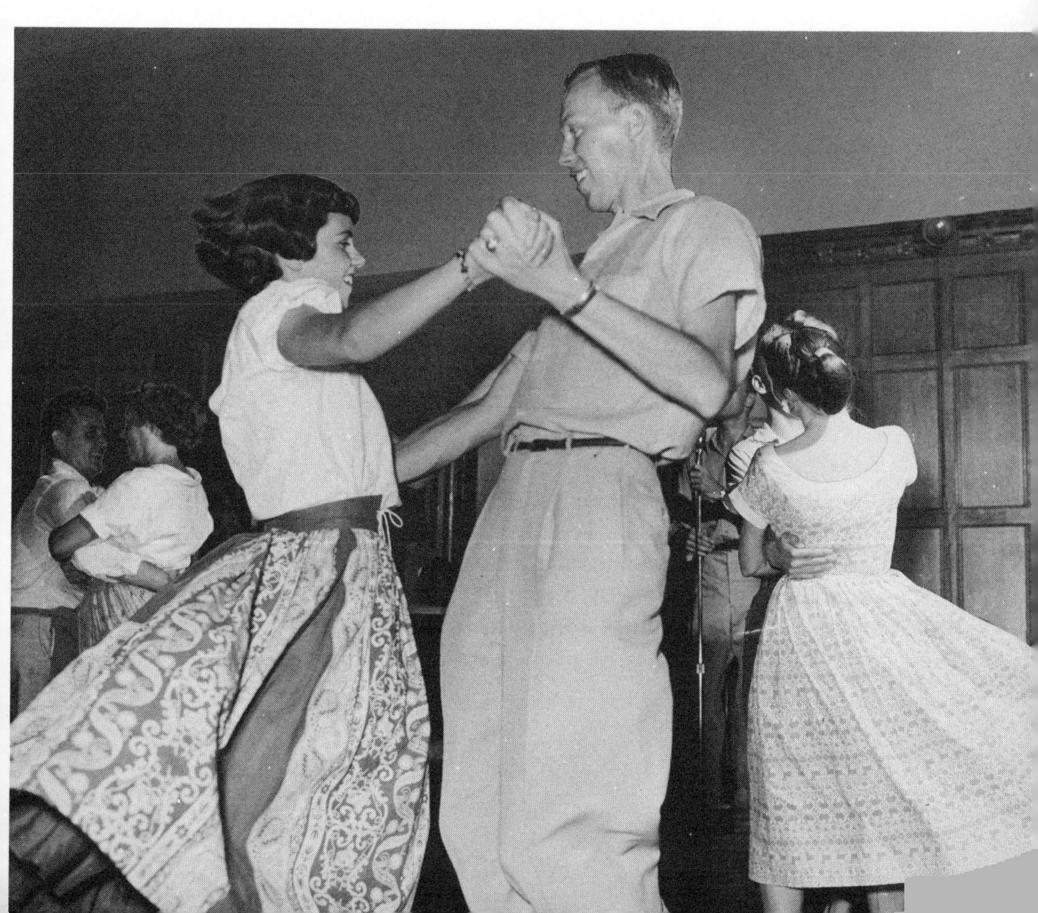

Progressive muscular relaxation

Relaxation is the basic skill of deliberate rest. Most people think that they have relaxed when they stop all voluntary movement, but true relaxation can go far beyond this point. Your muscles remain partly tense at all times, even during sleep. You can easily learn to reduce this tension deliberately.

Here is one simple way to get the feel of deliberate relaxation:

Hold your neck a tiny bit stiffer, then stiffer still, then quite stiff, then as stiff as possible. Now relax it from top stiffness to quite stiff, to moderately stiff, slightly stiff, and normal. Continue exactly the same process one step further to reduce normal muscle tone or tension. This is deliberate relaxation.

You can apply this basic method most easily by lying down in a quiet, darkened room, closing your eyes, and relaxing one body part after another in rotation. Relax your right arm and hand, your right leg, left leg, left arm, scalp, face, back, and abdomen. Repeat, striving for a further degree of relaxation. A twenty-to-thirty-minute afternoon rest break using this technique actually replaces three to four times as much nocturnal sleep.

Relaxing in the face of worry or tension

If you have difficulty getting to sleep or suffer from undue worry and tension, a variation on the basic technique of progressive relaxation often helps. Follow the same procedure outlined above, but concentrate on smaller areas at a time. Instead of trying to relax a whole arm at once, relax the hand, then the forearm, then the upper arm and shoulder. Or carry it down to even smaller divisions if you must.

Thorough relaxation at night makes insomnia completely harmless. You get as much rest from bedbound relaxation as from sleep. The key point in avoiding problems arising from poor sleep is to remain unconcerned as you continue to rest.

Brief tension-breaking pauses

A considerable amount of the fatigue associated with intellectual work results from tension. Very brief rest breaks can keep the muscular element of tension from building up, and considerably relieve the resulting fatigue. One simple method is to sit in a straight chair with both feet flat on the floor and both hands resting on your thighs. Close your eyes and let your head loll forward on your chest. Relax part by part as discussed above. After relaxing various body parts as much as possible on one round, raise one hand to shoulder height and let it fall back into place like a limp dish-rag. Repeat with the other arm. Continue part-by-part relaxation in this fashion for one to two minutes, whereupon you will usually be able to resume your work with renewed vigor.

CHAPTER 8

Your Health Heritage

A few hours after you were a mere gleam in your father's eye, your life took origin in the merging of two cells: a sperm cell from your father and an egg cell from your mother. At that instant, a presumptive blueprint

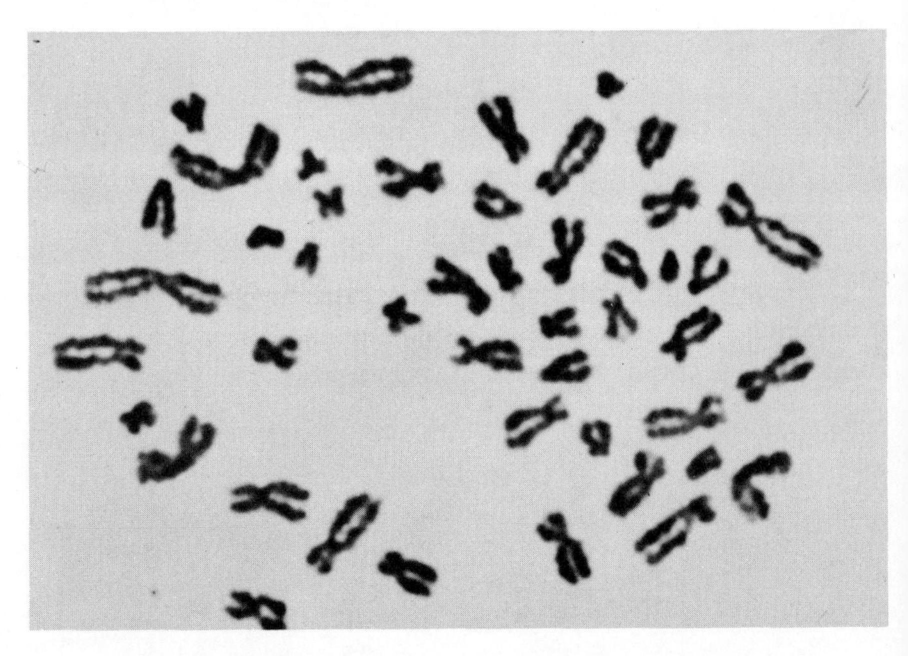

Figure 23. Human Chromosomes. *Used by permission of J. H. Tjio, Ph.D.*

of your future being was fixed. The basic design of your body, your intellectual potentialities, and many of your key reaction patterns were already ordained, subject only to modification by later environmental pressures.

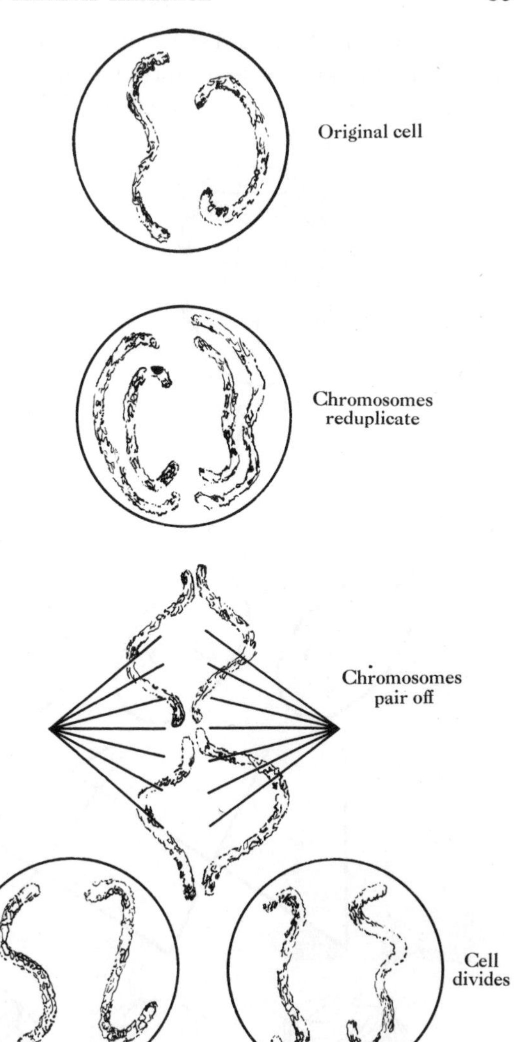

Figure 24. Cell division, simplified by representing only two chromosomes. Note that each daughter cell has chromosomes exactly like those of parent cell. *Adapted with permission from* Genetics of Human Heredity, *J. Ben Hill & Helen D. Hill. Copyright 1955, McGraw-Hill Book Co., Inc.*

CHROMOSOMES

How was this tentative blueprint established? Within the egg cell were twenty-three tiny strands of inheritance-ordaining substance known as *chromosomes*. Another twenty-three such strands came with the sperm cell. When the egg and sperm cells merged together, the resulting single cell had forty-six chromosomes. Those chromosomes governed the pattern of your growth and development from that moment forth. One cell became two, two became four, and so on up into the millions. Each dividing cell first produced a brand-new set of forty-six chromosomes, then walled off the new chromosomes to form a daughter cell. The same process is occurring right

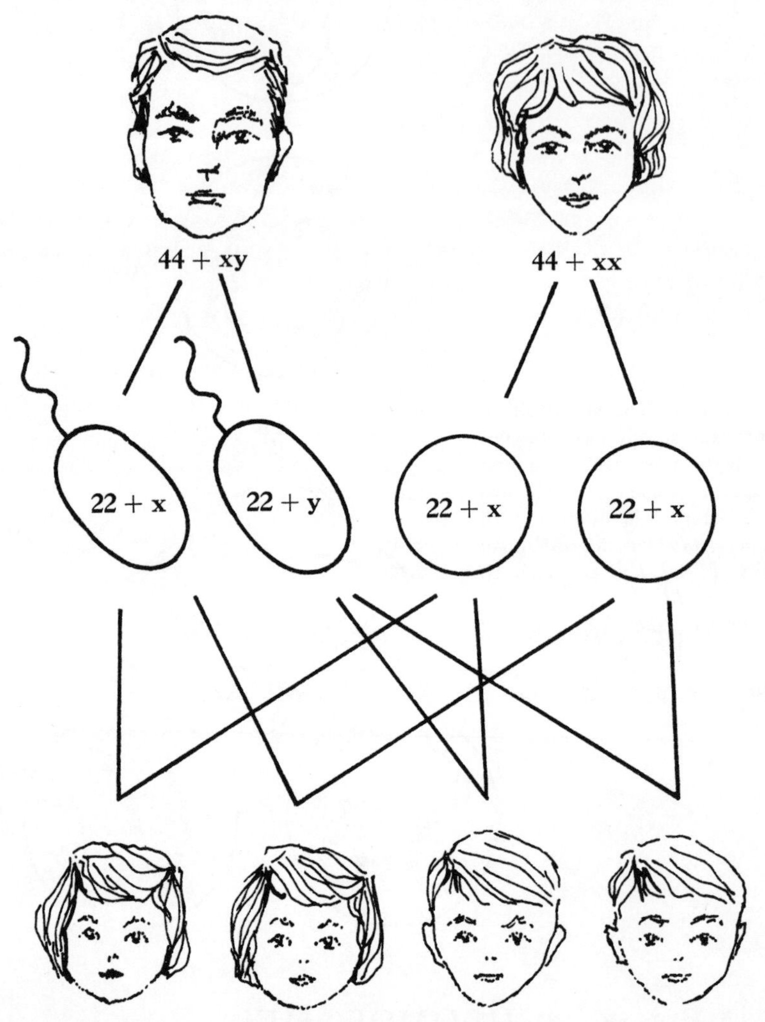

Figure 25. Determination of sex. *Adapted with permission from* Genetics: A Survey of the Principles of Heredity, *A. M. Winchester, 2nd Edition. Copyright Houghton Mifflin Company 1958.*

now, wherever your body cells are reproducing themselves. Every new cell except your own developing egg cells or sperm has its full complement of forty-six chromosomes, essentially the same as those with which you started.

Through those chromosomes, the traits you have inherited exert their sway.

When you form a sperm or egg cell it gets a set of twenty-three chromosome from your forty-six. Each chromosome is generally identical with that contributed by your father or that contributed by your mother, but only very remote chance makes the entire set correspond to that derived from one or the other of your parents. The representative of each of the twenty-three sets is determined entirely by chance, with the chromosome contributed by each of your parents equally likely to be selected.

Forty-four of the chromosomes in a human cell always consist of matching pairs. In the female, the other two also match: both are X-chromosomes. In the male, there is one X-chromosome and one smaller, male-determining Y-chromosome. Half of the sperm cells a man makes contain X-chromosomes. The other half contain male-determining Y-chromosomes. Egg cells always contain X-chromosomes only. If a sperm cell carrying a Y-chromosome fertilizes the egg cell, the baby will be a boy. If a sperm cell carrying an X-chromosome fertilizes the egg cell, the baby will be a girl.

GENES

Units of inheritance, apparently arranged in lines along the chromosomes, determine many of your important physical and mental characteristics. These units are called *genes.*

Some genes assert themselves only when they are present in the chromosomes contributed by both the mother and the father. They are called *recessive* genes. Other genes assert themselves whenever present in the chromosomes contributed by either parent, regardless of whether the chromosomes contributed by the other parent carry the same or different genes. They are called *dominant* genes.

Completely recessive genes determine several human traits, such as the absence of body pigment found in albinos. Chromosomes from both sides of the family must carry albino genes before lack of body pigment results. You can thus assume that any albino has the double albino (aa) genetic pattern. A nonalbino could be carrying albino genes from one side of his family or could have nonalbino genes (AA) from both his parents. You can be reasonably sure that he has a mixed genetic pattern (Aa) if he has an albino parent or begets an albino child. You can never be completely certain that he has a double nonalbino (AA) pattern.

In human genetics, many genes which ordinarily act as dominants occasionally fail to make themselves manifest. Genes for brown eyes generally win out over genes for blue eyes, for instance. A brown-eyed person might have a double brown (BB) or mixed (Bb) genetic pattern, while a blue-eyed one ordinarily has double blue (bb). An occasional gray- or green-eyed person actually carries brown-eye genes, however, so light-irised parents occasionally have dark-eyed progeny.

Although such incomplete dominance and other complexities of human genetics enter to some degree, you can ordinarily consider the genes which determine several normal characteristics as dominant or recessive. Nonred hair is dominant over red hair, while several genes determining dark hair are dominant over those determining light hair. Genes determine curly hair or straight hair, with wavy hair the result of mixed curly-straight inheritance. White forelock and piebald skin are dominant over uniform hair or skin color.

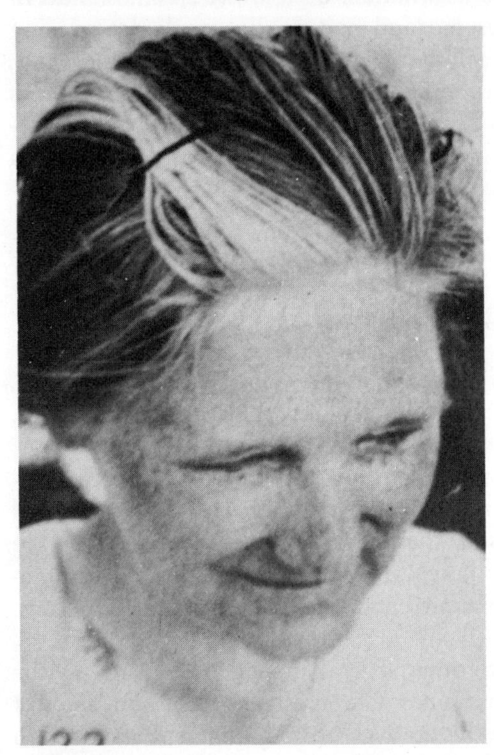

Figure 26. The white forelock, also seen in three generations of this person's progenitors. *From Sundför,* Jour. Heredity 30(3):67–77. 1939.

Multiple Alleles

More than two genetic determinates sometimes compete for the same position in the chromosomes and affect the same human characteristic. The gene determining your blood group (AB, A, B, or O) is a good example. Type A and type B are both dominant over type O, but not over each other. Thus the various possible genetic patterns lead to corresponding blood types as follows:

Genetic Pattern	Blood Type
AB	AB
AA	A
AO	A
BB	B
BO	B
OO	O

If you ever need a blood transfusion, doctors must match the blood very carefully with your own. Transfusion with mismatched blood causes chills, fever, and sometimes serious illness or death. Blood which does not match your own precisely with respect to other genetically determined qualities (of which there are at least eight) may also cause transfusion reactions, although generally milder than those caused by A B O mismatching.

When uncertainty arises as to who sired a certain child, as in lawsuits involving paternity, geneticists use three genetically determined blood-typing procedures (ABO, Rh, and MNS) to settle the issue. They often can make a definite statement that a certain man is not the father of a certain child. They can never state absolutely that he is the father, but their reports on the probabilities involved sometimes make the likelihood of error quite remote.

Rh Factor

One complex series of genetic determinates, all vying for the same position in one chromosome, leads to your Rh blood type. About 85 per cent of white Americans are Rh positive, the other 15 per cent being Rh negative. Rh factor problems can cause serious disease in a newborn infant if several conditions have been met.

••• An Rh positive man must impregnate an Rh negative woman.

••• The unborn child must inherit genes which make him Rh positive.

••• The mother must have had certain chemical elements of Rh positive blood circulating in her blood stream on one or several previous occasions. Two or more previous pregnancies or several blood transfusions of Rh positive blood usually are required to meet this condition.

••• In the course of these exposures, the mother's internal organs must have been conditioned to form chemical neutralizing agents or antibodies which combine harmfully with elements in Rh positive blood.

••• These antibodies must reach such a concentration in the mother's blood that many of them reach the infant's blood stream.

If these conditions are met and no medical treatment is given to prevent it, the infant becomes seriously ill soon after birth. However, you do not need to consider your Rh status in selecting a mate, as many students believe. If your marriage involves the one kind of serious Rh mismatching, namely an Rh positive husband with an Rh negative wife, the chances that an Rh problem will arise in any one pregnancy are less than one in fifty. Proper medical care during pregnancy will almost always detect an impending Rh problem before the child is born, and treatment is highly effective.

Sex-Linked Genes

You will recall that the male-determining Y-chromosome is smaller than the X-chromosome, and does not correspond precisely with it. This permits some genes to manifest themselves more frequently in one sex than in the other. Most sex-linked genes are recessive genes located in that portion of

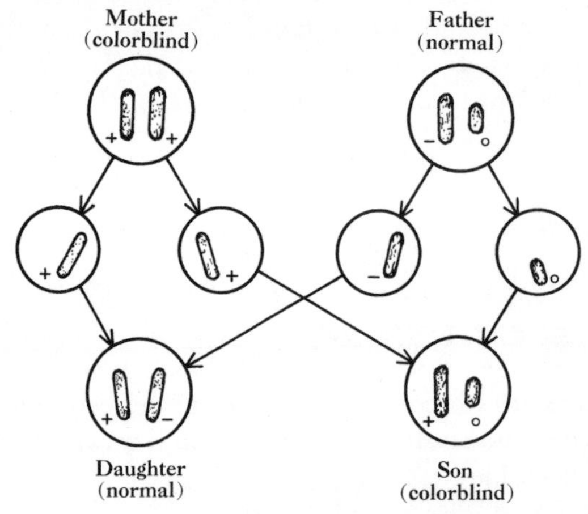

Figure 27. Transmission of colorblindness. *Adapted with permission from* Elements of Genetics, *3rd Edition, by Edward C. Colin. Copyright 1956. McGraw-Hill Book Co., Inc.*

the X-chromosome for which there is no matching section in the Y-chromosome. They can assert themselves whenever they are present in the single X-chromosome of a man's cells. They can assert themselves in the female only when present in both the X-chromosome derived from the mother and the X-chromosome derived from the father.

When a man or boy displays a sex-linked characteristic, he can only have inherited it through his mother. His father, who contributed only Y- rather than X-chromosome, has nothing to do with it. His mother's father and his maternal uncles give the best clues to the possible genetic constitution of his mother's X-chromosomes and thus to his chances of inheriting any sex-linked characteristic. Red-green color blindness is a good example of a trait carried in this way.

Deformities or Disease and Individual Genes

Several deformities of the extremities result from dominant genes. A few rare diseases [1] are also inherited in this way. Recessive genes may be concerned to some degree with epilepsy and with diabetes (see below) and with certain rare diseases.[2] Sex-linked genes lead to hemophilia and possibly to other rare disorders.

One caution regarding heritable conditions: the absence of the trait in one generation or one member of the family does not mean that it will not assert itself as a dominant trait. Many heritable human deformities fail to occur uniformly. Some strike 98 per cent of the people who carry dangerous genes, some strike half or less and still act as dominant traits—that is, they assert themselves when the deformity-producing gene has come from only one side of the family. If the presence of some serious heritable deformity makes you wonder about the wisdom of reproduction, get advice from a qualified human geneticist.

FAMILY RESEMBLANCE AND INHERITED CAPABILITIES

Your offspring probably will resemble you to a certain degree in many important characteristics not conveyed through single genes. Take height, for instance: tall parents are more likely to produce a tall child than are short parents, but if a very tall person marries a very short one their children will usually be more or less average in height rather than sharply grouped into talls and shorts. Apparently a number of different genes (besides environmental factors) are involved in determining height. The action of these genes averages out within the individual, and still leaves plenty of room for variation among brothers and sisters.

Multiple-gene inheritance also seems to determine some qualities of the mind. Ability to learn seems to be inherited in much the same way as height: intelligence is most likely to match the average of the two parents, but

[1] Polycystic kidney, Von Recklinghausen's disease, polyposis of the colon, and Huntington's chorea.

[2] Muscular atrophy, amaurotic idiocy.

varies somewhat around this norm. "Resemblance with variation" reveals itself in most sibling comparisons like this one: [3]

	% Bright (IQ above 113)	*% Average* (IQ 91–113)	*% Dull* (IQ below 91)
Brothers and sisters of brightest 4% of group measured	62.3	31.1	6.6
Brothers and sisters of average 4% of group measured	22.1	54.6	23.3
Brothers and sisters of dullest 8% of group measured	3.7	40.1	56.3

Certain specific capacities, such as mathematical or arithmetic ability, musical talent, and artistic potentiality seem to be governed by different genes than those concerned with general intelligence.

Can You Inherit Tendencies Toward Certain Diseases?

Genes control bodily configuration. Genes control or influence many important bodily functions. Some body configurations or ways of functioning dictated by genes make you more subject to certain types of breakdown than others. A tendency toward some diseases or toward freedom from them may, therefore, run in the family. Whether the disease actually occurs depends on various factors other than heredity. Genes conditioning your response to certain tars might conceivably make tar-induced cancer more likely, for instance, but you will still remain free of the disease unless your body is exposed to those tars. What you eat and how you live undoubtedly affects your chance of getting diabetes or of having heart disease regardless of your hereditary predisposition with regard to these conditions.

Cancer

Apparently some families carry a heritable tendency toward specific cancerous or precancerous conditions. A woman's chance of getting a cancer of the breast or of the uterus is about twice the national average if she has one or more close relatives with these disorders. Relatives of leukemia victims had a markedly increased chance of this disease (which recent research suggests to be associated with the presence in their cells of a tiny forty-seventh chromosome). Any one type of cancer is sufficiently rare that the vast bulk of predisposed relatives escape difficulty, however.

[3] J. A. Fraser Roberts, *An Introduction to Medical Genetics,* Oxford University Press. London: Humphrey Milford, 1940, p. 238.

Diabetes

If anyone in your immediate family within two generations has had diabetes, your chance of having the disease is distinctly above average. A diabetic tendency on both sides of the family increases your chance of having trouble more than a tendency confined to either maternal or paternal relatives.

Asthma, hay fever, infantile eczema, and hives

Some allergists regard familial predisposition as an important factor in asthma, hay fever, infantile eczema, and hives. Since these conditions are very common, up to a third of a child's relatives can suffer one or the other of them without evoking any concern about a family tendency. If you find that more than one-third of your prospective children's close relatives have suffered from some allergic disease, you may want to discuss an allergy-preventing infant-feeding program and other such precautions with your doctor.

Heart disease

Your family background makes you either more or less subject to heart disease. Probably only part of this tendency is due to inherited qualities, the rest being due to family dietary and living customs.

Tuberculosis

Although tuberculosis itself is not heritable, family background influences your chance of getting the disease. The most important point seems to be exposure to the victim's germs. Inherited factors such as body build and bodily response to infection may also play some part.

Mental illness

Schizophrenia in one of a pair of one-egg twins, whose genetic patterns are identical, makes schizophrenia in the other twin much more likely than in the case with two-egg twins, who are genetically only brothers of the same age. Children and grandchildren of victims of severe mental illness are somewhat more likely to be hospitalized for mental illness than people without such a family background. However, other factors besides inheritance enter into this situation. Mental illness and personality defects which often precede mental illness place strains upon everyone in the household. Increased alertness in the families of the mentally ill leads to detection of degrees of mental illness which might escape notice in other families. Furthermore, the impaired self-confidence, social stigma, and other strains resulting from the common idea that mental disease is inheritable may themselves be a reason for many extra mental breakdowns in families already touched by mental illness. Certainly, family background seldom if ever conditions anyone so strongly toward mental illness that a suitable environment will not overcome his predisposition.

COMMUNITY CONTROL OF REPRODUCTION

The responsibility for care of children born with severe handicaps usually devolves upon the community rather than upon the parents alone. Once these children have been born, our legal and moral codes prohibit any course other than their continued care. However, no one has an inalienable right to reproduce. Under the law, reproduction is a privilege granted by the state through marriage. The government can legally withhold this privilege, and enforce its control in other ways besides by denying marriage.

Community efforts to improve the stock (or at least prevent grossly defective issue) have generally taken three forms. Eugenic sterilization of people with seemingly heritable defects has been performed in several states, most notably in California. Laws prohibiting individuals with certain conditions from marrying (and thus presumably from reproducing, at least with the state's blessing) are on the books in many states. Research into human genetics and public education on the subject also receive sponsorship by both official and unofficial agencies in many states.

Although our knowledge of human genetics seems to have reached the point where scientific efforts to control reproduction should make sense, our past experience has revealed some of the hazards of overly vigorous action in this sphere. A great many states still have laws prohibiting epileptics from marriage, for instance, while most experts today do not feel that an epileptic's children have a sufficient chance of becoming wards of the state to justify this restraint. Many of the people sterilized for mental deficiency apparently had forms of brain damage now known to be due to uninheritable disorders. Community programs for control of genetic defects seem wise, but only when based upon solid and thoroughly confirmed fact.

CHAPTER 9

Hormones and Development in the College Years

EVEN THOUGH YOU ARE FULLY ADULT IN MOST RESPECTS, YOU PROBABLY STILL face many of the physical problems and rapidly changing functions of late adolescence. You may grow several inches after college entrance age. Some college students continue to grow measurably until they are twenty-three or twenty-four years old, often gaining an inch or more after age twenty-one. Moreover, many of your body measurements continue to change even after you have reached your final height. Chest x-rays show measurable growth of the rib cage up to age twenty-five. Internal organs also grow at their own rate, not necessarily in exact proportion to your height or weight. Your bones and muscles get heavier after they have achieved their full length, which makes ideal weight at any height increase by about one pound per year from age eighteen to twenty-five. Your eyeballs continue to grow until age twenty-five, which makes overshort, farsighted eyes improve and overlong, nearsighted eyes get worse. Sexual maturation continues well into the twenties, too, with both sex organs themselves and accessory characteristics such as breast, body hair, and beard often developing further during this period. Hormones produced by your endocrine glands play a large role in producing and regulating all of these changes.

Cell Growth and Endocrine Glands

Starting as one fertilized cell, you have grown into a complex being with billions of cells of thousands of different types, each working in conjunction with all the others to maintain your life and well-being. If you had continued to grow at the rate established in your slowest, final month as an unborn baby, you would weigh 2,000,000,000 times as much as the earth. Your body's system of growth control kept you from such a fate. It kept your body parts in good proportion to one another. It still impels your cells to replace injured or worn-out neighbor cells, and simultaneously prevents them from growing beyond the established bounds of maturity.

Your body controls its explosive initial growth, channels growth into nearly-perfect proportioning, and controls cellular growth during many years of self-repair mainly through the endocrine glands. These tiny bits of tissue make specific chemical compounds, known as hormones, which penetrate with the body fluids to every part of every organ. Hormones reach all the body's cells, many of which have no connection whatever with nerves or other body cells. Minute quantities of hormone spur the cells to action or lull them into quiet, the way a sniff of skunk scent drives a man to flight and the merest whiff of roasting turkey makes him feel at peace.

Endocrine Glands Have Other Crucial Functions

Endocrine glands have many functions besides control of cellular and physical growth. They control your body's use of fuel, the balance between water, salt, and certain other chemicals in your tissues, and the level of your blood pressure. They govern the bodily alterations required for pregnancy and reproduction. They seem to be deeply concerned with your mechanism of fighting infection, with allergy, and with all kinds of inflammation from itching scalp to arthritis of the toe. Here is a rundown on the important endocrine glands from top to bottom.

The pituitary gland

Your pituitary gland may well be the most important 1/50 of an ounce of tissue in your body. From its bone-ringed crater just beneath your brain, it controls almost all of your body's important process either directly or indirectly. The part of the brain located just above the pituitary gland (the hypothalamus) has a great deal of influence over certain of its functions, and provides the main liaison between the nervous and the endocrine systems. The front two-thirds of the pituitary gland is really a separate entity from the back one-third: it develops from different origins, contains entirely different types of cells, and has entirely separate functions.

The anterior pituitary gland

The front two-thirds of the pituitary gland controls growth. You need just the right amount of pituitary hormone during your growing years to keep from becoming either a midget or a giant. Your pituitary gland also helps to govern the cell growth by which injured and worn-out cells are replaced after maturity.

The anterior pituitary gland controls your other principal endocrine glands. It makes hormones which keep your thyroid and adrenal glands

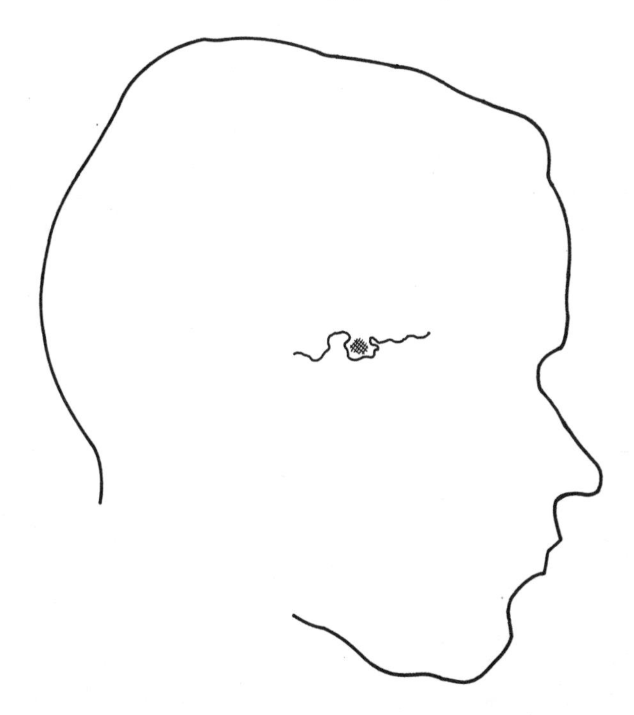

Figure 28. Location and size of pituitary.

active. It makes hormones which signal the ovaries to nurture a pregnancy or continue the menstrual cycle. In a sense, it is the king of kings, the master gland which controls other glands and through them many of your body's most vital functions.

The anterior pituitary gland also governs the breasts in production of milk. One type of anterior pituitary cell seems to influence body build and blood pressure. Probably the gland has other important functions, too, which we do not understand at present.

The posterior pituitary gland

The back one-third of the pituitary gland helps you to conserve your body's supply of water. If it does not function properly, you pass four to six times as much urine as normal (a condition known as "diabetes insipidus"). The posterior pituitary also exerts control over your blood pressure. Its hormones signal the uterus to contract after childbirth, keeping down a new mother's loss of blood.

The thyroid gland

Your thyroid gland usually weighs one ounce or less. It lies in front and at the sides of your windpipe. The thyroid gland controls the rate at which your body burns fuel and thus spurs or holds back almost all body functions.

Mild thyroid disorders frequently cause an easily corrected form of abnormal fatigue in college students. At the end of the adolescent growth spurt, the production or the use of thyroid hormone often drops below

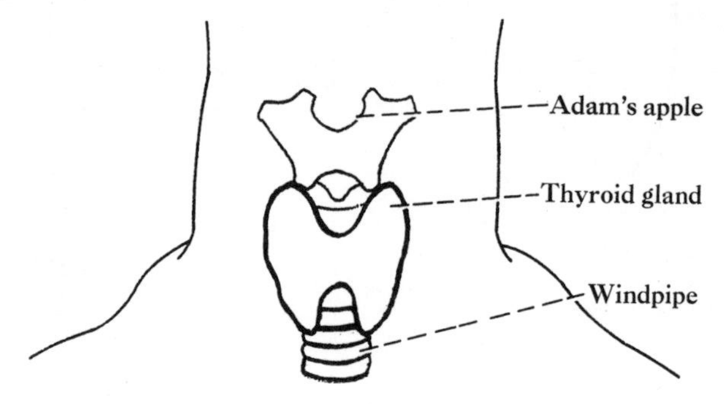

Figure 29. Location and size of thyroid gland.

normal for a year or two, especially in women. Although fatigue is the most common complaint, many victims also have coarse hair, moistureless skin, and either nervous irritability or torpor. Thyroid-deficient women tend toward irregular, scanty, or heavy menstrual periods. Inexpensive, painless, and convenient medical treatment entirely restores normal physical and mental functions in thyroid deficiency, so a physician's evaluation is definitely worthwhile whenever such a disorder might be present.

Unsightly enlargement of the thyroid gland commonly stems from lack of iodine in the food over a period of years. This type of goiter occurs very frequently in the interior areas of the United States because most food grown in this country lacks iodine. You can substantially decrease your chance of getting such a goiter if you use iodized salt on your food.

The parathyroid glands

Four tiny bodies buried in the thyroid gland really function as a separate entity from it. These are the parathyroid glands. They control your body's use of calcium and phosphorus. Calcium and phosphorus must be kept at precisely controlled concentrations in your tissues to maintain bony structure, to allow nerve fibers to function, and to avoid kidney stones.

The adrenal glands

Your two adrenal glands weigh one-third of an ounce each. The outer portions make a variety of hormones concerned with sexual functions (especially in the male), with blood pressure, with inflammation and other infection-fighting mechanisms (some of which occasionally miscarry to

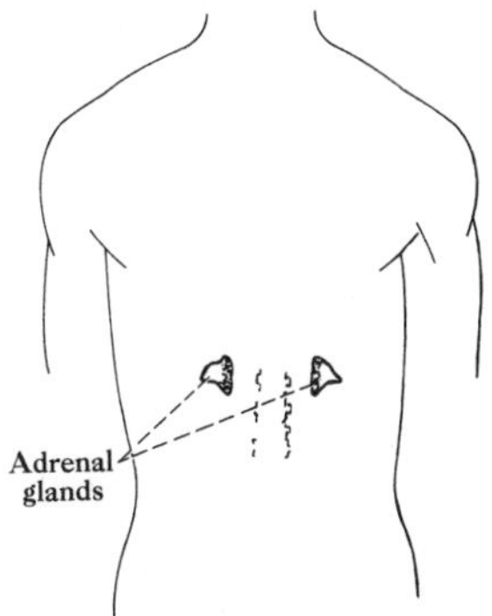

Figure 30. Location and size of adrenal glands.

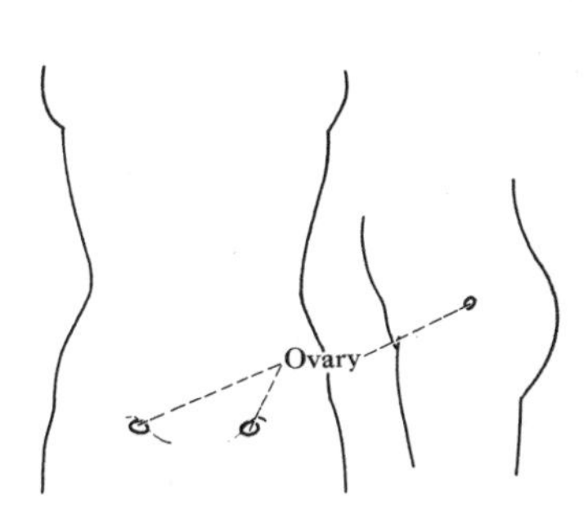

Figure 31. Location and size of ovaries.

produce or aggravate disease), and with control of your body's salt resources. The inner portions are stirred into action whenever you suffer strong emotion. The adrenalin which then flows into your blood stream gives you a temporary boost in blood pressure and blood sugar, closes down blood vessels to your skin and surface parts, dilates your pupils, and speeds passage of material at the lower end of your bowel. Psychologists talk about this response as preparation for fight or flight—more blood to muscles and less to the easily injured skin, more ready fuel and less burden of potential sewage, etc.

The ovaries

Besides fulfiling their role in reproduction, the two ovaries also serve as important endocrine glands.

The ordinary menstrual cycle

Egg cells form in fluid-filled pockets within the ovaries. The walls of these fluid-filled pockets make important female sex hormones. While an egg cell is actually forming, the hormone produced is estrogen. It makes the lining of the uterus thicken in the first stage of preparation for a pregnancy, besides helping development of the breasts and exerting other long-range feminizing effects. At about the fourteenth day, the egg cell pocket bursts and the egg cell erupts. Usually this bursting is painless, although

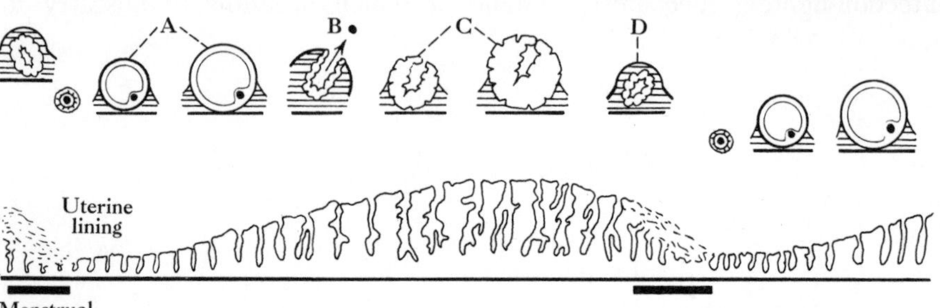

Figure 32. Ovarian hormones and the menstrual cycle. Estrogens produced by the ovarian follicle (A) make the uterine lining thicker. After the follicle ruptures (B) and turns into a corpus luteum (C), it forms progesterone which stimulates the uterine lining to develop succulent glandular structure. If pregnancy does not occur the corpus luteum degenerates (D) and the uterine lining thins down by sloughing its surface layers in menstrual discharge. *After Corner in Arey:* Developmental Anatomy, *6th Ed. 1959. Philadelphia. W. B. Saunders Company.*

it occasionally causes mild discomfort and tenderness low in the abdomen for a few hours in certain individuals. The lining of the pocket in which the egg cell formed changes character after ovulation. The lining cells form a yellow body on the surface of the ovary, and produce a different hormone called *progesterone*. Progesterone acts on the lining of the uterus to make it form a succulent glandular surface upon which a fertilized egg cell can flourish. If a pregnancy occurs, the yellow body enlarges somewhat and remains active until the baby is born. Its hormones are vital to the continuing pregnancy. If pregnancy does not occur, the yellow body soon stops functioning. The thickened, glandular lining of the uterus comes away as menstrual discharge. Another egg cell pocket ripens, and a new ovarian cycle begins.

The infertile-type menstrual cycle

During the first few months of menstruation, almost all periods occur without an egg cell being cast loose and without formation of a yellow body. The uterine lining thickens and sloughs because of varying estrogen levels. As the years go by, more and more ovarian cycles result in formation of a fully mature egg cell and a complete estrogen-progesterone cycle. By college entrance, most women form a living egg cell about three months out of five. The infertile cycles may be noticeably different in character, usually with less discomfort and more flow.

Discomfort during menstrual periods

Most women report some discomfort during menstrual periods. Lower abdominal cramps are frequent, generally on the first day of the cycle. Nausea and vomiting sometimes occur, and fainting or giddy spells are also frequent. These complaints usually clear up within a few hours and do not signify any serious disorder. Mild disturbances often yield to simple measures of preventive hygiene like these:

1. Extra rest *the day before* menstruation is expected, which does much more good than rest after complaints develop.
2. Avoiding cold showers, chilling during swimming sessions, or undue cold exposure the last day or two before anticipated menstruation.
3. Use of napkins instead of tampons for feminine hygiene, except for special dress-up or sporting occasions.

Too many young women write off ten or more days a year in disability because they regard menstrual discomfort as "just something you have to live with." If menstrual discomfort interferes with your ordinary activities or causes substantial distress, you should certainly see what your doctor can do to help it. Abruptly increasing difficulties after menstruation is thoroughly established also deserve attention, even if they are not disabling.

The menopause

Menstruation usually ceases at about age forty-five. Less female sex hormone is formed in the ovaries thereafter. The abrupt decrease in hormone supply may cause certain complaints. Hot flashes, brief spells of mental fogginess, occasional dizziness, and sometimes a feeling of something crawling on the skin are the most common forms of physical distress. Psychological disturbances such as extreme depression are often blamed upon the menopause, too, but the vast bulk of such disorders seem due to the emotional and social adjustments of the menopausal time of life rather than to hormone deficiencies. Menopausal symptoms almost always respond to inexpensive medical treatment, and usually subside to the point where further care is unnecessary within two years.

Many people falsely believe that the menopause signals the end of sexual satisfaction for a woman. This is not true. Driving urge toward sexual activity disappears after the menopause, but sexual satisfaction in marriage is frequently enhanced and never abruptly destroyed.

A woman can tell roughly when to expect her menopause by taking these facts into account:

1. The menopause usually occurs between age forty-five and fifty.
2. If menstruation begins early, the menopause is usually late; if menstruation begins late, menopause is usually early.
3. Most women tend to resemble their mothers in duration of menstrual function.
4. Married women can expect two to four more years of menstruation than spinsters.

The placenta

An unborn infant not only derives nourishment from his mother through the organ which forms his attachment to the inside of her uterus but also forms hormones there which circulate through all parts of her body. These placental hormones affect the uterus and the ovaries in ways essential to continued pregnancy, and also prepare the mother's body in many ways for the processes of birth and lactation. Laboratory tests for early pregnancy are based on the fact that certain animals (frog, rabbit, or mouse) react in easily detected ways to the placental hormones in a pregnant woman's urine. These tests usually become positive quite early in pregnancy.

The testicles

Like the ovary, the testicle produces both reproductive cells and hormones. The hormones bring about the deep voice, bearded face, hairy body, and other characteristics of the adult male. Apparently they also affect growth, strength, and temperament to some extent: eunuchs, whose testicles are removed before adolescence, tend to be abnormally long-legged, somewhat lighter in musculature, and somewhat more even-tempered than their still-male brethren.

The male menopause

Testicular function generally decreases in the late fifties or early sixties. Loss of sexual interest or capacity result. A few men suffer dizzy spells or other complaints while their hormone picture is changing.

Extra facial hair in women

Some women develop heavy hair on the upper lip and chest. Perfectly normal levels of perfectly normal adrenal hormone cause this effect: no testicular or strictly male hormones are responsible. Femininity or sexual adequacy are not affected; hormone treatment is unnecessary. If you wish to rid yourself of unusually heavy hairs for cosmetic reasons, your doctor can suggest appropriate measures.

Other Endocrine Glands

A number of other bodily organs contain cells which either have or might have endocrine functions. The pancreas contains islands of specialized cells which make a hormone essential for proper use of sugar in your body. This hormone's relationship to diabetes mellitus receives further discussion in Chapter 22. Parts of the stomach and intestine make hormones which induce increased secretion from the liver and other digestive glands. The kidney apparently makes hormones which affect blood pressure and circulation. The thymus gland, located behind the upper part of your breastbone, probably has some endocrine functions. From its location and appearance, the pineal body (a small structure attached to the brain's upper surface) has long been considered an endocrine gland, even though no definite hormone production or glandular function can be attributed to it.

CHAPTER 10

Sex and Marriage for Collegians

AS A COLLEGE STUDENT, YOU PROBABLY HAVE TO DEAL WITH THE SEX URGE right now. A strong sex urge is perfectly normal in both men and women of college age, and few of them are in a position to requite it fully. An acceptable way of dealing with sexual pressures can improve your immediate efficiency and contentment, and also can help you to keep sex in proportion with your other aims in working and planning for the future. Several safe and proper approaches other than marriage grant you such relief.

EFFECTS OF THE SEX URGE

The sex urge tends to express itself mainly in psychological yearnings. The physical attractions of members of the opposite sex become greatly enhanced: the homely become acceptable, the acceptable attractive, and the attractive almost irresistible. The importance of physical attraction compared to economic, social, and intellectual virtues is temporarily exaggerated. The victim is plagued by obsessive thoughts of sex play and participation or means of achieving same.

Few people realize how deeply the unrequited sex urge influences them. In one informal experiment, for instance, several young husbands looked at the Rorschach ink blots immediately after a long period of separation from their wives. The blots positively crawled with sexual symbols—breasts, feminine silhouettes, and so on. A few weeks later, after resuming their marital relationships, these same men reviewed the blots and found almost no sexual images. An unrequited sex urge enters all thinking processes, including decisions on everything from choice of companions to choice of career and viewpoints on everything from Shakespearian comedy to rock-and-roll. Although these effects seem somewhat more intense in young men than in young women, both sexes are influenced by biological pressures to some degree.

Specific genital discomforts also plague victims of an unrequited sexual urge, especially if previous experience has fully awakened bodily response. Aching, twitching, crawling sensations, and heaviness seem the commonest complaints.

RELIEF OF THE SEXUAL URGE

Relief of the sexual urge through an actual sexual climax occurs through nocturnal emissions, through masturbation or petting to the point of climax, and through sexual intercourse.

Nocturnal Emissions

Most unmarried men of college age have occasional erotic dreams with seminal emission. Erotic dreams of diving fighter planes, stampeding cattle, or other symbolic crescendos of excitement are just as normal as dreams involving the sexual situation itself. Barring other forms of sexual release, most college men have one or two nocturnal emissions each month. You can have many more or many less without feeling concern, since this is a perfectly normal and harmless phenomenon.

Masturbation and Petting to the Point of Climax

Some form of sexual self-relief is almost universal whenever circumstances prevent normal, healthy men from fulfilling their biological desires. The practice of masturbation when either circumstances or appropriate moral restraint prevent adequate sexual intercourse does not point toward mental illness, and is mentally and physically harmless. Sexual self-stimulation also occurs fairly frequently in perfectly normal young women, often without their awareness of its nature (as when the quivering of muscles in a certain strained posture conveys pleasure without specifically genital sensations).

Petting to a point of climax often provides considerable release of sexual tension even though the climax is emotional rather than physical. Petting to the point of orgasm provides release similar to that of masturbation but may impose considerable strain on both parties' self-control. Pregnancy can also sometimes occur without actual entrance of the male organ into the female if seminal material is deposited in the vicinity.

Sexual Intercourse

Several cogent health arguments support the social taboos on premarital and extramarital relationships. Couples who wait until after marriage find that sex can be a symbolic sacrament of biological union which effectively welds the union of husband and wife, while less patient or less faithful pairs usually find intercourse merely a mutual, a friendly, or a contractually compensated service. Couples whose sole excursions into the sexual sublime have been in each other's company get a very helpful degree of continually reinforced identification through sex which other couples mainly miss. Of course, many couples build a successful sexual adjustment in marriage on the contract principle: "You satisfy me and I'll try to satisfy you" or "You provide for me financially and I'll provide for you sexually," for instance. However, such an attitude makes sex a household arrangement instead of an emotional relationship. Both sex and the relationship are poorer as a result.

To this major argument for premarital chastity you can add lesser ones like the danger that biological pressures will push you into a lifelong union with a poorly selected partner, the possible emotional and physical damage to the woman of an inconsiderate introduction to sex, the burdens of anxiety and guilt, the hazards of disease or pregnancy. While each individual must make up his own mind, these points add up to a substantial argument against premarital intercourse (in addition to religious and moral constraints which we will not discuss here).

Indirect Relief of the Sexual Urge

Any activity in which you can completely immerse yourself helps you to forget or offset sexual pressures. Captivating, creative experience of any sort serves as a means of sublimation. If you find sexual pressures or preoccupations disturbing, you may gain considerable relief by throwing yourself wholeheartedly into such an avocation or interest.

SEX IN MARRIAGE

One of the greatest fallacies prevalent in America today might be expressed:

Sex is instinctive.
Instinctive acts do not have to be learned.

Ergo: You do not have to learn anything about sex to be a satisfactory participant.

The fallacy, of course, lies in adding new qualifications to the conclusion. Perhaps you do not have to learn anything about sex to procreate, any more than you have to learn table manners in order to eat. However, you have to learn a great deal in order to realize your potential for getting or giving satisfaction, whether you pick up the necessary knowledge through trial and error, unintentional absorption, or deliberate acquisition.

Premarital Instruction

Some high schools and many colleges offer courses in preparation for marriage. These courses generally spend considerable time on sociological and emotional aspects of the relationship. As discussed at length in Chapter 3, close personal relationships involve heavy demands and responsibilities, for which many people of college age are not yet entirely prepared. Since sex is ideally an integral part of the relationship rather than a mechanical service or sport, emotional maturity and properly welded personal association are necessary foundations for sound sexual adjustment in marriage.

Preparation for marriage courses usually offer comparatively little guidance in the field of sexual technique. You usually can get good library references from the instructor and may be able to arrange a conference for further discussion if necessary. Your religious adviser may be better qualified

Figure 33. Lively exchange of ideas in a prep-for-marriage course. *Gary K. Cowell.*

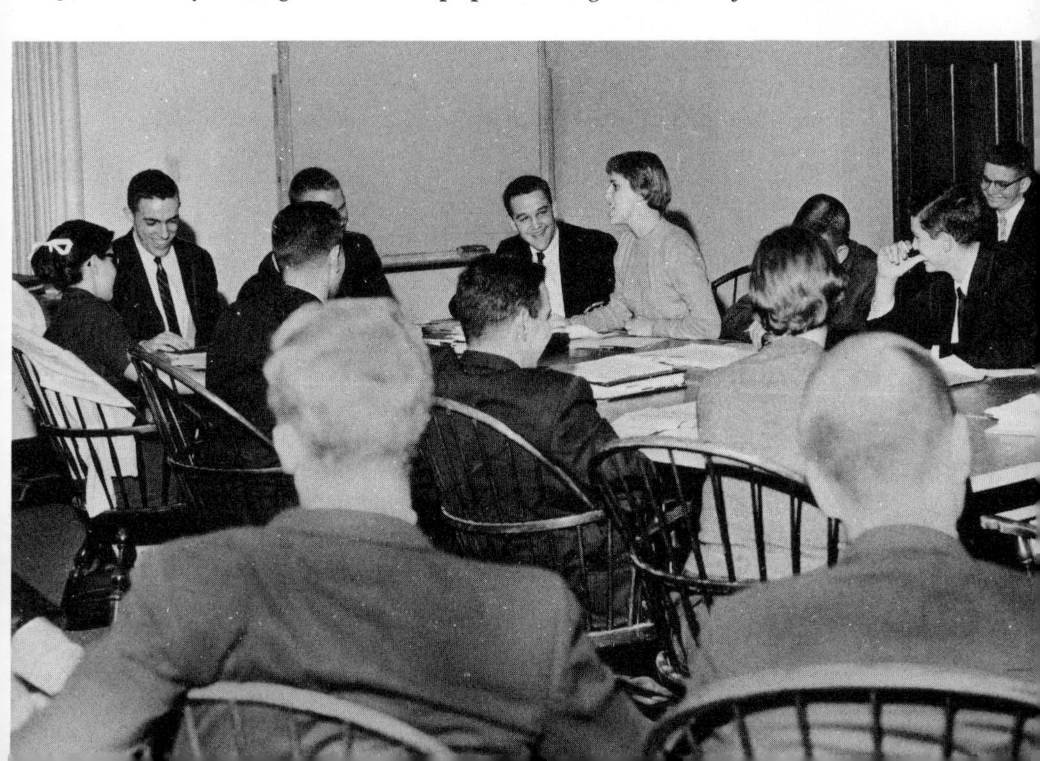

for counseling in this respect than you would expect. A good marriage counselor can advise you with regard to physical as well as emotional aspects of the relationship. Your personal physician can probably recommend suitable readings and answer your questions competently.

The Honeymoon

The early weeks of marriage are more valuable as a period of learning and adaptation than as one of sexual delight and satisfaction. Even couples with considerable prior experience may find their approach requires revision in the more intensively emotional interplay of married sex. The virginal bride seldom develops her capacity for satisfying sexual climax in less than two weeks, and generally does not reach her ultimate level of responsiveness for between six weeks and a year or more. The inexperienced groom seldom has developed very adequate sexual control. Attempts to achieve immediate, keen sexual satisfaction generally lead to disappointment.

You have a much better chance of forming a sound sexual adjustment in marriage if you forget the romantic but totally false notion that love guarantees mutual sexual satisfaction. During the early weeks of marriage, a couple's first aim should be to achieve sexual union without discomfort to the woman, which can be absolutely assured through suitable measures. Their second aim should be to learn how to maintain the man's sexual excitement without precipitating his sexual climax. Only after thorough mastery of these basic sexual achievements, which may take anything from a few days to several weeks, should they attempt to explore the deeper realms of sexual delight. By making haste slowly, any couple can achieve a thoroughly comfortable and pleasant introduction to connubial bliss.

MARRIAGE AS A RELATIONSHIP

Marriage involves considerable new responsibilities and burdens along with considerable new satisfactions and emotional supports. Several principles can help you reduce marital stress, meet marital stress better, and promote the emotional welding of sound marital union. If you understand what goes into making a sound marriage beforehand, you may be able to improve considerably the ease and thoroughness of your marital adjustment.

Basic Stresses and Supports in Marriage

Although superficial and often trivial situations trigger most open arguments in marriage, certain big issues commonly provide the basic marital unrest and tension which makes these minor matters seem important.

What is a marriage?

Different concepts of marriage itself lie beneath many marital conflicts. Any contract whose terms have different meaning to the participants generates later friction. Marriage is a contract, but few couples agree beforehand on exactly what each individual's responsibilities and rewards will be. The legal position which makes man the master is cleary anachronistic. The general principle of equality gets lip service from everyone, but proves either useless or downright harmful in practice. The doctrine of "fifty-fifty" is useless because you can never equate qualitatively different tasks, rewards, or needs. It is harmful because "fifty-fifty" makes marriage a perpetually renegotiated agreement between individuals instead of a communally functioning merger. The viewpoint on which you will base your behavior and your emotional response in situations of marital conflict probably bears little relationship to either man-the-master or "fifty-fifty," probably has never been clearly defined, and quite possibly differs sharply from that of your future spouse.

How do you feel about your family?

Most in-law problems and many conflicts in the field of child-rearing arise through different concepts of the family and of family responsibility.

Figure 34. Is this really "the whole family," or does the blood bond involve dozens of others? *Wide World Photos, Inc.*

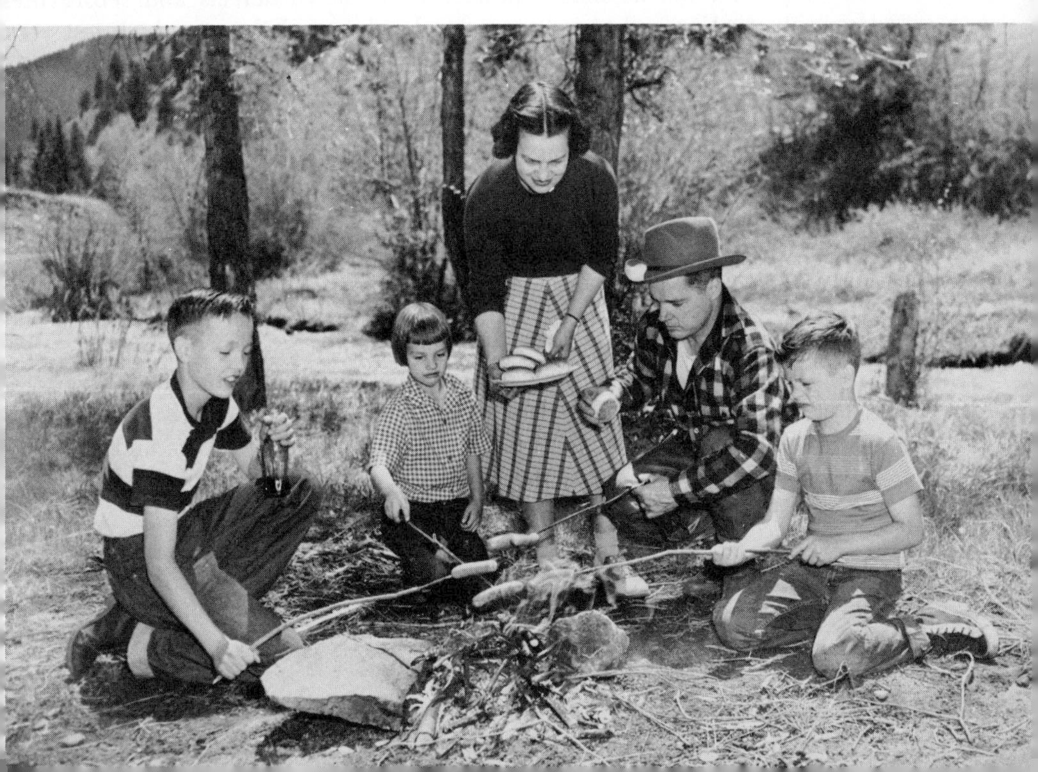

Some people view the family as including every cousin, and regard their responsibility to other members as quite heavy. Others view the family as including only parents and children, perhaps even parents and children who are members of the same household, and feel highly limited responsibility. In your relationship with both your own family and your in-laws, you tend to apply your own standards of family responsibility. These may differ sharply from those your spouse recognizes.

Family feeling enters numerous issues. Should you spend part of your vacation time visiting parents? Should you devote one evening a week to them if they live in your home town? If your uncle needs an operation, can you impose financial burdens on your own household in order to help him meet the expense? What about piano lessons for Junior, or college tuition for his sister Sue? Are these adequate reasons for parental sacrifice?

Unless a husband and wife fully appreciate each other's viewpoint on family feeling, such matters cause considerable conflict and resentment through the years.

Are you ready to give emotional aid and comfort?

The emotional relationship of marriage imposes both burdens and threats. You assume many virtually psychotherapeutic responsibilities with marriage. You accept a constant obligation for giving considerate aid to the other person *in difficulties which arise out of conflict with you,* as well as in emotional upheavals imposed by financial, household, familial, and sexual responsibilities. The simple fact of a personal relationship without reserve, in which you can no longer protect your known defects and sensitivities from observation and assault, imposes burdens and threats which test your personality strength.

Emotional benefits you can expect from marriage

Exactly the same bonds through which marriage imposes emotional burdens and threats also give substantial emotional support. Considerate aid is a two-way street from which both parties actually benefit in understanding and fellow feeling. Responsibilities give a feeling of purpose and achievement to your life. The systematization necessary to meet those responsibilities gives security-boosting structure. A relationship without reserve gives intense personal satisfaction in itself, and increases the satisfactions of most shared experiences. Your personality grows and strengthens through such a relationship whenever you can achieve and maintain it.

How to Reduce Marital Stresses

A clear-cut formulation of your own and your partner's viewpoint toward marital and familial responsibilities may help substantially in preventing or reducing marital stress. Most couples can discuss these matters quite rationally as principles or in hypothetical cases, while they cannot be rational once conflict arises. Points to settle, before marriage if possible, certainly include these:

• • • Do you believe in division of responsibility and authority (e.g., wife responsible for household operation with undisputed authority to manage the household budget, husband responsible for securing funds with undisputed authority in that sphere)? If so, exactly what areas should each partner handle? What degree of authority does he have over the other person's activities (or inactivity) in the field?

• • • How much time and effort do you feel should be devoted to keeping contact with parents and other relatives? Exactly which relatives would you feel obligated to help in a financial emergency? Which would you pay funeral expenses for? If providing special instruction like music lessons involves giving up your planned vacation trip, or if helping your child through college means going into debt yourself, do you think your obligation as a parent will demand that you provide such opportunities?

• • • What about religion? Are you fully agreed on the religious training you will give your children? Do you plan to observe regular religious exercises in your household?

• • • Do you expect to get strong backing and help from your marriage partner in dealing with your own personal problems? If so, do you recognize that at least momentary mastery or dominance is frequently a part of such help, and are you willing to accept same? Likewise with couple rather than individual problems: do you expect to defer to the other person's greater strength in crises which you cannot readily handle yourself? Can you take over masterfully in crises which your partner cannot handle? Discuss several cases in which each might occur.

How to Meet Stresses Better

Every married couple needs some means of handling differences and upheavals. Several points seem worth raising:

• • • Marital difficulties and upheavals call for a constructive approach. The biggest single service most couples get from a marriage counselor

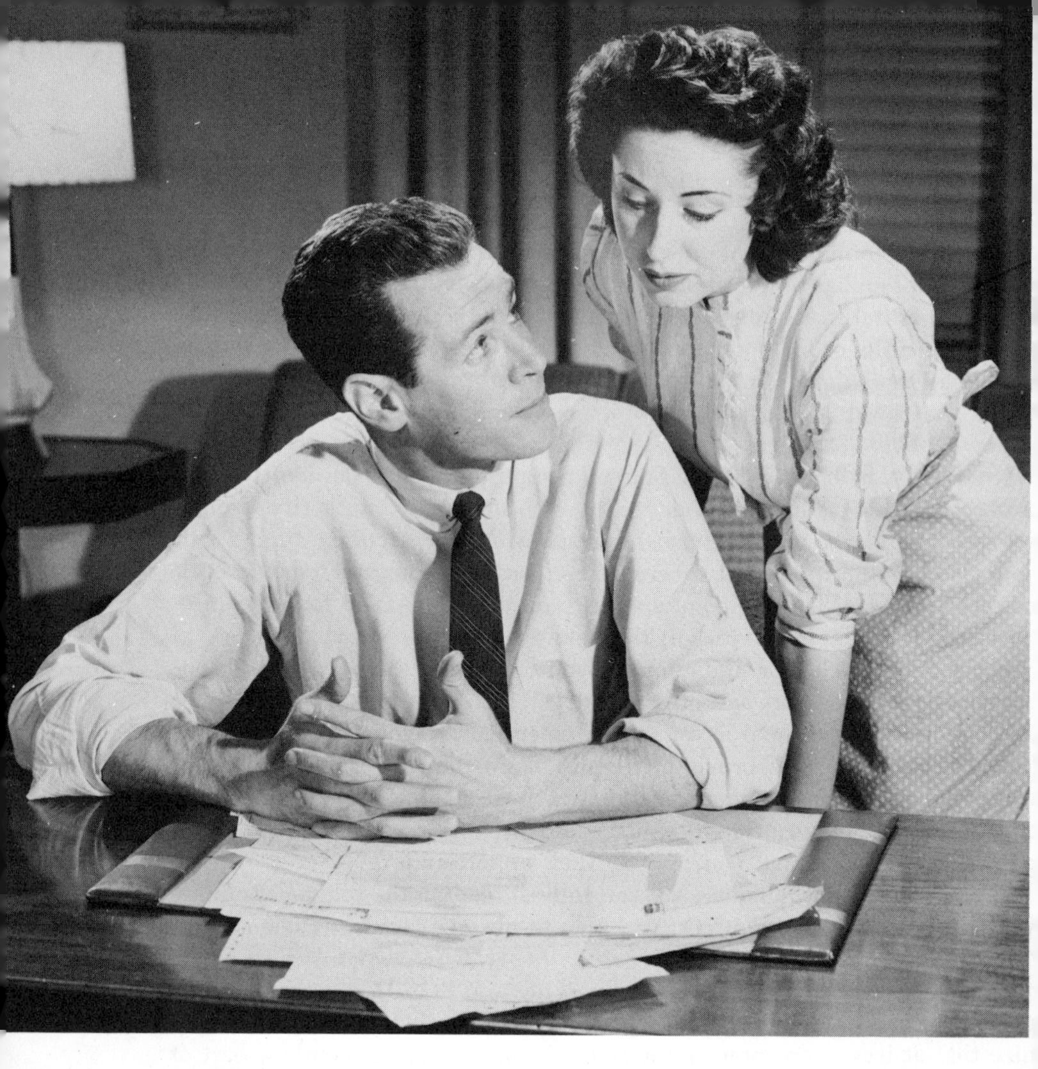

Figure 35. "Let's work out a budget" accomplishes more than "You've run up too blasted many bills!" *Ewing Galloway.*

consists of a change from futile who's-to-blame arguments to where-do-we-go-from-here thinking.

• • • The issues precipitating marital difficulties and upheavals seldom constitute the main area of conflict. Often they symbolize deeper issues. A disagreement over where to spend a vacation may symbolize the broader dominance issue which causes perennial but unmentionable strain in the sexual sphere, for instance. Sometimes spats result from a chip-on-the-shoulder attitude with completely unrelated origins, as when a husband blasts his wife for overcooking his steak when he is actually upset about his child's school problems. In such instances, the most constructive procedure usually is to make peace by giving in if necessary on the inconsequential item with an eye to later review of major spheres of your life together (household management, sex and parenthood, use of leisure time, dominance, family relationships, etc.).

• • • The value of a soundly working marriage deserves continual re-emphasis as an antidote to petty arguments and pique. For every four marriages, one couple seeks a divorce. Marital discontent seems even more common: many couples stay together for reasons of convenience or commitment without a really good marital adjustment. A good marriage stems from vigorous effort, not from the mere nature of wedded life. Especially in the early, stormy years of marriage, most husbands and wives profit by occasionally writing a forecast of what their life would be like in ten or twenty years with a sound marriage or after a divorce. Certainly the difference far outweighs in importance most causes of marital discord.

• • • Lastly, husbands and wives can try to pick the right time or set the proper atmosphere for settling conflict-ridden issues. Certainly, the time for raising complaints is not the moment when you are stinging from previous defeat or insult, and feeling distinctly mean. The proper atmosphere is friendly, but not so friendly that you appear to be taking advantage. It is sufficiently relaxed for calm discussion. It is free from the likelihood of untimely interruptions, and cheerful but not hilarious in mood. Like diplomats setting the stage for a productive conference, most married couples need to spend considerable time and effort on selecting or creating a proper moment so that a difference-settling parley can be calm and productive.

Community Help with Marriage Problems

For every four marriages in this country today, there will be about one divorce. Many other marriages end in separations or survive periods of estrangement only with considerable difficulty. Even if your own marriage never approaches the breaking point, you must help meet the cost of deserted wives and abandoned children, of court actions and social work investigations, and of the excess delinquency and mental illness which arise in broken homes.

Most communities have found that a little effort to save marriages saves vast later heartache and expense. The courts would rather help you patch up a marriage than grant a divorce. Family service agencies would rather work with you during each early marital upheaval than see you go into the divorce court. Educators and social workers would rather encourage delay than allow too-young couples to marry in haste.

Although you may not need these agencies yourself, they help you meet your responsibility as a community member more fully and with less expense than that involved in last-ditch, inescapable welfare commitments.

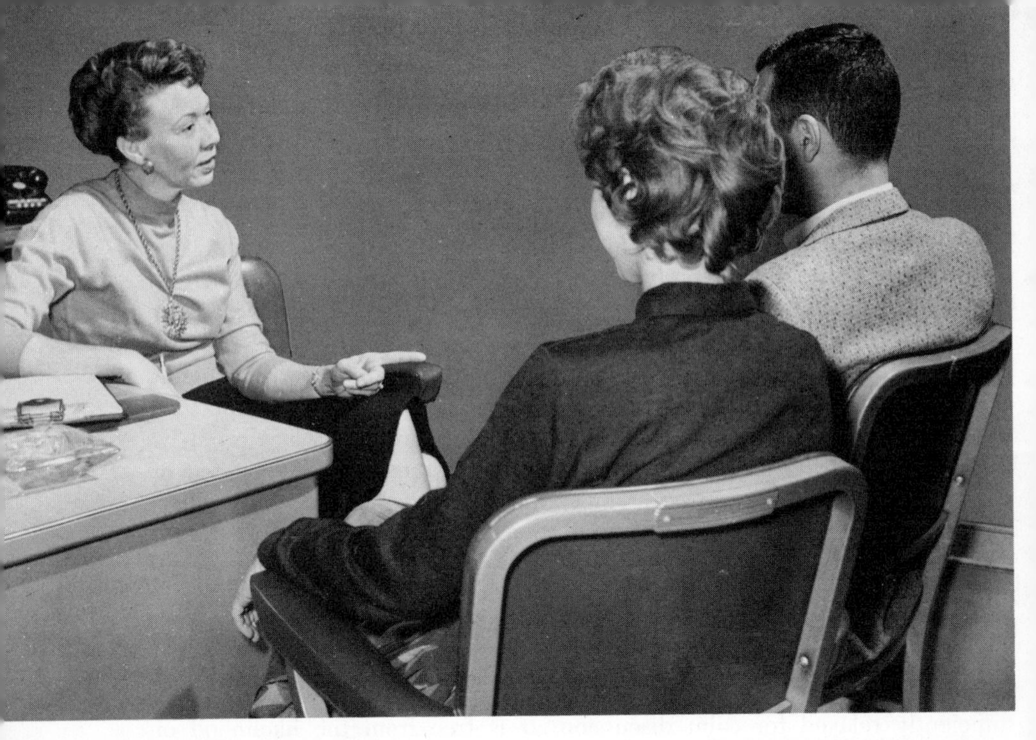

Figure 36. Marriage counseling at the University of Iowa. *Wide World Photos, Inc.*

Progressive programs to aid failing marriages and to prevent as many inappropriate marriages as possibly deserve wholehearted support, whether they are carried out by the courts, by health and welfare divisions of the various government levels, or by voluntary agencies.

How to Promote Marital Union

Although all marriages are contracts, the best ones work more like mergers. If you can achieve functional identification (see Chapter 3) the emotional rewards life brings to each partner reflect intensively upon the other. Neither partner cares whether he is receiving his just due, since the rewards the other person receives mean as much to him as his own. Likewise with the performance of tasks: the marriage is a mutual endeavor in which it really makes no difference who does what, not a cooperative one in which the good and bad must be carefully parceled out.

You can build the merger-identification viewpoint in marriage by taking several steps:

1. Provide intellectual and emotional environs for each other's betterment and aggrandizement without intramarital competition.
2. Try to recognize and meet each other's continually changing emotional requirements rather than fall into a static pattern. This is particularly im-

portant with regard to dependency, where both parties alternately need to feel supported and need to feel needed.

3. Seek a good over-all sexual adjustment as a couple instead of ecstatic satisfaction for each individual in each sexual episode. Even with excellent sexual adjustment, the woman's main gratification in many sexual contacts will derive from the satisfaction she gives her partner rather than from sheer fleshly delight. The romantic myth that lovers ultimately achieve uniform, mutually ecstatic satisfaction imposes a heavy burden of marital strain. Sex need never be a burden and is generally a blessing to most marriages, but the idea that it provides consistently intense delight leads to considerable unnecessary disillusionment, false accusations, and feelings of inadequacy.

4. Learn the art of compassionate concern. When your bride burns the roast or your groom wrecks the family car, you should be able to commiserate without stirring further anger or distress. True identification makes you feel a share of the blame along with the feeling of loss, just as if you had actually participated in causing the tragedy. It makes you continuously conscious of the other person's feelings and situation so that you react with him instead of as an independent being.

5. Finally, try to share the profoundly unifying experiences of parenthood and child-rearing as soon as your situation and biological providence permit. Marital discontent is twice as frequent in childless marriages. While this may partially result from hesitance to have children when the marriage is poor, it also results in part from lack of the symbolic merging and intensely mutual endeavor involved in having and rearing children.

COURTSHIP AND MARRIAGE DURING COLLEGE

Four health considerations enter strongly into the question of marriage during your years of college or postgraduate study. These involve your capacity to select and promote the best possible marital union at this time of life, your ability to control fertility, your capacity to manage the burdens of self-support and domestic responsibilities on top of school chores, and the extra strains on marital adjustment in the shifting situation of a primordial career.

Are You Both Ready for Marriage?

Virtually every college student is physically ready for marriage. Few couples regard financial independence as essential, so economic readiness is rarely an issue. The key question in evaluating your readiness for marriage is whether you have developed sufficiently in personality to choose a marriage partner wisely and to build a sound marriage. Some college freshmen have already reached that state, some will never reach it, and most arrive during or shortly after their four college years. Perhaps these questions will help you evaluate your own position:

• • • Does marriage seem like an escape from parental demands and various pressures, or like a new venture which you would take on even if it would not change any of your current relationships or responsibilities?

• • • In your last argument or disagreement with your roommate or family, were you able to control yourself sufficiently to do what you now know would have been best for the sake of the future relationship?

• • • If you write down your six main objectives in life and your six main interests, are you sure that those lists will be approximately the same six months from now?

• • • What part did your parents play directly or indirectly in your choice of college and major?

Your prospective partner's personal maturity also affects your chances of marital success. How would he or she rate on each of the questions above? Can each of you see why these points are important to successful marriage?

Birth Control

Even if religion places no restriction upon birth control practices, unplanned pregnancies occur fairly frequently. Students who have read of "95 per cent efficient methods" often do not realize that efficiency is rated by ability to reduce fertility from its unimpeded level, not by ability to forestall conception until the couple decides to have a baby. Thus a 95 per cent effective method allows one pregnancy every 200 months even if properly and uniformly applied. If you want to defer pregnancy for five years with such a method, nature will therefore thwart you roughly 30 per cent of the time. Any married couple's plans therefore must take into account at least some possibility of an unexpected pregnancy, even if their religious beliefs permit use of any available contraceptive technique.

Marriage as an Extra Burden

When you get married, financial responsibilities and domestic duties take many more hours each week than they previously occupied. While some of these tasks provide a change from the intellectual grind of school work, they are still burdens when superimposed on an already saturated schedule.

The Graduation Shift

Lastly, most couples who marry in college or professional school find that they have to endure an extra adjustment phase after graduation. The relationship between fellow students or between student and sponsor-wife is different from that between a business or professional man and his wife. The dependency situation, the wife's recognition through her husband's achievements instead of her own, her frequent need to subjugate her own wishes and needs to the good of his career, different and much sharper division of responsibility with more of the dull household chores falling to the wife, and many other changes test the flexibility of the initial adjustment.

CHAPTER 11

Parenthood

MOST COLLEGIANS KNOW EXACTLY WHERE BABIES COME FROM. WHEN IT COMES to practical situations involving pregnancy, labor, and early motherhood, however, they may lack necessary details. For instance, would you know what to say in the following situations?

• • • An unmarried girl confides that she is considering desperate action because she missed her last menstrual period and is therefore sure that she is pregnant.

• • • Shortly after a strenuous golf game, a young wife's first pregnancy ends in miscarriage. You find her crying in her hospital bed, overwhelmed with feelings of guilt. "If only I hadn't overexerted myself!" she exclaims.

• • • One of your neighbors is expecting a child, and is quite worried about getting to the hospital in time. "How soon do you have the baby after labor begins?" she asks.

• • • You visit a new mother who would like to breast feed her infant, but is worried about the effects on her body.

If you can meet the problems of pregnancy and labor matter-of-factly, you will save yourself and your associates considerable emotional distress. This section covers many matters on which you personally may need to make decisions, such as when to start visiting an obstetrician and natural childbirth *vs.* medicinal anesthesia, besides many you will often hear discussed, like criminal abortions and miscarriages. Let's take up these problems as they arise in the course of pregnancy.

FERTILIZATION AND PREGNANCY

Most women's ovaries produce about eight fully ripened egg cells each year during their reproductive period. Their other menstrual cycles are infertile (*see* p. 105). In any one month, only one egg cell is generally pro-

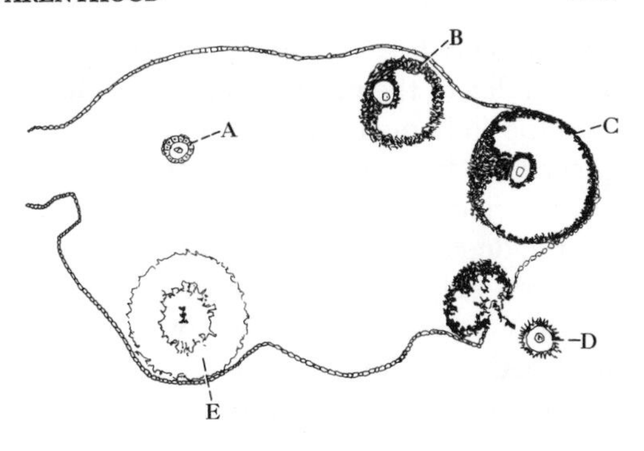

Figure 37. Schematic diagram of egg cell development. From one of many primary follicles (A), a hormone producing follicle (B) develops and matures to stage (C) over a period of about two weeks. The mature egg cell (D) then breaks loose from its follicle and the follicle develops into a corpus luteum (E) which secretes hormones different from those produced by the ovarian follicle and performs an indispensable function in pregnancy. *Adapted with permission from* Human Embryology, *by Bradley M. Patten. Copyright 1953. McGraw-Hill Book Co., Inc.*

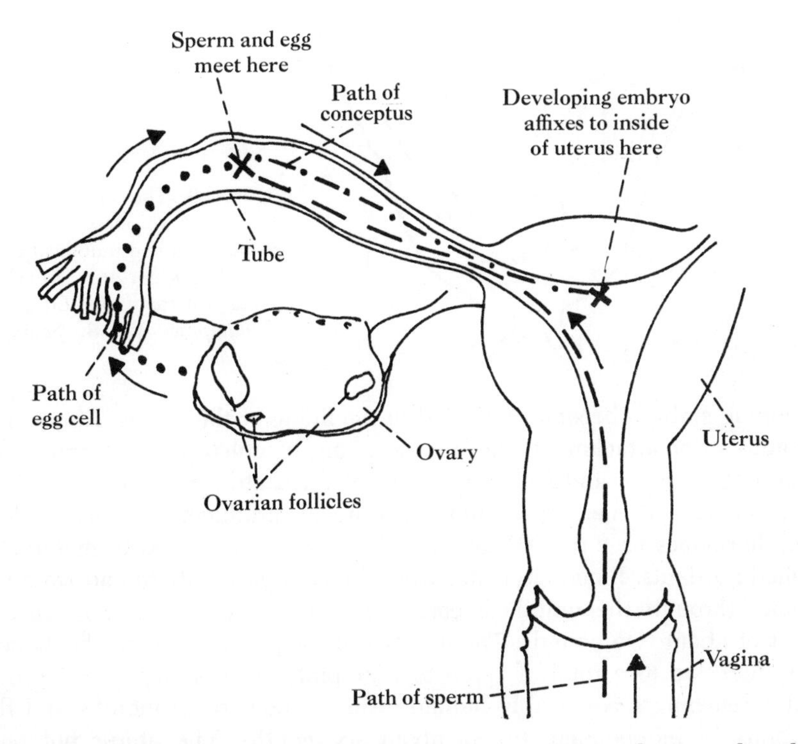

Figure 38. Movement of sperm, egg, and conceptus as pregnancy begins. *Adapted with permission from* Physiology and Anatomy *by Esther M. Greisheimer, 7th Edition. Copyright 1955. J. B. Lippincott Co.*

duced. This breaks free of its pocket of ovarian juices at about the fourteenth day of the menstrual cycle. Although it may not always move directly into the Fallopian tube (sometimes floating free in the abdomen and being picked up by the tendrils at the tube's funnel-like end) the egg cell ultimately finds its way into that narrow passage. If one of the millions of sperm deposited in the vagina moves sufficiently vigorously to reach the egg cell before expiring, fertilization occurs, generally about one-third of the way down the tube. The product of conception floats freely in the tube as it begins to develop, reaching a mulberry-like stage with perhaps 32 cells before arriving in the uterus. Forty-eight to 72 hours after fertilization, the

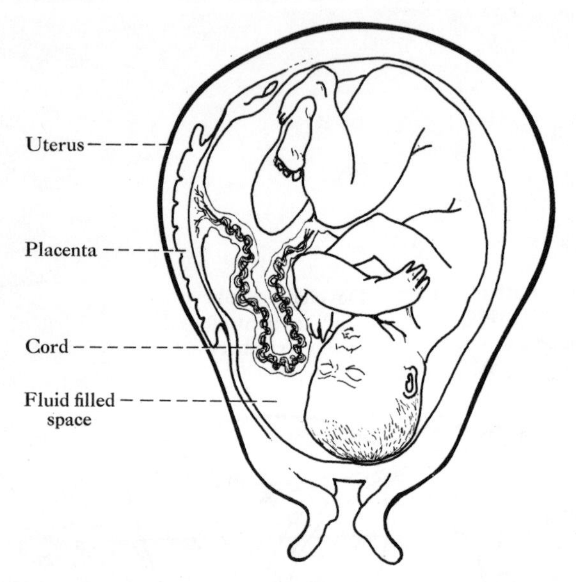

Figure 39. The unborn baby's attachment to mother's uterus via placenta and umbilical cord. *After Ahlfeld, in Arey:* Developmental Anatomy, *6th Ed. 1959. Philadelphia. W. B. Saunders Company.*

developing embryo becomes attached to the lining of the uterus. Almost immediately after attachment, the uterine lining completely incorporates the developing embryo, and from that moment forth attachment is quite firm. The placenta and membranes develop quickly, producing pregnancy-governing hormones (see p. 106) and aiding the embryo's access to maternally supplied nutrients. Blood circulates from the embryo's body to and from the placenta through the umbilical cord. Ultimately, the placenta reaches a weight of about two pounds. The fluid within which the embryo floats normally increases to a total of three to four pints. The embryo itself grows rapidly, reaching recognizably human form in about three months and the possibility of independent life in about six months. The uterus not only stretches but actually grows to accommodate the child, weighing two ounces initially and about two pounds at term.

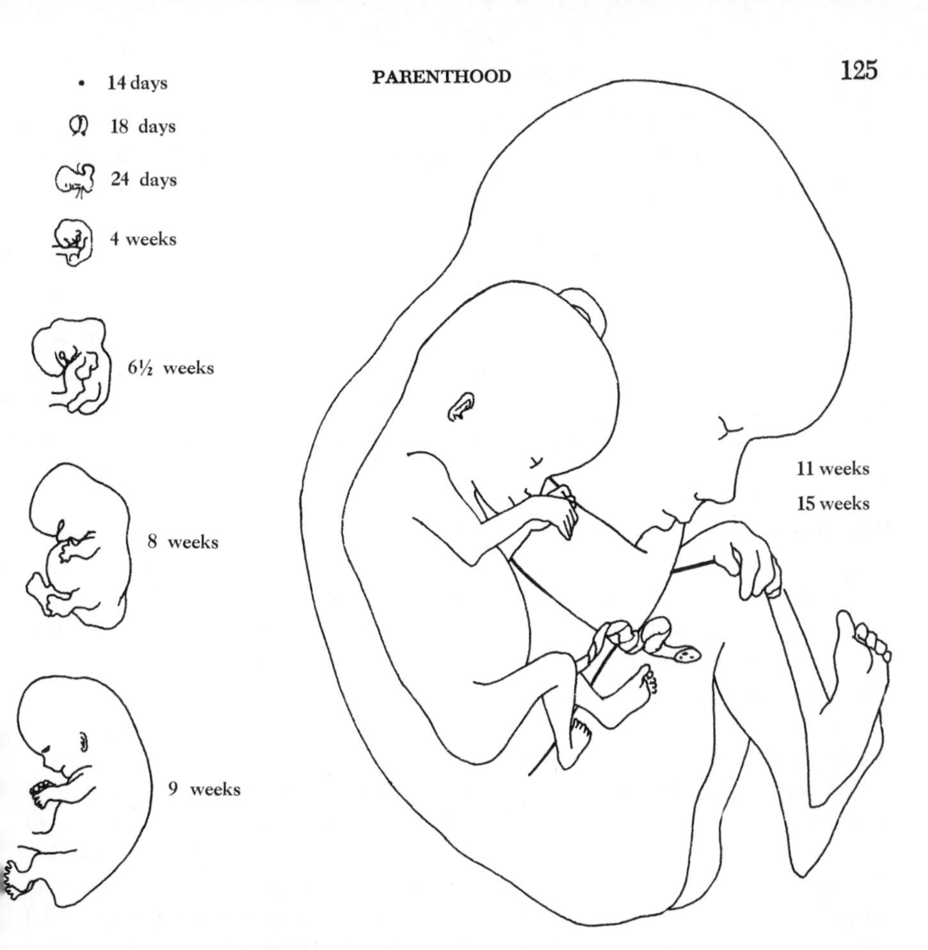

Figure 40. Explosive growth during early embryonic life: drawings at actual size. *After Arey:* Developmental Anatomy, *6th Ed. 1959. Philadelphia. W. B. Saunders Company.*

Twins

Fraternal twins occur when two mature egg cells break loose from the ovaries during one ovulational period, and both become fertilized. Such twins have independently determined genetic patterns and are simply siblings of the same age. Identical twins occur when the fertilized egg cell splits into two independent embryos at a very early stage in development, usually when only two or four cells are present. Such twins have identical genetic background. If a prospective mother has fraternal twins in the family, she is somewhat more likely than average to produce such twins. A family background of identical twins on either the maternal or the paternal side makes such twins more likely. However, the family influence is not very strong: even mothers who have already had one set of twins and thus have proved themselves genetically predisposed have only twice as much chance as other mothers of producing twins with each later pregnancy.

Determination of Pregnancy

When you want to know whether you are pregnant, nothing short of complete examination with laboratory tests suffices. A missed menstrual period is suggestive, but far from definite evidence of pregnancy. Between one-half and two-thirds of the single girls who pay for (and think they have gotten) a criminal abortion were never pregnant at all. Every doctor knows of hasty marriages followed in a few months by an operation for ovarian cyst. Menstrual delay often spurs couples into marriage, leaving perpetual suspicion of fraud when regularity resumes. If you need to know whether pregnancy exists, make an appointment with a competent physician who can almost certainly settle the issue with a complete examination and some laboratory tests. Hormones found in the urine during early pregnancy produce characteristic changes in a frog, mouse, or rabbit making laboratory diagnosis quite exact [1] within four weeks after fertilization occurs, or not more than two weeks after the first missed period.

Where crucial decisions do not hinge upon the presence or absence of pregnancy, most patients do not want to undertake the extra expense of laboratory tests to settle the issue early. Your doctor usually can determine by physical examination alone whether pregnancy is present when menstruation is about six weeks overdue. That is the proper time for the first obstetrical visit unless vomiting or other complaints create earlier need.

Criminal Abortion

Intentional interruption of pregnancy for reasons other than medical necessity constitutes criminal abortion. This is undoubtedly the commonest illegal operation performed in this country. Three-fourths of the customers are married, mainly women with several children who feel that they have a big enough family.

Abortions performed out of medical necessity by a competent surgeon involve virtually no risk. However, the bulk of criminal abortions are performed by people posing as doctors, nurses, or midwives, but actually without scientific training. Deadly infection or hemorrhage frequently result, as they would from any operation performed by a traveling reprobate with

[1] Although technically rated at 95 to 98 per cent accurate, almost all errors occur in late pregnancy or in the presence of abnormalities clearly distinguishable from pregnancy on physical examination.

dirty, makeshift tools. Aside from moral issues involved, the legal prohibition against abortion makes it almost certain that anyone willing to do the job is either incompetent, highly unreliable, or both.

Medicines sold illicitly for the purpose of producing abortion likewise have considerable dangers. Doctors do not use drugs for legal abortions because none works effectively in safe doses. Most materials sold for the purpose are either ineffective, very dangerous, or both.

Spontaneous Abortion

Lower abdominal cramps and vaginal bleeding in the early months of pregnancy generally mean that spontaneous abortion is threatening. The victim should lie down quietly and summon medical aid. Prompt care for any febrile illness, for kidney or bowel disorders (as signified by burning on urination and frequent passage of urine or by diarrhea), and for major injuries is especially worthwhile during early pregnancy.

When abortion occurs despite adequate treatment, the mother virtually could never have influenced the outcome in any way. Abortion occasionally follows severe maternal illness or injury, but more commonly stems from congenital defects incompatible with life. The minor jostlings, ailments, or injuries people sometimes blame for abortion actually have no bearing whatever. Perhaps the best viewpoint toward spontaneous abortion is that it proves fertility and clears the deck for further reproductive efforts. Certainly, it neither punishes past failures or prejudices future results.

Weight Gain During Pregnancy

When a baby is born, the mother usually loses a total of about twenty pounds. The baby weighs seven pounds or so, the placenta and membranes two to three pounds, the amniotic fluid three or four pounds, and the uterus about two pounds extra. Considerable extra fluid dilutes the blood in the last few months of pregnancy (making any bleeding at or after birth less hazardous), and disappears soon after the baby arrives. If weight gain during pregnancy does not exceed two pounds a month, permanent body substance will not be increased. Very large babies, which often make for somewhat more difficult labor, also are less frequent.

Restrictions During Pregnancy

Most doctors do not require drastic curtailment of physical activity during pregnancy. The extra weight and abnormal posture of advanced pregnancy may cause somewhat limiting backaches or fatigue. Douches, tub baths, and swimming sometimes are restricted during the last few weeks so that water will not carry germs up into the vagina just before the onset of labor (which is difficult to predict precisely in advance). Sexual intercourse likewise may be interdicted for the last few weeks.

HOW BABIES ARE BORN

The normal birth passage leads from the uterus through the vagina to the exterior. Nobody understands the exact mechanism which makes labor begin. Once it starts, contractions of the muscular uterine walls push the

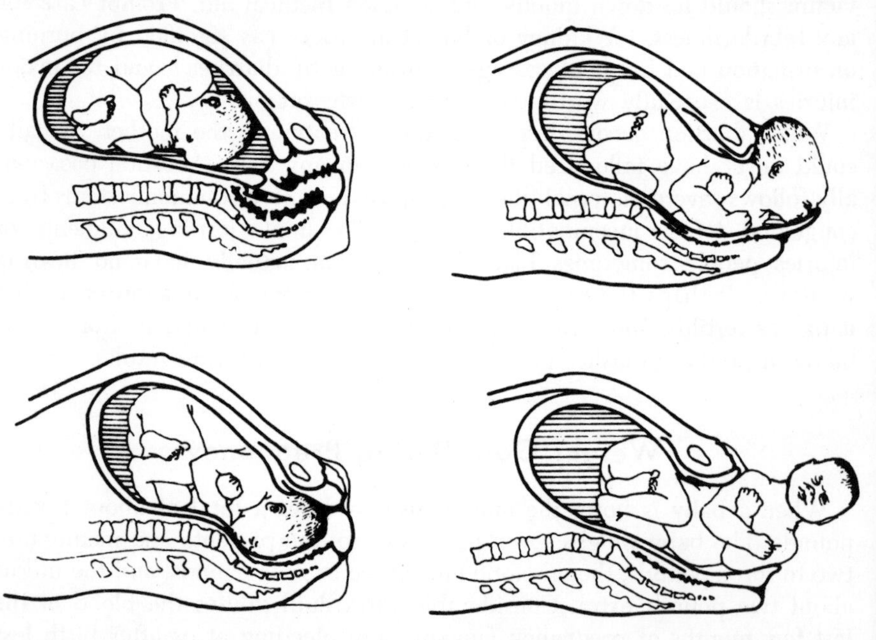

Figure 41. Childbirth. *From Eastman, N. J.* Williams Obstetrics, *11th Ed., 1956. Courtesy of Appleton-Century-Crofts, Inc.*

baby down into the vagina. Instinctive but voluntary squeezing with the abdominal muscles supplements uterine contraction to complete birth. On the average, the process takes about thirteen hours for first babies and at least several hours thereafter.

Part of the fluid-filled membranous sac around the baby pushes through ahead of him, acting as an opening wedge. The crown of the baby's head usually comes next. Some babies deliver rump first in what is called "breech presentation." Less than one in a hundred wedge crosswise or in other positions from which normal delivery is impossible.

The baby ordinarily continues to get oxygen and nourishment from the mother for a minute or so after birth. Then circulation in the umbilical cord ceases and the placenta comes loose from inside the uterus. This process usually takes about ten minutes, and involves loss of half a pint to a pint of blood. Whether the cord has been cut or not, the baby must get air into his lungs soon after circulation through the umbilical vessels ceases. Delivering the placenta or cutting the cord is much less urgent.

False Labor

In the last ten days of pregnancy, most women have rhythmic uterine contractions which sometimes cause intermittent discomfort or pain. These may occur in episodes easily confused with labor. This process of false labor involves actual contractions of the muscular uterine wall, but the contractions differ in nature from those occurring in true labor. Discomfort generally centers just under the umbilicus and is likened to menstrual cramps in severity. Contractions last thirty seconds or so, and usually occur at intervals ranging from five to thirty minutes without any set pattern. Perhaps one-third of women without previous experience and a substantial number who have already had children cannot distinguish these cramps from true labor pains, requiring either medical examination or brief hospitalization for these false alarms. This is not evidence of undue concern or sensitivity.

Prematurity

Labor may sometimes start early, producing an infant not yet fully qualified for independent life. Infants weighing less than 2,500 grams (5.5 lbs.) at birth are considered premature, and have a substantially higher death rate during the first few weeks of life than better developed infants. Brain injury during birth (since the sheltering skull bones have not fully developed) and failure of immature breathing mechanisms to supply brain tissue with enough oxygen cause nervous system damage in some premature infants. However, even considerable prematurity leaves at least 70 per cent of the infants totally free of any mental or physical impairment. Most infants with brain damage have distinct and definite evidence such as paralysis of certain parts, so that you need feel little concern that a seemingly normal premature infant will have lingering aftereffects of his early birth. Moreover, a great deal of medical research is now being done on the hazards of prematurity. You can certainly expect some progress in this field during the next few years.

Preparation for Baby's Arrival

Probably the biggest single step you can take to assure yourself of getting to the hospital on time is to keep your household clean and well organized. Most women have plenty of time for a leisurely ride to the hospital after early twinges of labor put them on notice, but quite a few do not have time to make the house spic and span because Mother is coming to take care of the baby, iron their bed jacket, and write out menus for husbands who won't use them anyway. If you are worried about getting to the hospital on time, get your household organized and your labor will take care of itself.

What to Do When Labor Begins

Labor usually starts with cramplike pain centering in the low back and working gradually around to the lower abdomen. Pain sometimes spreads to the thighs and hips, too. Early cramps last ten to thirty seconds and usually occur about every twenty minutes. They gradually increase in frequency and duration, although this progression is never as regular as clockwork. In well-established labor, contractions usually last about one minute and occur about every five minutes. When the mouth of the uterus begins to open up, the blood-tinged mucus plug which normally occupies its opening comes loose and appears at the mouth of the vagina as so-called "bloody show." In some cases, the fluid-containing pocket of membranes ahead of the baby's head breaks, leading to the uncontrollable passage of a considerable volume of liquid, often accelerating during a contraction.

If contractions seem progressive, if any bloody show appears, or if the waters break (with or without pains), the time has probably come for medical attendance. Call your doctor as soon as any of these signs develop. A stack of old newspapers or diapers in the back seat of the car may save considerable mess. The expectant mother should ideally ride in the back seat where she will have room to lie down in case of bleeding or precipitous birth, although the emotional crisis involved is usually such that she stays in front where she can be close to her husband.

Any bleeding in the latter stages of pregnancy with or without pain calls for very prompt medical attention. If you cannot reach your doctor immediately, go to the hospital where you can get skilled aid until he can be located.

Managing Precipitous Birth

Back-seat deliveries happen more often in cartoons and movies than in real life. When delivery seems imminent, the prospective mother can usually hold back for five or ten minutes by panting rapidly during pains. This prevents the grunting-, bearing-down type of abdominal straining which extrudes the infant. If the mother lies down, the baby will not be harmed by a fall if he is born unaided. Rub the baby's back with your hand or with a piece of cloth if he does not breathe or cry soon. This works better than the traditional spanking. Otherwise, leave well enough alone and continue to the hospital. Delivery of the placenta, cutting the cord, and treatment of any tears will wait. Lasting harm to either mother or child almost never results.

Pain Relief *vs.* Natural Childbirth

Uterine contractions usually cause pain ranging from discomfort during early labor to considerable pain just prior to birth. Several measures give effective relief:

1. Sedative, amnesia-inducing or pain-relieving drugs can assuage the discomfort of labor as soon as it begins to become troublesome. Recent studies showing that the percentage of infants who do not breathe promptly after birth is much higher after the use of these drugs in high dosage has led to some moderation in their use, but some degree of relief can almost always be provided with complete safety.
2. Injections into the pain-carrying nerve pathways of anesthetic agents like Novocaine give complete relief at no risk to the infant, although the mother runs some slight risk of adverse reaction or aftereffects. In skilled hands, this risk is very slight compared to the emotional aftermaths of a completely unrelieved labor.
3. Natural childbirth. Some mothers take specific training in muscular relaxation throughout their months of pregnancy to reduce or eliminate discomfort so they can participate actively and consciously in the birth of their child. This training probably puts to work psychological forces very similar to those involved in hypnotism, long known to be sufficiently intense in certain subjects for complete pain relief even during surgical operations. While nobody claims that labor is not genuinely painful or that womankind exaggerates the severity of discomfort, a great many women achieve completely comfortable labor and delivery either with no medicinal agents or with reduced amounts of anesthesia by the natural childbirth technique.

Breast Feeding

Most mothers who want to do so can breast feed their babies.[2] Since modern pediatric science can supply the infant with perfectly sound nutrition by formula, breast feeding is completely optional. The main advantages are:

1. Breast feeding speeds the return of the uterus and female organs to normal (usually about six weeks after the baby arrives).
2. If Mother is calm and willing, breast feeding supplies ideal forging of emotional bonds between mother and child.
3. Antibodies conveyed through milk give some protection against certain diseases.
4. Breast feeding involves less work and less expense than formula fixing.

The main disadvantages are:

1. Although a bottle can be substituted occasionally to give Mother an outing, breast feeding is quite confining.
2. Some women are repelled by the whole idea, in which case the emotional framework for the forming mother-child relationship is adversely affected by Mother's unwilling participation.

Note that several old wives' tales regarding breast feeding are without foundation. Breast feeding does not have adverse effects upon the figure, need not lead to accumulation of extra weight, and will not keep you from getting pregnant (although it often suppresses menstruation for several months).

MEETING PARENTAL HEALTH RESPONSIBILITIES

Your main aim in rearing children is probably to help them reach their maximum potential in physical, mental, and social development, which virtually echoes the definition of good health. Think for a moment about the specific tasks parents perform in child-rearing: selecting and preparing food, providing a good home, training the child to accept discipline and author-

[2] Over-all, only about 40 per cent who try succeed. However, doctors who repeatedly reassure their patients that they will produce enough milk and who leave the baby on the breast without supplying too much other food for a week or so find that almost all mothers ultimately produce enough milk.

ity, showing him what love and fellowship mean—all fundamentally concerned with physical, social, or mental aspects of health. How can you prepare yourself for these responsibilities, plus the even heavier ones that fall on you during times of illness or injury? Aside from the basic health knowledge your personal health course should supply, several specific points deserve consideration:

Help and Guidance for New Parents

A new baby seems so fragile and precarious that most new parents have trouble taking care of him in a relaxed way. They usually act as if the least error or omission might do irreparable harm. Actually, babies are pretty tough and resilient little creatures. Most brand-new parents in the college-attending social stratum err on the side of overprotectiveness and unduly active wrestling with problems rather than neglect, and on the side of spontaneity-curbing overuse of guidance materials rather than ignorance or misinformation. Several simple steps might help you to avoid these errors:

1. *Choose one principal child care adviser.* Most parents need someone to lean upon during the insecurities of a new baby's early months as much as they need child care information. A family physician or pediatrician in whom you have complete confidence gives such support, especially if you treat him as a personal guide instead of the purveyor of certain facts and services. You can give your child's doctor his proper place in the child-rearing constellation by choosing him well in advance of the baby's birth, asking his recommendation as to baby care books and other literature beforehand, and consulting him freely by telephone or in person during the infant's early months. Many modern doctors make special arrangements for such services on a monthly rather than a per-call basis, imposing an additional charge only when care of illness makes extra burdens. Well Baby Clinics, operated by most state and municipal health departments, offer similar supervision either free or on an ability-to-pay basis.

2. *Learn something about child development.* Most parents find books about child development reassuring at times. When your youngster starts sleeping on the floor underneath his bed at eighteen months or so, it is nice to read in the books that perfectly normal children often do this for a few weeks. When Junior gets into a particularly disruptive phase, you will take comfort from reading that this phase will soon be succeeded by a more tranquil one (although you must sometimes be careful not to read what comes next after that). If you understand that many apparent problems pass away without being actively combated, you can accept your child more freely and spend more time enjoying him.

On the other hand, many parents devote altogether too much attention to criticizing the exact rate at which their children develop certain abilities and skills. Your child needs considerable calm, noncritical acceptance. You

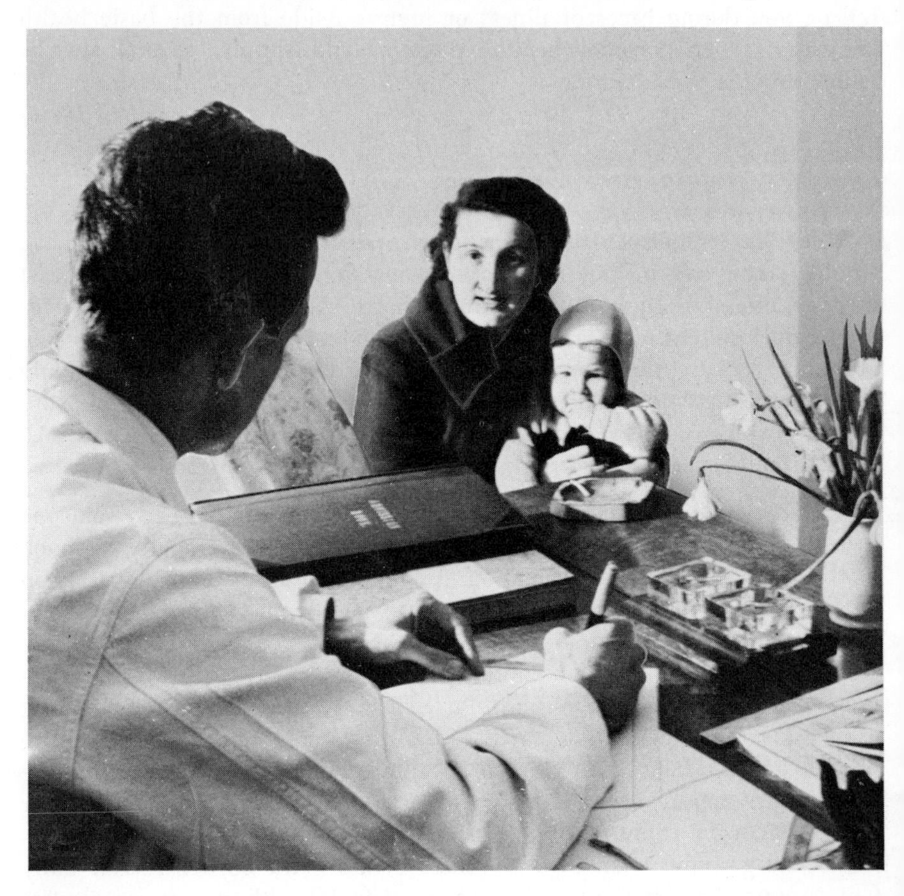

Figure 42. Mother, child, and doctor. They all should get to know one another. *Wide World Photos, Inc.*

unjustly punish him when you show concern over his failure to talk as soon as the book says or when you try to force toilet training simply because the neighbor's child was trained at your child's age. Leave it up to your medical adviser to appraise your child's development. As long as he says the child is making normal progress, don't worry about your child's apparent lags. Most children make progress somewhat unevenly: they may be far ahead in some things and far behind in others. You will do better to accept an expert's over-all appraisal than to consider each new accomplishment a race against a psychologist's chart.

3. *Treat child care literature as suggestions, not as gospel.* Child care books and articles can often offer valuable suggestions both for general care and for meeting specific problems. These suggestions sometimes fit in perfectly with your needs. However, the particular combination of temperaments and situations with which you find yourself faced as a parent is unique. Suggestions which are perfect for nine cases out of ten might be wrong for you. Moreover, in child-rearing many problems concern themselves primarily with emotional relationships or involve influence achieved largely through those relationships. If you do not feel that the solution offered is exactly right for you, it probably acts as a barrier instead of as an aid to parental influence. When burdensome problems arise in the course of child-rearing you should go to the books, to your physician, or to your relatives and friends for commiseration and ideas, but you should clearly reserve the final decision and entire responsibility for yourself.

Discipline

Comfortable acceptance of family discipline not only helps make later family life more pleasant, but also prepares your child for comfortable acceptance of the many restraints necessary to civilized life. Family discipline erects the models on which most people ultimately build their reaction to initially external pressures of many sorts—religious codes, legal restrictions, moral restraints, and social standards. Although your own temperament and situation do much to determine the details, certain general principles almost always apply.

1. *Discipline should be consistent.* If everyone who cares for a child follows approximately the same rules and metes out roughly the same type punishments and rewards at all times, the child's general security and comfortable acceptance of rules are promoted.

2. *Rules should be simple.* Most children have trouble keeping detailed or concept-involving regulations straight. Simplify rules, even at some price in extra stringency (e.g., "Stay inside this block, without crossing any curbs" even if one or two houses which would otherwise be in bounds are excluded). Put rules in terms of place instead of concept (e.g., "You can play with things in *this* drawer, but not in any other cupboard or drawer in the house" instead of "These things are yours"). Consolidate items to which a rule applies (e.g., by putting stored boxes in your basement together in one place, throwing a sheet over them and saying "Keep away from that").

3. *Displace rules with principles as soon as possible.* When you begin to know the reason for rules, you inevitably want to govern your behavior in a

way calculated to achieve desired ends instead of meekly obeying externally imposed regulation. At times your own application may be less perfect than that which would have been imposed on you—almost every child gets less sleep than he needs for a few years after his parents stop compelling him to go to bed at a certain hour, although he knows that he should get plenty of rest. However, your quest of self-determination is an inevitable part of the process of growing up and will not be denied. Any effort to compel obedience for very long after pressure to self-determination develops generally leads to rebellion with more extreme, even self-destructive disobedience. Nobody is wilder than the preacher's daughter gone astray.

In encouraging your own children toward comfortable acceptance of discipline, you need to learn the difficult art of letting go. When you start with a new baby, you cannot easily make discipline too rigid. The security of an imposed living pattern is good for most infants, and they usually accept it fairly well. However, you have to let your children grow up even when you know that they will make mistakes if left to set their own course. "Enough rest" instead of "eight o'clock bedtime," financial responsibility instead of parent-managed purchases, reasonable restrain in sex and social life instead of constant chaperonage—all these changes have to come before the child's internal pressures toward self-determination overthrow your rules, not because he is absolutely ready for self-determination but because he can no longer accept the total dependency of rigid parental control.

4. *Punish the act but support the person.* Your main lever in discipline is the other person's concern over your opinion of him, often intensified by his importance to you as a source of love. You mold his behavior best by keeping this lever sound. You can put discipline in constructive terms so far as his self-respect and recognition is concerned whether your point itself is positive or negative (e.g., "We'll all think more of you if you can manage table manners better" or "People think more of you if they can trust you not to reveal confidences"). You can reveal continued love for the person even as you discipline the act (e.g., "If we didn't care about you, we'd just let it pass, but you'll get along better in the future if——").

Atmosphere in Child-Rearing

Physical, social, and emotional atmosphere are important aspects of child-rearing to consider at college age, while you are molding your career, setting the stage for marriage, and revising your personal and familial relationships. Many parental responsibilities can be met much more easily through providing proper atmosphere than through direct and immediate action. For example, very few parents can ordain their child's choice of playmates or of games, but you govern your child's associations to some extent by your choice of neighborhood and school, and you encourage certain types of play by providing suitable grounds and equipment.

Children respond very keenly to an atmosphere of emotional calm or tension. Children sense emotion in a more direct and primitive manner than adults, without depending heavily on words and gestures. For example, I have often seen a frightened child in a medical office calm down abruptly after his distraught mother left the room. This direct sensitivity to emotional tension enters into handling marital differences. Many parents have allowed internecine strife to smolder for years because "we didn't want to fight things out in front of the children." Although an amiable means of settling differences is ideal, even an occasional pitched battle may be better than the constant domestic tension of unresolved conflict in its effect upon emotion-sensitive children. Such children are both disturbed and confused by the emotionally loaded atmosphere. They wonder whether their own behavior or presence on the scene might be at fault. They frequently feel insecure and unloved.

Most psychologists agree that the basic patterns of friendship and love which form the basis for most later intimate personal relationships develop around models either seen or experienced in early childhodod. The examples you give your child at home teach him the benefits and nature of love as well as the techniques of amiability. These are priceless gifts. Remember their worth when the pressure of time makes you choose between relaxed conviviality with your family and harried pursuit of further material advantages for them.

Instruction

Although discipline and atmosphere do more to teach your children how to get along in this world than actual instruction, several points seem worth considering. You make life easier for your child by supporting those authorities whom he must recognize: many a parent disparages the schools, individual teachers, the police, and others whom the child must obey, then wonders why the child shows too little respect for them. Every child needs some basic information on sex, reproduction, and other matters on which the school gives inadequate or too-slow instruction. Even if your own knowledge in these fields is imperfect, your child is better off getting them from you than from the gutter (which usually supplies all the basic facts before age twelve). Perhaps most important of all, a parent needs to maintain a permissive atmosphere in which the child feels free to ask questions about anything which is perplexing him, with certainty that he will not be punished or made the butt of later jokes for having done so and that his inquiry will be taken seriously.

In Case of Illness

When something goes wrong with one of your children, you will probably get professional guidance in helping restore his health. However, you can still play an important part in speeding his recovery. Two roles you will play might affect your present activities or plans.

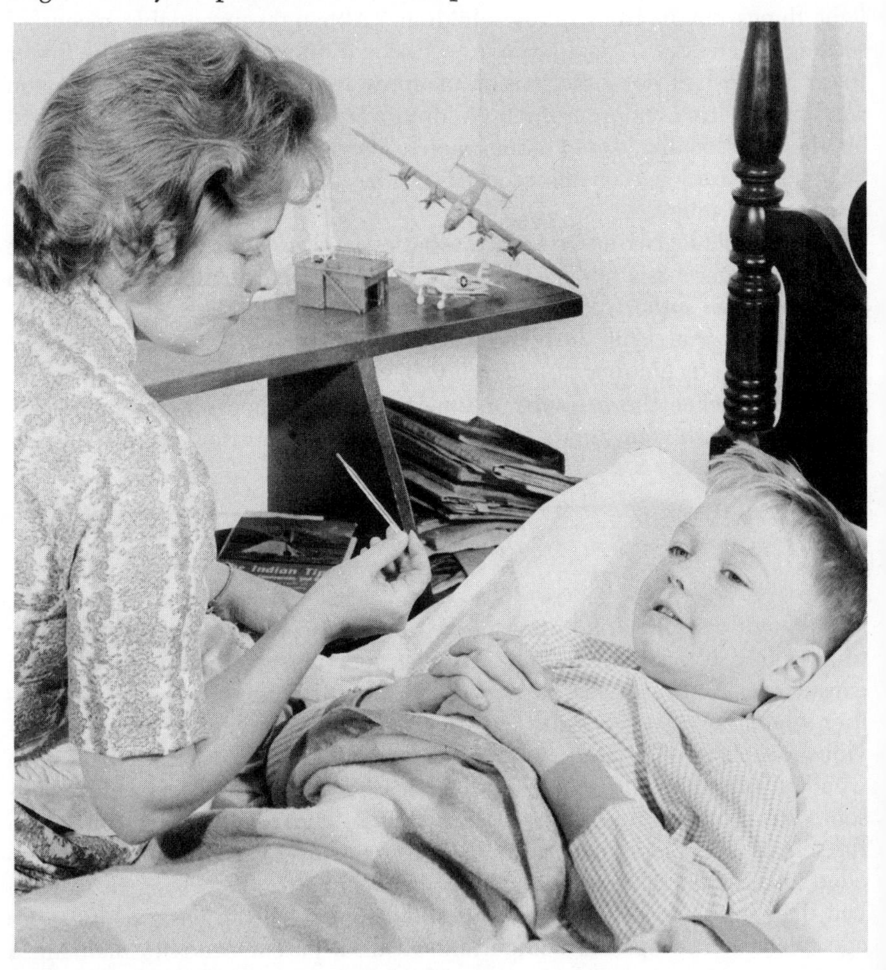

Figure 43. Johnny feels better because Mother is there. *Ewing Galloway.*

1. *Skill in home care of illness helps a lot in rearing a family.* A course or some readings in the field of home nursing can prove very helpful if you can find time in your college program for it. Children's Bureau pamphlets such as "Your Child from One to Six" and "Your Child from Six to Twelve" include valuable information on common diseases. You can obtain them from the Department of Health, Education and Welfare, Washington 25, D. C. at nominal cost, and quite possibly from your state department of health for nothing.

2. *Your children will need your personal support frequently in case of illness, accident, or upheaval.* In this age of the working mother, many women build their career plans around the idea that a child becomes relatively independent at school age. While this assumption may sometimes hold true so long as everything goes well, its validity ceases abruptly with any illness, injury, or upheaval. Children (and even adults) often need to resume a degree of dependency in times of stress. While it is hard to feel useful when you are merely keeping yourself available, the fact that a parent is always ready and willing to give aid sustains any child. Emergency guidance and support is of critical importance on a few occasions in almost every child's life. You should not neglect it in weighing the advantages and disadvantages of the various types of work mothers can do.

CHAPTER 12

Your Complexion, Skin, and Nails

COLLEGE MEN AND WOMEN CAN USUALLY CONTROL SUCH COMMON DIFFICULTIES as comedones, pimples, minor blemishes, and dandruff through properly chosen grooming techniques. Maintaining a smooth, attractive skin and relatively flake-free hair may sometimes require medical aid, but more commonly calls only for simple hygienic measures.

OIL GLAND PROBLEMS

Your skin remains resilient partly because it constantly bathes itself in oil. Glands within the skin continually pour out a thick lubricating material. However, these sebaceous glands frequently become plugged, especially during your young adult years. The resulting disorders frequently annoy or disfigure college students.

Comedones

Comedones or blackheads form when sebaceous glands plug up sufficiently that dried skin oil piles up within the gland openings and becomes discolored. Soap and water cannot dissolve this material from its protected pit. Hot cloths stimulate the skin glands to further oil production and therefore should not be used to soften the comedo. The only way to get rid of a comedo is usually through pressure, but the common technique of pinching the skin between two fingers affords many opportunities for germs to invade the affected skin glands and often bruises or damages the skin. When you plan to empty a comedo, wash your hands thoroughly and cleanse the affected area with soap and water or rubbing alcohol to reduce the likeli-

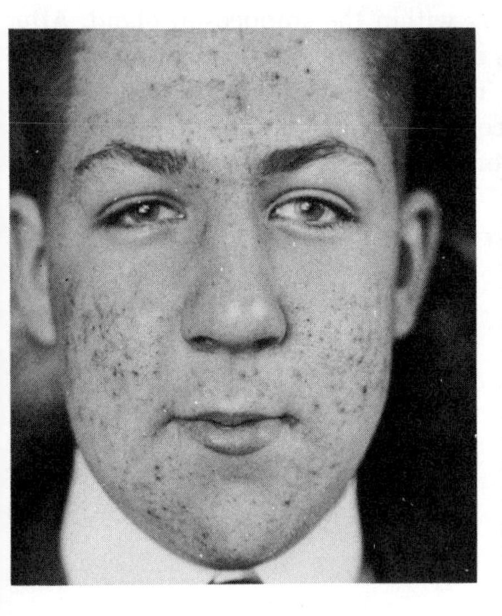

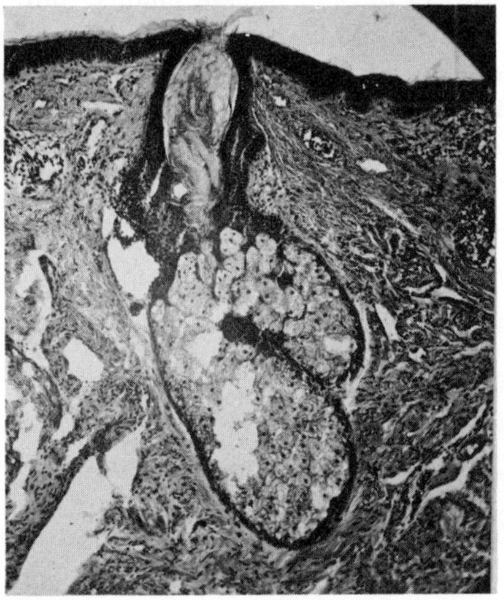

A B

Figure 44. (A) Blackheads and their appearance. (B) Blackhead-plugged pore. Opening from pouch-like gland to skin surface (top of photo) is twice as wide as normal. In this photo the originally blackish core within shows up light-colored and strandish.

hood of infection. A needle whose point has been passed through the flame of a match and a blackhead squeezer which has soaked in rubbing alcohol make suitable germ-free aids. You usually can empty out a small comedo by centering the hole in one end of the blackhead squeezer over it and pressing straight down into the skin. If this fails, it is perfectly safe to gently lift off the surface film from the blackhead with a flamed needle and try again. Do not slide the squeezer along the skin, since this is almost as rough on skin glands as pinching. If direct pressure fails, wait a few days for further ripening.

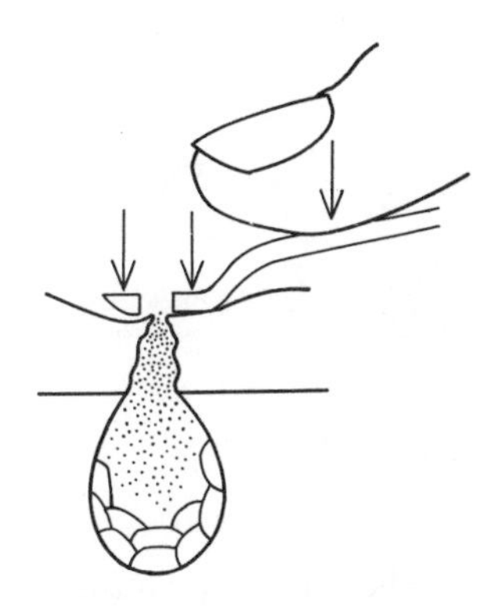

Figure 45. Use of blackhead squeezer.

Pimples

Pimples also start as plugged sebaceous glands. The plugging occurs when piled-up surface skin cells crowd into the gland opening. Germs, which are always present in skin glands, multiply within the stopped-up gland. After a slow build-up period of three weeks or so, they reach sufficient numbers to stir your bodily defense mechanisms. Tiny blood vessels in the vicinity flare open. Germ-devouring white blood cells pour into the affected gland, and puff it out with a whitish accumulation of pus.

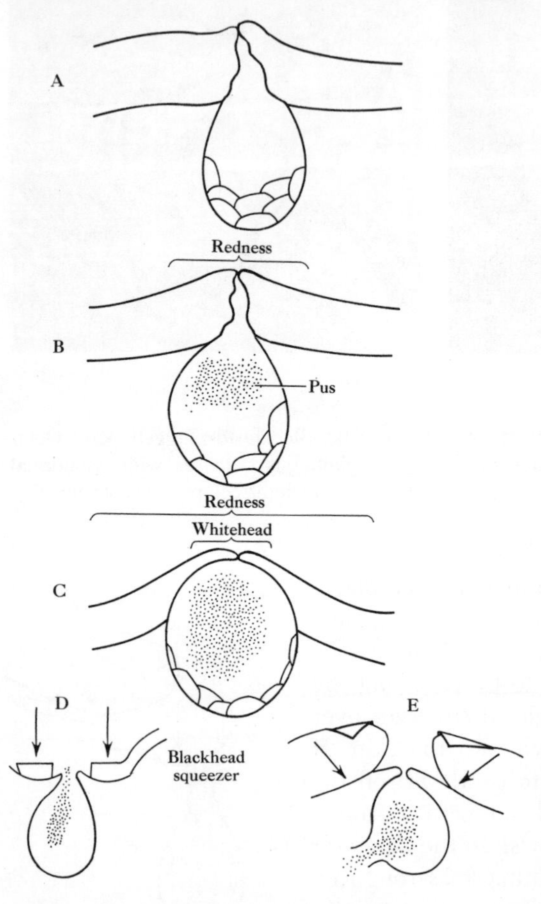

Figure 46. Formation and relief of pimple. Gland opening plugs (A), ever-present germs cause accumulation of pus (B), which stretches skin into whitehead (C). Pus best released through skin surface or with blackhead squeezer (D). Pinching between fingers may make pimple burst inward (E) and lead to deeper sore.

The chemical consistency of skin cells and the nature of skin oil determine your liability to pimple formation. Your diet has a great deal to do with both of these factors. Fried foods, including sandwiches with fried meat centers and fried-at-the-factory items like potato chips and doughnuts, increase pimple formation. If you have any tendency to form pimples, you will probably do better if you limit yourself to one serving or less of such foods each day. Chocolate is a great offender, and excess sweets of any kind do some harm. On the other hand, daily scrubbing with soap and a washrag helps to wash away excess oils and pore-clogging skin-cell accumulations, often making pimples less frequent.

Even occasional pimples sometimes lead to disfiguring scars and pits unless they are opened in the gentlest possible manner. A pimple is ready to open when a whitish center forms, representing pus beneath a film of dead surface skin cells. This pus can be emptied out in the same way as a blackhead. Attempts to squeeze pimples between the fingertips or to open them before a whitehead forms occasionally make the pus sac break inward with later formation of a much larger, scar-promoting sore.

Frequent or deep-seated pimples deserve a doctor's care, both for their own sake and to minimize permanently disfiguring scars or pits. This disorder is called acne, and can almost always be brought under control by proper and persistent medical treatment. In most cases, doctors can also help such aftereffects of acne as unsightly scarring, pitting, or thickening of the skin. Young men or ladies who are self-conscious about such states can often get much more help than they realize, and at much less cost than they anticipate.

Sebaceous cysts

A plugged sebaceous gland often continues to make skin oil even though here is no opening through which that oil can escape. The gland blows up like a balloon, usually to a size between that of a pea and a walnut. Such a sebaceous cyst may occur at any age, and in people who are not subject to comedones or acne. Sebaceous cysts occur most commonly on the scalp or trunk, but can develop in other areas as well. If you get a sebaceous cyst on

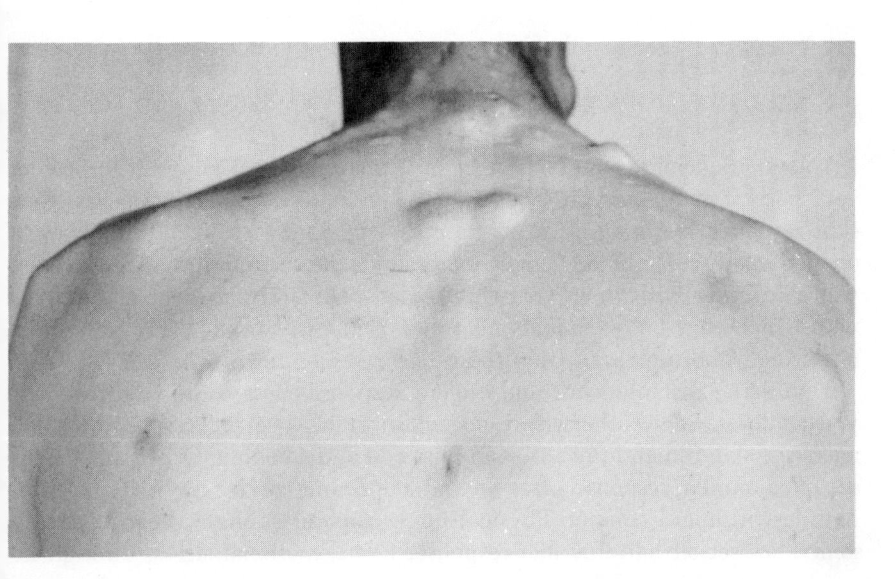

Figure 47. Sebaceous cysts. *Photograph Department, Minneapolis General Hospital.*

your scalp where it is often irritated by your comb, on your face, or in a location subject to clothing pressure, your doctor can remove it without hospitalization or disability.

DANDRUFF

In the scalp, natural skin oils or oily hairdressings often make the dead cell shells which continually flake off from your skin stick together in visible sheets or globs. The protecting stand of hair in the vicinity holds these flakes and lets them conglomerate still farther. The result is dandruff.

Frequent shampooing controls most mild cases of dandruff. Saponified coconut oil is a nonirritating and inexpensive form of liquid soap which makes an excellent shampoo. Pure soap shampoos seem to be especially effective as compared to detergent shampoos among the commercial preparations. Soft water for both shampoo and rinse is very important to preserve hair luster and prevent after-shampoo itch.

If you have troublesome amounts of dandruff, several further preventive or hygienic measures besides shampooing usually help. Thorough brushing and scalp massage help knock surface cell shells loose before they conglomerate into dandruff flakes. More sparing use of hair dressings and substituting light, nongreasy preparations may prove beneficial. Or you can ask your doctor to prescribe a scalp lotion for you: he can save you a lot of expensive experimentation with drugstore and barbershop preparations.

SKIN IRRITATIONS

Your skin's keen responsiveness to any apparent threat allows it to protect your body from many types of assault. When injury or infection occurs, your skin responds by bringing extra nourishment to the scene through newly opened microscopic blood vessels. Body fluids filter through the blood vessel walls, carrying with them the white blood cells and chemical neutralizers with which your body combats microbes. Redness, swelling, and sometimes blistering or oozing result from these responses.

Your skin's instantaneous and violent responsiveness causes difficulty for you at times. Some otherwise innocent substances set off responses which make the skin red and raw, or even blistered and weeping. Other substances set off a similar response after an initial priming period even if they are harmless in initial contact. Physical forces such as sunlight, heat, and cold sometimes set off harmful skin response. Even emotional stress, through its effect on the nerves which control skin functions, may cause blemishes or distress. Inept skin responses thus cause many common disorders, from poison ivy and cosmetic eruptions to sunburn and stress-related facial blemishes. Your skin's reactivity influences many everyday decisions, from choice of bath and beauty products to protective measures used on the beach.

Fundamentally Harsh Substances

If you come into contact with sufficient amounts of certain common substances, your skin will respond in a way which generates distress even if you have never encountered the offending substance before. Everyone gets skin eruption from sufficiently concentrated poison ivy oil, for instance. Repeated contact may add further sensitivity to this basic response, but it is not strictly necessary. Likewise with certain soaps and solvents, and with many substances used in industry.

Poison ivy, oak, and sumac

Although the plants take different form in different parts of the country,[1] oil from the leaves or roots of any variety of poison ivy, oak, or sumac causes redness, swelling, and in some cases blistering when it comes into contact with the skin. Nobody is immune to this effect, though some people do not react to the amounts of oil ordinarily encountered from brushing against ivy leaves.

The first time you get a poison ivy eruption, the itching, redness, and blisters appear seven to ten days after contact. Thereafter, the response usually takes twelve to twenty-four hours, and often become progressively worse. Further significant facts:

1. Poison ivy eruptions often spread beyond the area of actual contact with the plants, but fluid from the blisters has nothing to do with this spread. Less intense contact with the plant oil at the time of original exposure or bodily reaction in neighboring areas not directly involved cause the apparent spread of poison ivy eruptions.
2. Highly sensitive people do not necessarily have to touch a poison ivy plant to get an eruption. They can get into trouble with minute quantities of indirectly transported plant oil. One of my patients, for instance, used to get

[1] At least some of these variations are purely the result of soil and climate. One dermatologist collected plants of supposedly different species from all over the country, only to find that they all looked the same when he grew them in his own back yard.

an eruption of her hands and arms whenever her youngsters played out in the woods. They rolled in the ivy, she handled their clothing, and the oil she got on her hands from her children's trousers was enough to kick off a rash. Even the smoke from burning ivy plants affects some ivy victims.

3. Washing with yellow soap upon your return from the woods is time honored, but completely futile. The irritating ivy oil does its damage inside five minutes. Washing does no good after this brief interval.

Preventing ivy eruption

You can usually avoid poison ivy eruptions. These simple precautions are highly effective:

1. Learn to recognize the local brand of poison ivy, oak, or sumac.
2. Use protective clothing, and remember that ivy oil may coat its surface on your return from the woods. Gloves are a big help when handling brush, but you should launder them frequently and use rags or leaves when you take them off to keep from getting any adherent oil on your fingers.
3. Ask your doctor to recommend protective tablets, lotions, or creams if you are highly subject to poison ivy and are going into the woods.

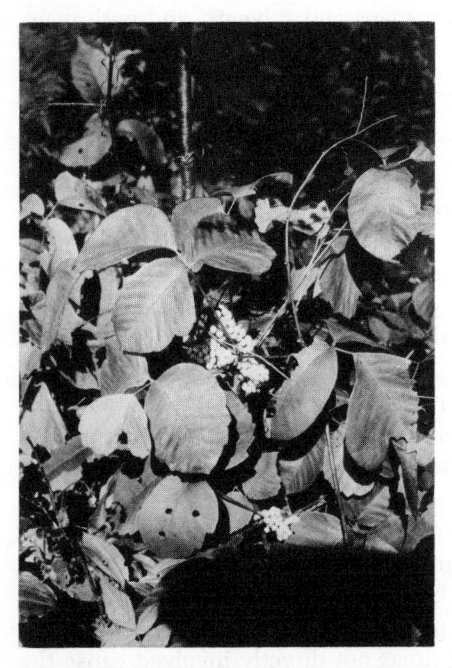

Figure 48. A midwestern poison ivy plant. *From* Diseases of the Skin, *Ormsby and Montgomery, 8th edition, 1954. Philadelphia. Lea and Febiger.*

Soap and detergent eruptions

Many of the soaps and detergents you might use for your hands, face, or clothing can set off a skin rash. Dishwashing and other household soaps or detergents are particularly likely to be harsh, often causing dry, sandpaper-like skin and sometimes causing severe eruptions or painful splits at the knuckles or folds. Toilet soap may cause eruption of the hands or face through allergy to its perfume content as well as through the chemical harshness of soap itself. The tiny amounts of washday detergent which cling to your clothing can also cause tiny, dry, harsh granules over the backs of the shoulders, arms and chest. Affected spots are usually redder than the surrounding skin, but often not strikingly so. Most patients do not complain of itching or burning, although after the condition has healed they realize in retrospect that it did impair skin comfort. This rash, which is very common among college students, usually becomes more pronounced when warm weather gives a bridge of perspiration to float the detergent across to the skin surface.

Preventing soap and detergent rash

Household rubber gloves to keep hands soft are cheaper in the long run than lotions and creams to repair soap and detergent damage. If you find gloves clumsy, your doctor can recommend potent protective lotions or creams. If soap makes for minor blemishes and skin discomfort of the face or hands, a switch to unscented, pure white soap usually helps. In some cases, less irritating medicinal skin cleansing detergents are worthwhile. Mild detergent-caused eruption of the shoulders and back usually disappears when clothing is washed with mild soap flakes or powder and rinsed three times in soft water. Any eruption of consequence or any rash which persists in spite of lessened exposure to harsh soaps and detergents deserves a doctor's care. Often such rashes prove to have some other underlying cause, and are merely aggravated rather than initiated by cleansing agents.

Sensitizing Substances

Many substances which will not cause skin irritation on first exposure can still bestir violent reaction in a few people after repeated contact. Sometimes sensitization occurs over long periods: I once treated a man for a skin rash which he developed after over twenty years in the baking trade, but which still proved to be due to hard wheat flour. Sometimes sensitization takes only a few days or weeks. Once present, however, sensitivity to a given substance tends to continue or to become worse rather than to improve. The rash clears if you avoid further exposure to the offending substance, but further contact even after an interval of many years usually causes further eruption.

Cosmetic eruptions

Among the thousands of substances and ingredients people use as grooming aids, many can cause skin eruptions. Lipstick, hand cream, powder or pancake makeup, eyebrow pencil, hair tamer, nail polish, perfume, deodorants, antiperspirants, depilatories, scalp lotion or pomade, and after-shave lotion all can act as skin sensitizers.

If a grooming aid causes prompt eruption at the site of application, you usually figure out for yourself what causes the rash and switch to a different preparation. However, cosmetic rashes often have one or more of three characteristics which you may find confusing unless you are forewarned:

1. A cosmetic rash may appear abruptly after you have used the offending preparation for months or years without difficulty. Sometimes, this is due to a change in chemical composition of the product: the "new improved formula" or "exciting new shade" may not be for you. In other cases, your body gradually acquires sensitivity by prolonged or frequent contact with the offending substance, but the rash appears only after sensitivity reaches a critical point. To cite one case: a young lady complained of itching and redness behind the earlobes which began abruptly a few weeks before she sought aid. The eruption was caused by perfume which she dabbed behind her ears. She had only one bottle of perfume to her name, though, and had used it for eight months without previous difficulty.

2. A cosmetic rash frequently does not flare until twelve to 24 hours after the offending preparation is used, and sometimes appears gradually over a period of weeks.

3. A cosmetic rash may involve areas of the body other than those to which the offending preparation has been applied. Fingernail polish often causes eruption of the eyelids. Shampoo often causes rash behind the ears instead of on the scalp.

Ways toward clear, unirritated skin

You can probably use a broad array of grooming aids without injuring or irritating your skin. These two approaches will help you to use cosmetics and grooming aids without suffering harmful effects:

1. Find one or two manufacturers whose products agree with your skin, and stick to them. The more different chemicals you bring into contact with your skin, the more chance you have of developing sensitivity to one of them. All shades of lipstick of a certain brand are usually made with the same base and the same perfume, while different brands have different bases and different perfumes. Your skin is therefore exposed to many less chemical sensitizers if you stick to a few basic brands.

Good-quality cosmetics are often less sensitizing than bargain brands, since the manufacturers can afford costly substitutes for allergy-producing ingredients. Products labeled as "hypoallergic" are not required by law to meet any exacting standard, and may or may not be less sensitizing to your skin than others. Several manufacturers specialize in preparation of individually compounded nonallergic cosmetics: if you have difficulty finding a standard brand which leaves your skin clear and unblemished, you may find their services worthwhile.

2. *Replace harsh chemical depilatories, antiperspirants, and deodorants with milder methods.* While any method of removing unwanted hair involves some element of risk, the danger of nicks and infections from shaving is less than the danger of skin sensitivity from depilatories. You can shave off unwanted hair without making future growth heavier or darker. In one experiment, college girls shaved one leg frequently for a year, then let the hair grow. It was indistinguishable from the growth on the other leg. Lathering with plain soap and careful use of a clean, sharp safety razor is effective and safe. Armpits can also be shaved with relative safety. A little rubbing alcohol or an aftershave shower helps control any shave-accentuated tendency toward boils.

You can control unwanted perspiration or its aftereffects in several safe ways. A number of my patients have feet which perspire until the skin is waterlogged to a dead-white hue, sore as blistering hide (and often mistakenly treated as athlete's foot with home measures). Milder degrees of overactive perspiration cause itching and burning without visible change. Usually these problems yield to thorough drying, dusting with talc or prickly heat powder, and a clean pair of white cotton socks under the regular pair every day. After the skin has healed, rubbing alcohol applications help to keep it dry. Leather soled or ventilated shoes also help, since rubber soles trap the sweat.

Medically prescribed antiperspirant tablets can control perspiration for four to six hours. They help heal sweat-damaged feet and are very useful to people who perspire excessively under the nervous strain of public speaking or performance. Commercial antiperspirants cause skin sensitivity quite commonly with protracted use. Except on rare occasions when protection against moist but clean armpits are worth the risk of later raw and itching ones, you will probably find the control of normal amounts of bodily perspiration unnecessary. A thorough bath gives positive odor protection for four to six hours of any ordinary social activity, anyway.

PHYSICAL FORCES

The physical forces which frequently affect your skin include sunlight, pressure, heat, and cold. Many other forces, such as x-rays, radioactive emanations, radio waves, and sound waves have effects on the skin in intense concentration, but not at the levels you ordinarily encounter.

Sunburn

Ultraviolet light, not heat, is the ray which causes sunburn. This ray is present not only in direct sunlight, but also in skyshine and in the diffuse glow of an overcast day. Radiation is very intense on summer days between 10:00 A.M. and 2:00 P.M. Moisture in the earth's atmosphere filters out most ultraviolet light at seasons and at times of the day when sunlight strikes at a considerable angle.

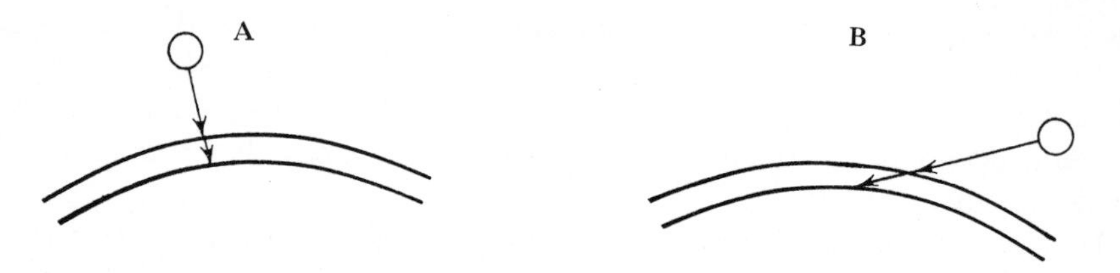

Figure 49. The summer sun at noontime must penetrate only a thin layer of atmosphere (A) compared with the early morning, late afternoon, or wintertime sun (B).

The skin's reaction to ultraviolet light comes on slowly over a period of six to twelve hours. Any immediate redness you notice during sun exposure is due to the heat rays rather than the ultraviolet. This heat response is not necessarily proportionate to impending ultraviolet response, so the presence or absence of pinkness is a poor index of sun exposure (especially on overcast days when heat rays drop off much more sharply than ultraviolet).

How your skin builds sun resistance

The same ultraviolet rays which cause sunburn stir protective responses against further sun exposure. Probably the most important of these responses is a thickening of your skin's outer coat of dead skin shells. Average depth of your skin's outer layer goes from eleven to thirteen or fifteen cell layers after frequent sun exposure. These extra layers of dead skin shells filter out a great deal of ultraviolet light before it ever reaches the living cells. Tanning, which results from an increase in brownish pigment in cells within the living skin-building cell layer, affords a further barrier to penetrating rays.

From the standpoint of physical health, a suntan is of dubious value. Sunlight spurs production of vitamin D within the skin, but your need for vitamin D falls off sharply as growth ceases. The amount of butter or oleomargarine you eat almost certainly fulfils your vitamin D requirement. No other substantial tonic effects stem from sun rays. However, young adults always have spent and probably always will spend lots of time in the sun, so knowledge of sun exposure hazards and how to avoid them is definitely worthwhile.

Gradual sun exposure

Gradual sun exposure permits you to acquire a protective tan without sunburn. Start with exposure to skyshine in a spot shaded from the direct sun. Expose each body surface for two minutes during the midday period, or somewhat longer when the sun's rays are oblique. Check with a mirror for redness six and twelve hours later. If no reaction occurs, increase exposure by two minutes the next day, and continue stepwise increases until you reach fifteen minutes of indirect sun. If you still get no redness or discomfort, switch to direct sunlight for two minutes, and follow the same routine. Add two minute exposure to each surface whenever no reaction has occurred. If slight redness follows a given sun exposure, keep your sunning period unchanged the next day. If burn or discomfort occurs, cut back your sun time.

Suntan oils and lotions

The main use of suntan oils and lotions is in increasing the period of sun exposure required to produce a burn. Most preparations filter out about 6/7 of the ultraviolet light reaching your skin, so that you can stay in the sun seven times as long with lotion as without it. These preparations will not allow a person whose normal skin response to sun is thickening rather than tanning to get a browner skin, though.

Lifeguards and other people who have intense sun exposure need extra protection against sunburn on body prominences like the nose, shoulder blade ridges, and ears. Yellow petroleum jelly is much more efficient for this purpose than ordinary suntan oil, since a very thin layer blocks off about 19/20 of the ultraviolet light impinging on its surface.

Skin Responses to Pressure and Abuse

Your skin responds to repeated pressure by soreness, blister formation, or thickening into callus. Sometimes callus forms in the shape of an inverted pyramid, so that pressure on its surface drives it against the tender skin nerves like a wedge: then it becomes a corn.

Proper shoe-fitting

If your shoes do not press upon your skin or crease it, you will never get blisters, calluses, or corns. Repeated pressure, not rubbing, is the main problem.

Many shoes which feel comfortable in the shoe shop do not really fit perfectly in daily use. Nor can you depend entirely on the shoe salesman, whose business is to sell shoes, to preserve your foot health. These three steps will lead to proper fitting of any oxford or low-heeled shoe:

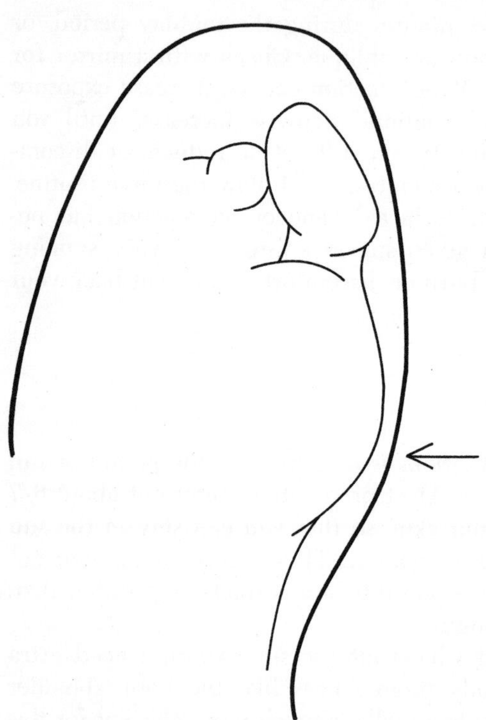

Figure 50. Foot in proper length shoe.

1. Choose shoe length by the location of the ball of your foot, not the tips of your toes. The ball of your foot should fall precisely at the sharp inward curve in front of the shoe arch. One foot is often larger than the other. If so, shoes should fit the larger, not the smaller foot. Some feet have sufficiently elastic arches that they lengthen half a size or more under the burden of body weight. It is wise to check shoe size with your weight on the foot before making a final decision.

2. Check width across the front of the foot from ball to little toe. The shoe should neither bulge out beyond the edge of the sole nor be too loose so that slack folds appear when it is pressed from the sides. Most feet spread one unit or more of width under the burden of body weight, so check while standing up.

3. Check heel width and retention. If the heel is too broad or if you can push the heel end of the shoe up and down more than an eighth of an inch with gentle pressure, a snugger heel fit is necessary. Your shoe salesman can correct for slight looseness of the heel with a felt butterfly. Greater looseness calls for a shoemaker's services either in taking up the heel or in fitting molded heel counters.

Special preventive measures

Calluses and corns form very commonly over the first joint of the little toe and on the sole of the foot behind the base of the second toe. At these points, the underlying bone ends press the skin against the confining leather and spurs formation of callus or corn. Properly fitted shoes may relieve this pressure by spreading the weight more evenly across the front of the foot. If proper shoes alone do not do the trick, check with your doctor for further suggestions.

High heels, flattie shoes, and foot troubles

Despite the fact that some mainly male occupations strongly predispose toward flat feet, men have five times as much chance of escaping foot troubles as women. By age forty, only one out of ten college women will have trouble-free feet, while half the men will still happily qualify.

Most foot experts blame the difference on female fashions in footwear. A high heel shifts the bulk of the body weight from the strong, well-padded heel to the more delicate front part of the foot. To be exact, a low heel leaves 70 per cent of your weight on your heel when you are standing and through most of your walking stride. A $2\frac{1}{2}$ inch heel puts 70 per cent on the front part of your foot instead. It is not remarkable that this $133\frac{1}{3}$ per cent overload leads to a heritage of miserable bunions, corns, and calluses. At the opposite extreme, most flat shoes are so flimsy that they give little protection or support to the feet. Arch strains frequently result.

Perhaps fashion should dictate footwear on special social occasions. But shouldn't foot comfort and lifelong freedom from foot miseries take control during the pavement pounding of everyday life?

How to avoid blisters

Blisters are the result of unaccustomed, repeated pressure on small skin areas. Friction is not responsible.

You can prevent most blisters by spreading point pressure. Work gloves operate in this way. Heavy socks during athletic or other foot-pounding events are worthwhile. Many ardent golfers and hikers fit their walking shoes while wearing two pairs of heavy socks.

How to trim your toenails

You can trim your toenails best just after a soaking bath or warm foot soak. Cut straight across, leaving at least 1/8 inch of white nail beyond the quick. This keeps the nail corners from becoming imbedded in the adjoining flesh, and prevents painful and disabling ingrown nails.

HEAT, COLD, AND YOUR SKIN

Your skin helps you to adjust to heat and cold through perspiration and shifting patterns of circulation which either bring more blood close to the surface or shunt it through deeper tissues. In the process, it protects itself from injury through a wide range of temperatures. Aside from burns and frostbite, which will be considered in another chapter, skin disorders due to heat and cold mainly consist of prickly heat and chapping.

Prickly Heat

The mechanisms by which you control your skin circulation develop slowly throughout childhood. Infants and children frequently respond to excessive warmth with almost microscopic spots of extreme flushing instead of with more intensive and diffuse increase in near-the-surface circulation. The resulting rash looks like red pepper scattered on moist skin and creates considerable itching and burning. In infants, cornstarch or talcum powder seems to help prevent prickly heat in moderately warm weather. Somewhat stronger preparations, which your doctor can recommend, work well in more intensive heat. Children of school age often get prickly heat when overdressed for the warmth of their environment, as when they wear the sweater Mother gave them for outdoor warmth into an overheated classroom. Suiting clothes to the temperature usually solves this problem (unless an overcautious teacher has sent the youngster home as a possible measles victim in the meantime).

Chapping

Chapping stems from loss of moisture in the skin. It occurs mainly in body or facial areas where the normal, moisture-retaining oil coating of the skin has been repeatedly removed by washing, licking, or the like. Cold exposure plays some part, and the dryness of heated air in wintertime is also a factor. In most cases, anointment with any pleasant substitute for skin oil relieves chapping. Humidifying the heated air to cut loss of skin moisture may also help. Extensive involvement of the body may force you to decrease the frequency of your baths.

EMOTIONAL STRESS AND YOUR SKIN

Many college students get temporary skin blemishes when under emotional pressure. These blemishes look something like pimples, but each spot comes and goes much more quickly (often in a day or less) and does not come to a head. Spots frequently itch or burn, especially while in the process of developing.

A few people get severe skin rash, often of the face, hands, feet or genitals, whenever under emotional pressure.

These skin changes come about through imbalance in the sympathetic nervous system. The sympathetic nervous system controls most of your body's automatic processes, including physical elements of emotion, adjustment to heat and cold, and changes in circulation to meet varying work loads. Its control of the skin's blood vessels permits the flush of excitement, the pallor of fear, and various stress-induced rashes.

Some victims find that their "nerve bumps" disappear with a little extra rest or a slight change in schedule or situation. A few people find such rash almost valuable as a red flag which signals the need for some rearrangement in their living pattern to avoid more serious consequences. However, the rash may prove sufficiently aggravating to justify medical measures. If so, a doctor can give considerable aid.

CHAPTER 13

Better Teeth

ONE OF MY PATIENTS HAD A SIMPLE PHILOSOPHY REGARDING TEETH: LET THEM alone until they need to be pulled, then get them out and use dentures. His dental bills were remarkably low, but his smile was a snaggletoothed horror for ten years before he was toothless enough for plates. Toothaches made him miserable for many weeks during his tooth-shedding years. The indigestion he suffered because of inadequately chewed food cost him more than better dental care would have cost. And he still wound up with artificial teeth, which work about as well as artificial legs—they do the job, but nobody claims they are as good as the originals.

A less extreme program of neglect makes even less sense. Unless you plan to let your teeth go to pot, every breach in your tooth care program costs you considerable extra money and misery. An ideal program of preventive dental care involves a few minutes a day at home, perhaps an hour twice each year in the dentist's or hygienist's chair, and only moderate dental expense. A less intensive program involves money and time for fixing more and larger cavities, fitting bridges or partial dentures and treating infection of gums and tooth sockets. These more than make up for the time and money saved by skipping preventive care. A halfway program costs more and involves more discomfort than either whole-hog prevention or whole-hog neglect. Generally speaking, the very best in dentistry costs less in time, misery, and money than any available alternative.

THE IDEAL DENTAL PROGRAM

You can prevent between two-fifths and three-fifths[1] of all cavities by using fluorides to toughen your dental enamel and by controlling the growth of mouth bacteria. Prompt dental care will clear up cavities rapidly, comfortably, and inexpensively.

[1] The higher figure only if fluoridated water is available from birth.

Cavities are the result of a definite chain of events. Mouth bacteria multiply rapidly whenever food particles or substances are available to nourish them. As they multiply, these bacteria lead to the formation of acid. The acid eats through your tooth enamel. Once the hard tooth enamel has been pierced, acids eat even more rapidly into the softer underlying tooth structure, forming cavities.

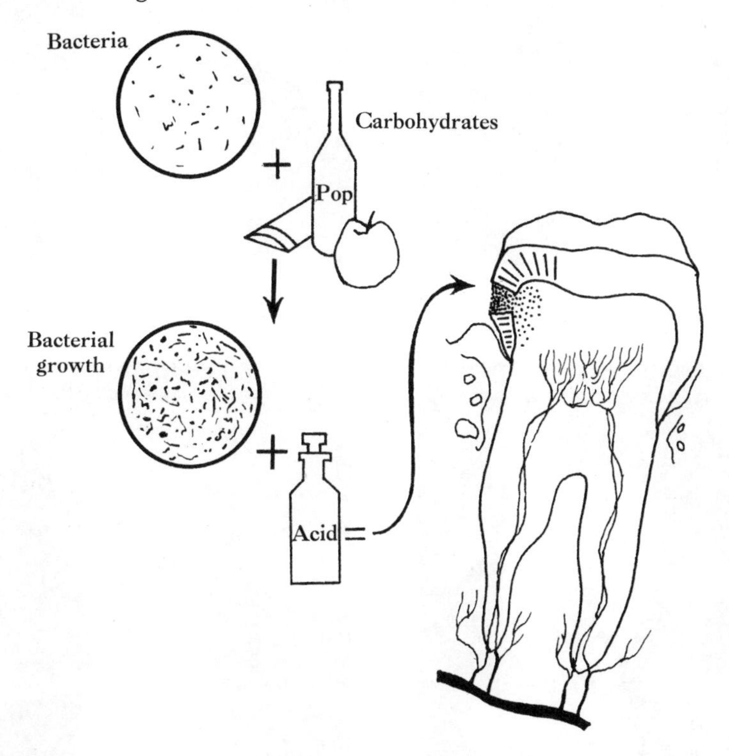

Figure 51. The chain of events which causes cavities. *Adapted from* Dental Health for Teachers, *Minnesota Department of Health.*

The chain of events which leads to cavity formation and growth is subject to attack at several points.

Diet and Cleanliness

Mouth bacteria feed mainly on food particles or sugar solutions in the mouth. You can keep down their multiplication by depriving them of these nourishments. Two main steps keep bacterial multiplication to a minimum and reduce cavities by about one-third:

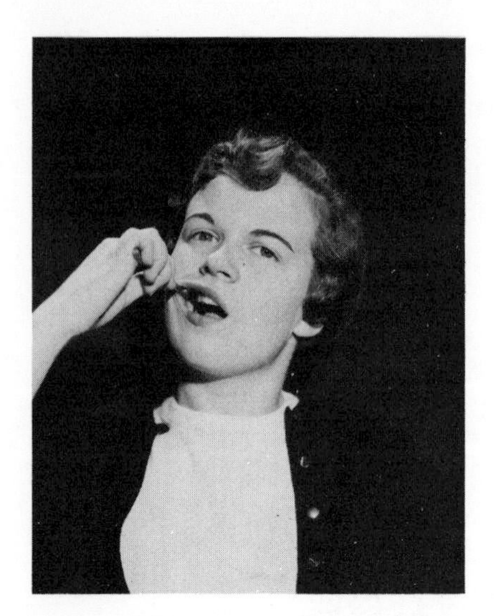

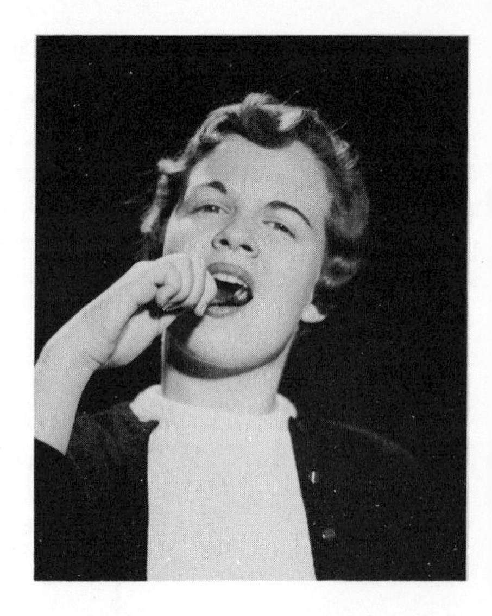

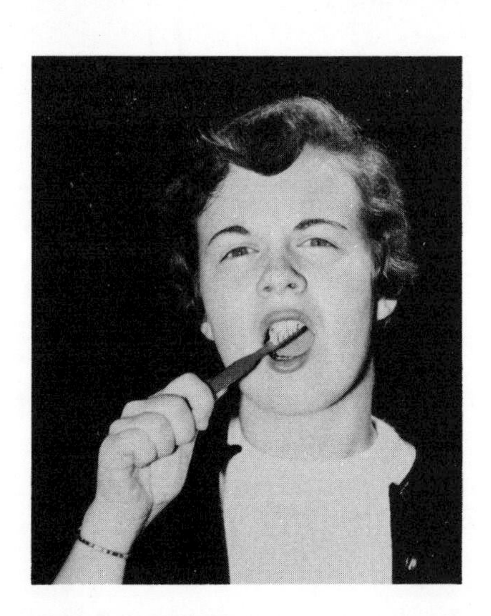

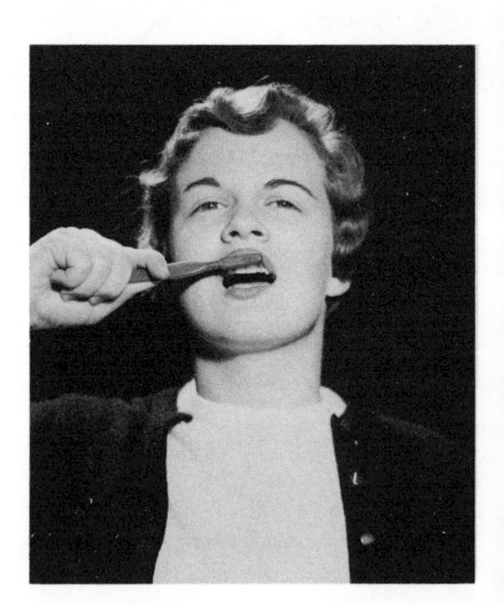

Figure 52. One effective toothbrushing technique. *Courtesy American Dental Association. From* Toothbrushing, *copyright 1957 by the American Dental Association.*

A) Clean the outside surfaces of the upper back teeth by firmly rolling the bristles of the brush down over the gums and teeth toward the grinding surfaces.
B) Clean the inside surfaces of the upper and lower back teeth by firmly rolling the bristles of the brush over the gums and teeth toward the grinding surfaces.
C) Clean the inside surfaces of the upper front teeth by drawing the bristles downward and forward over the gums and teeth toward the biting edges.
D) Clean the outside surfaces of the upper and lower front teeth by firmly rolling the bristles of the brush over the gums and teeth to the biting edges.

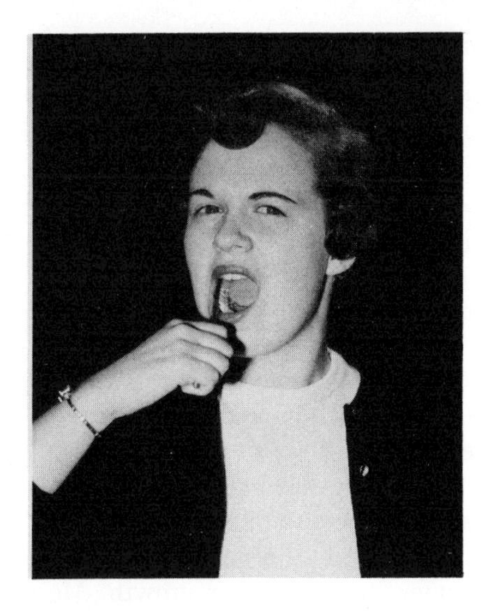

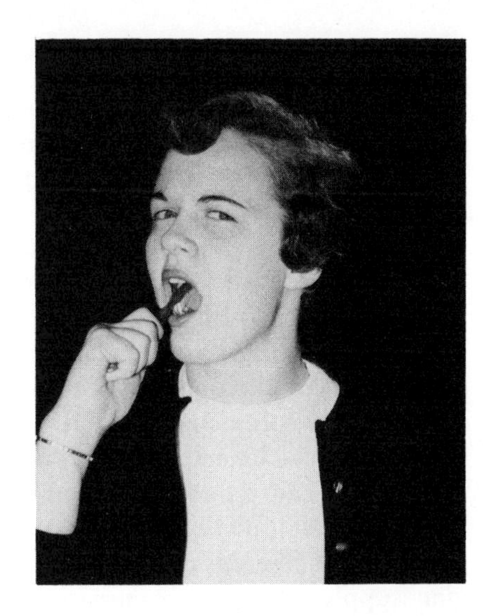

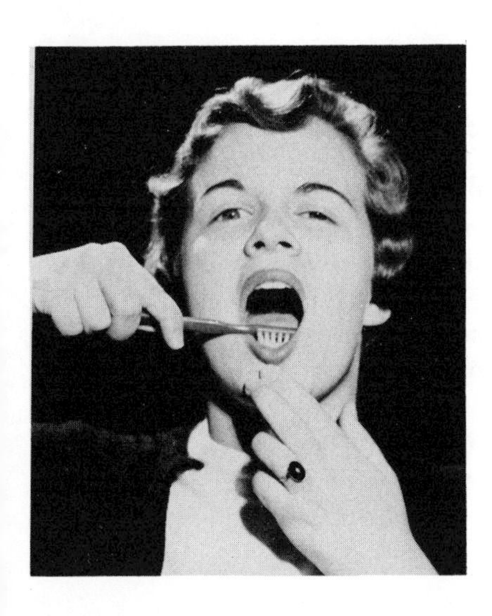

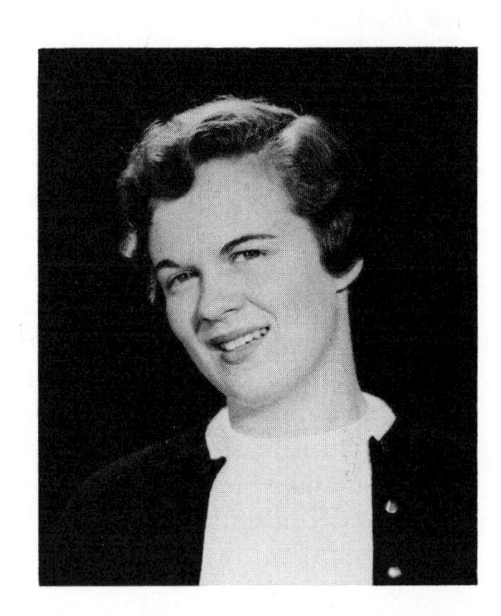

E) Clean the outside surfaces of the lower back teeth by firmly rolling the bristles of the brush up over the gums and teeth toward the grinding surfaces.
F) Clean the inside surfaces of the lower front teeth by drawing the bristles upward and forward over the gums and teeth toward the biting edges.
G) Clean the grinding surfaces of the teeth by forcing the bristles of the brush well into the grooves and vibrating the brush backward, forward, and sideways.
H) Clean, well-cared-for teeth are an asset to health, beauty, and personality. The care and time you devote to your teeth now will benefit you throughout life.

••• Food particles and substances cannot spur bacterial growth if you remove them from the mouth promptly. You remove many food particles and substances with proper toothbrushing. Strokes should start well up on the gum and roll toward the crown of each surface of each tooth. If you try to brush your gums with most strokes instead of your teeth, you will get better results. Take at least ten strokes in each area of both the outer and inner surfaces. If brushing is not practical, you can remove some food particles and other bacteria-nourishing substances after each meal, snack or beverage by thorough mouth rinsing. If you swish two or three swallows of water between your teeth and around your mouth immediately after eating, you hinder bacterial growth considerably.

••• You can reduce the number of opportunities your mouth bacteria have for rapid growth by avoiding excess sweet snacks and sugar-containing beverages. A few sips of pop, a bite of candy or a piece of ordinary chewing gum supply plenty of bacteria-feeding sugar for a spurt of growth. Most people find it easier to avoid excess indulgence in sweets than it is to brush their teeth or rinse out their mouths after each such exposure.

Fluorides

Fluoride ions are important chemical building blocks for cavity-resisting tooth enamel. Your body can build a more resistant outer layer for each tooth when it has fluoride ions available for use. Even if fluoride was not available when your body manufactured your tooth enamel, that enamel can soak up fluoride ions placed on its surface under certain circumstances, thus gaining resistance against cavity formation.

Pure fluorine is a gas, but its simple salts such as sodium fluoride and stannous fluoride dissolve readily in water to make easily consumed or applied solutions. Most drinking water contains small amounts of fluoride, but natural concentrations are seldom sufficient for full decay-preventing effect.

Fluoridated Water

If you grow up in a town where the drinking water contains at least 1.0 to 1.5 parts per million of fluoride salt, your tooth enamel forms out of cavity-resistant chemical compounds. You will have between sixty and seventy per cent less cavities than people who did not have the benefit of fluoride-containing water. About one-fifth of United States citizens reside in communities which add fluoride to their water supplies for this purpose.

A few communities have thirty to fifty times as much fluoride in their wells as is put into deliberately fluoride-supplemented water. At these very high levels, some undesirable effects sometimes accompany the beneficial cavity protection. The enamel is often stained with brown or blackish blotches. In a few extreme cases, bone and joint changes have been attributed to excessive fluoride exposure.

This unfortunate result of high fluoride consumption will never result from fluoride-supplemented water supplies. You would have to drink five to twenty gallons of water every day for 3,000 consecutive days [2] before fluoride-supplemented water would do you any harm. That is thirty times the normal intake, or about one glassful every five minutes while you are awake. The water itself would make you sick before the fluorides caused harmful effects.

If you live in a community which has no fluoride in its water supply, you can obtain fluoridated drinking water in many groceries or drugstores or can add fluoride compounds (prescribed by a doctor or dentist) to your drinking water. You can keep commercial or home fluoridated drinking water in the refrigerator, make beverages with it, and otherwise encourage its use while your children are forming permanent teeth under their gums, which is mainly during pre-school and school years. This approach is much more expensive and bothersome than community water fluoridation, but it is equally effective.

Fluoride Painting

Another way to get the benefit of fluoride-hardened tooth enamel is by applying fluoride solutions to each surface of each tooth. A trained professional worker [3] can do the job painlessly. Most dentists advise four applications of 2 per cent sodium fluoride at about age three, seven, ten, and thirteen, or one application of 8 per cent stannous fluoride each year. Fluoride application seems to help adults who are subject to frequent cavities, too. The effect is not quite as great as that obtained by fluoridating drinking water while the teeth develop, but may still be appreciable.

Fluoride-Containing Toothpaste

If you could get as much good from brushing fluoride onto your own teeth as you get from professional application, fluoride-containing toothpaste

[2] Pelton and Wisan, *Dentistry in Public Health,* W. B. Saunders Company, Philadelphia, 1956, p. 106.

[3] In some areas, dental hygienists apply fluorides; in others only dentists are allowed to do so.

would be a simple, inexpensive way to prevent cavities. Fluoride-containing toothpastes have two obvious disadvantages when compared with professional fluoride application, though.

1. Materials must be less concentrated to assure safety in home use.
2. Even ideal toothbrushing technique gets relatively little toothpaste between the teeth and up along the gum line. Average toothbrushing methods probably miss the most important tooth surfaces.

In spite of these handicaps, early tests show fair results with fluoride-containing toothpastes (especially those using stannous fluoride), which seem to reduce cavity formation by 30 per cent in areas without fluoridated water. Fluoridated water and professional fluoride application are more thoroughly established methods, but toothpaste with fluoride may serve as a stopgap or supplement. The amount of fluoride contained in the commercial products is entirely safe even if you have used fluoridated water or had professional fluoride applications.

Benefits of Frequent Dental Care

The highest interest rate you will ever pay, either in money or in misery, is on delayed dental care. A person who needs ten dollars' worth of fillings and attention every six months will probably need about three hundred dollars worth of care to put his mouth in shape after three years of neglect.[4] Small cavities become big ones, restorable teeth are lost and must be replaced with bridges and appliances, and bacteria-harboring scales accumulate near the gum margins, making cavity formation even more rapid than before.

When a dentist treats a cavity, he does more than fill the hole: he stops a morbid process which would otherwise rapidly lead to further damage. Professional tooth cleaning also keeps tooth disease from making further progress by removing bacteria-harboring scales.

INFECTED TOOTH ROOTS, SOCKETS, AND GUM SURFACES

Your gum tissues and tooth sockets constantly fight off teeming mouth germs. Infection-fighting white blood cells continually arrive at the scene. These cells move freely between your tissue cells to find and devour germs.

[4] Average of estimates provided by several practicing dentists and confirmed as conservative by Dr. William Jordan, Chief of the Dental Health Division, Minnesota State Department of Public Health.

They usually die in the process. The accumulation of germ-stuffed, dead, white blood cells blocks the steady, efficient flow of fresh fighter cells unless pus can escape freely.

When infection occurs at the tooth roots or in the gum pockets around the tooth sockets, your body is at a disadvantage. Pus pours into pockets instead of away from the site of germ invasion. Loosening of the tooth sockets, spread of infective pus into the jaw, and formation of tender, bleeding gums or gum ulcers frequently result. Fortunately, you can usually prevent or stop these harmful results.

Periodontal Disease

You can save a great many natural teeth by proper home and professional care when infection of the lining of the tooth sockets causes loosening of

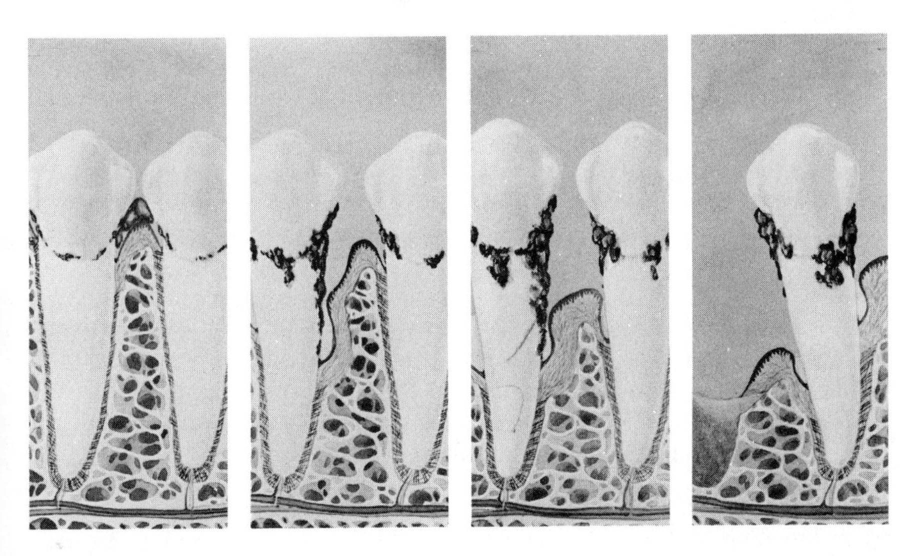

Figure 53. Disorders of the structures supporting the teeth are the leading cause of lost teeth in adult life. These diagrams show several stages of unchecked infection of the tooth socket linings. *From* Your Guide to Dental Health, *American Dental Association, copyright 1954. Used with permission.*

the teeth. Periodontal disease causes more loss of teeth than any other single dental disorder in adult life. You can forestall its ravages in three important ways:

1. Have a dentist or hygienist remove bacteria-harboring scales and deposits from the gum line frequently. Even though cavities become less

common as the years go by, the increasing importance of professional periodontal care makes regular dental attention every six months worthwhile.

2. Keep teeth clean and gums firm with proper brushing.

3. Eat foods which require considerable chewing each day. A soft, mushy diet definitely increases your tendency toward periodontal disease. Stick with steaks and salads instead of soufflé and soup for healthier gums and tooth sockets.

Abscessed Teeth

Infection at the tooth root causes a pocket of pus which presses on the surrounding bone. Sometimes headache, general aches and pains, loss of appetite, or slight fever are more notable than pain at the site of the infection. Swelling of the jaw, fever, and pain often follow at a later stage. Prompt and adequate treatment may save the tooth, which will otherwise need to be removed.

"Trench Mouth" and Other Gum or Mouth Infections

Sore or bleeding gums plague many college students. Four questions always come up in such cases:

1. Is toothbrush injury at fault? Many students who complain of slight soreness and occasional bleeding brush their teeth vigorously with a rotary or back-and-forth motion rather than in a rolling, down-from-the-base motion. Bristles may catch in the gum folds at the base of their teeth and rub them raw. Proper toothbrushing usually helps.

2. Is lack of vitamin C at fault? Lack of vitamin C severe enough to cause bleeding of the gums is very rare in the United States today. An occasional serving of citrus fruit, tomatoes or juice will prevent the profound deficiency required to cause bleeding gums.

3. Are virus-caused ulcers at fault? An ulcer is a gap in the lining layer of any inside or outside body surface, which exposes the underlying, normally protected layers. Gum and mouth ulcers look like whitish or grayish plaques or craters. The virus which causes them probably is present in most people's mouths at some time or other. College hours, college stresses, and the collegian's frequently unbalanced diet seem to be factors in letting the virus get a foothold, although some virus-caused ulcers occur without such indiscretions. If you have a tendency to get ulcers repeatedly, or if the ulcer persists for more than a week or ten days, your doctor may recommend further effective measures.

4. Could this be trench mouth? One particular combination of microorganisms frequently causes gum infections. Tenderness, bleeding gums, and sometimes gray-based mouth ulcers result. Trench mouth is not contagious, as was formerly believed.[5] Lowered resistance from inadequate sleep, poor oral hygiene, or poor nutrition seem to be the most important factors in precipitating an attack.

Whenever you have reason to suspect trench mouth, visit your dentist or physician promptly. He can perform the examinations and tests needed to make a diagnosis. If present, the disease usually requires prescription germ killers and dental instrumentation for cure.

DENTAL INJURY

Athletics, automobile accidents, and altercations are the big three causes of tooth injury. Mouth protection is important in any contact sport. Face masks or bars help considerably for football linemen. Mouthguards which fit over the teeth are more practical in sports like hockey and lacrosse where a broad field of vision is essential.

Dental injury from biting hard objects is fairly common among college students. The smart thing to do is use replaceable, relatively inexpensive tools and utensils rather than teeth for any other job but proper chewing.

People often make the tragic mistake of removing a tooth which has been knocked loose. Even if the tooth is hanging by a thread, it will sometimes become firmly rooted again if it is replaced. In some cases, a dentist can replace a tooth which has been knocked entirely free if the victim brings it to him immediately.

GROWING TEETH

Your first set of teeth erupt by age three. Permanent teeth erupt between ages six and twenty-one, usually displacing the primary set by age eleven.

Even though primary teeth will soon be replaced, they are very important. They help to maintain space in which the pursuing permanent teeth can erupt. Cavities and infection in or around the primary teeth can cause

[5] Pelton and Wisan, *Dentistry in Public Health,* W. B. Saunders Company, Philadelphia, 1956, p. 138.

discomfort, poor appetite, and other problems. Most dental authorities feel that a child should visit his dentist regularly from about age two and a half, and should try to keep cavities to a minimum with all of the measures discussed above.

One of the major dental health problems which develops during childhood years is malocclusion. Crooked teeth or teeth which do not meet in a proper bite are not merely a cosmetic problem: overload on certain areas

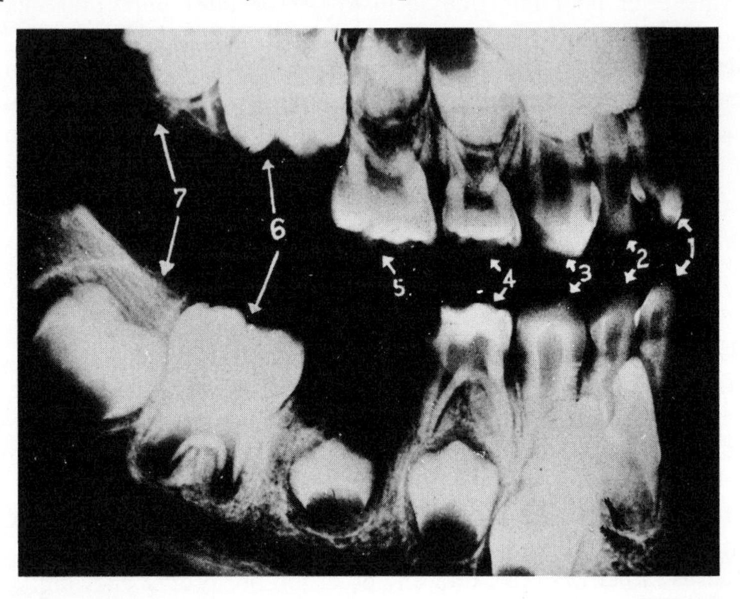

Figure 54. X-ray picture of the upper and lower jaws at 6 years of age. 1 to 5, primary teeth; 6, first permanent molars; 7, unerupted molars. Note the tooth buds in which permanent teeth are developing beneath each of the primary teeth. *From* Your Child's Teeth, *American Dental Association, copyright 1956. Used with permission.*

and abnormal pressures and strains lead to frequent and severe tooth problems in later life. Malocclusion often can be prevented by proper care of primary teeth, which helps to maintain space for the underlying permanent teeth. If primary teeth in the chewing area are lost, a space-maintaining appliance should be fitted by a dentist. Teeth which protrude or are otherwise malaligned should be corrected during the years of active growth. The sooner corrective measures are applied, the easier and less expensive they are.

The first molar teeth that erupt at age six are permanent teeth. Proper tooth care from the start will help them last a lifetime.

CHAPTER 14

Food Choice and Weight Control

IF YOU LET SCIENTIFIC NUTRITIONAL FACTS INFLUENCE YOUR FOOD CHOICES, you often gain extra physical vigor and disease-fighting resistance. Besides sufficient fuel, your body needs a variety of vitamins, minerals, fats, and proteins which you can provide only by consuming a well-chosen variety of foods. Nutritional deficiency sufficient to interfere with energy and resistance probably affects at least one-third of college students. Although only a physician can determine your nutritional status absolutely, these three questions might lead you to suspect need for his help:

1. *Does your vitality, mood, and appearance jibe with your age?* Compared with poorly nourished people, those who eat properly have more strength and tire less easily. Their firmer muscles help them sit and stand straighter, avoiding the slouched and sagging look of malnutrition. Their outlook on life is brighter, with less inclination toward the blues, less irritability, and less jitteriness. Lustrous hair and robust, fine textured skin contrast with malnutrition's coarse mane and sallow, dry, harsh hide. If fatigue, slouched posture, glum moods, or pasty skin belie your comparative youth, you might ask your doctor to review your diet with you.

2. *Does your diet measure up to nutritional standards?* Write down everything you have had to eat in the past twenty-four hours. After you finish reading this section, see how many servings you fall short of the ideal food program spelled out below. A nutritionally planned daily menu (e.g., in a well-run dormitory) may fall one or two servings short of the ideal pattern presented here without being deficient, but a diet planned without professional dietetic aid needs the provided latitude.

3. *Does two weeks on a demonstration diet make any difference?* Probably the best method for determining whether minor, hard-to-detect nutritional deficiencies impair your well-being is to see how you feel after two

weeks on an ideal diet. Over one-third of college students who have followed the program outlined below report back after two weeks with accounts of increased energy and improved mood. Why not give scientifically selected food a chance, and see how much it benefits you?

FOOD CHOICE AND PEAK ENERGY AND RESISTANCE

You can have the advantage of scientifically ideal nutrition at very little cost in money or inconvenience if you will apply the following principles.

Count Four-Five-Five

You can get enough of every substance known to be nutritionally necessary by putting emphasis on these five food groups:

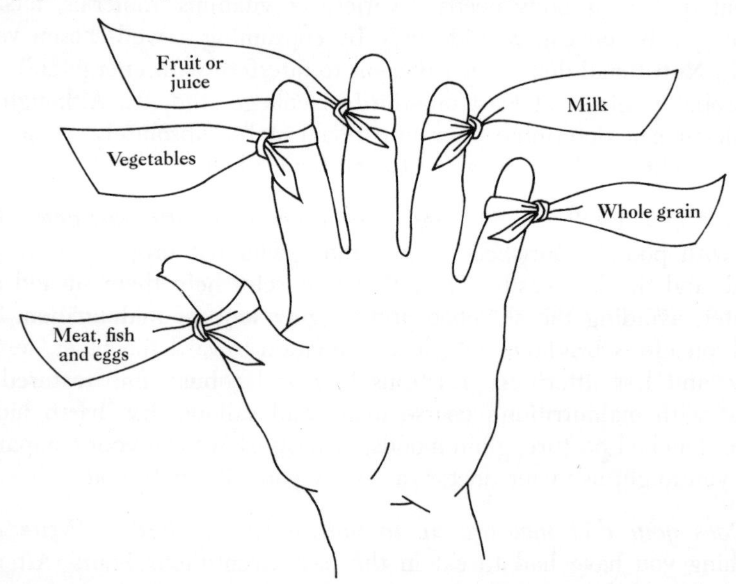

Figure 55. Five food groups to remember. *From* The Five Essentials for Nutritional Health *by Anna May Wilson, Today's Health, April, 1954.*

Meat, fish, and eggs

You need protein for building and repairing living tissue, for keeping the fluid portion of your blood inside the tiny capillaries whose walls act like sieves to smaller-moleculed substances, and for many disease-fighting functions. Meat, fish, and eggs are your body's main sources of protein. Dried peas or beans are cheaper substitutes which can replace part (but not all) of your animal protein requirement. Nutritional ideal: at least two medium or three small servings per day of meat, fish, eggs, or legumes.

Vegetables

Vegetables provide various vitamins, minerals, and necessary trace elements. Vary your vegetable choice among a list of at least eight, including green leafy and yellow ones. Three servings a day, including not more than one from the potato family, is ideal.

Fruit or juice

Probably the most important single substance your body gets from fruit is vitamin C (ascorbic acid). This vitamin is richly supplied in citrus fruits and tomatoes. At least one of the two servings of fruit or juice recommended daily should be orange, lemon, lime, grapefruit, or tomato.

Milk

A pint of milk yields numerous necessary substances sparsely supplied in other food sources. Vitamin B, calcium, and phosphorus are probably the most important. Other dairy products such as cottage cheese, cheddar cheese, and ice cream, can be used to meet a portion of your body's milk requirement if necessary. These foods are not exact equivalents of milk, however.

Whole grain

Grain-derived foods yield vitamin B and minerals as well as inexpensive, highly digestible fuel. They deserve an important place on your menu. Highly milled forms of grain such as polished rice and plain white flour have much less vitamins and minerals than cruder forms. Even enriched bread, which has extra vitamins added, lacks some of the nutrients found in whole grain. You get extra nutritional values at no extra cost in foods made from whole grain like whole wheat bread, rye bread, and oatmeal. Whole wheat bread, for instance, contains about twice as much iron, calcium, phosphorous, and vitamin B as white bread, as well as more protein. Incidentally, commercially prepared breakfast foods are no better or no worse than other forms of whole grain. They cost considerably more per unit of weight, which makes crunchiness and little noises rather expensive. Whether you take little letter O's or brown bread, your body needs three servings of whole grain every day.

Meat, vegetables, fruit, milk, and whole grain. One simple way to make your diet come out right is to count these items off on your fingers after each meal. After breakfast (or your midmorning snack if you split your morning meal) you should be able to count off four groups. After lunch or your midafternoon snack, count off all five again. After dinner, count off all five once more. Without the advance menu planning tacitly assumed by the Basic Four and other popular plans of nutrition instruction (but impossible for most college students) you can assure sound nutrition by this portion-counting technique. Count 4-5-5 every single day to keep your energy and resistance at a well-nourished peak.[1]

Preserve or Add Nutrients

How many dollars' worth of vitamin B has gone down the drain in your home? Vitamin B and certain other vital substances dissolve readily in water. If you cook vegetables by immersing them in hot water and then pour off the excess fluid, you lose a large part of their nutritional value. You are very fortunate indeed if more than half of the nutrient values your vegetables originally contained reached the table.

You can save these nutrients by cooking vegetables with a small volume of water so that they steam instead of soak. Use a pan with a tight-fitting lid or a pressure cooker. Or use the water in which vegetables have been cooked to make gravy. Nutrients are also preserved when you make stew or soup, because you consume the fluid elements in which the soluble vita-

The preparation or handling of vitamin C-containing foods also presents

mins dissolved.

a problem. Vitamin C is destroyed by oxygen from the air. If you squeeze orange juice today and leave it in an unsealed vessel until tomorrow, it loses substantial amounts of vitamin C. Cooking in an open pan or vessel speeds this process tremendously. For practical purposes, boiled orange

[1] People who learned nutrition on the Basic Seven plan will be wondering what happened to butter or oleomargarine, the main purveyors of vitamin D. The average American diet is so rich in dairy products that vitamin D deficiency is almost unknown in adults unless they are deliberately avoiding fats. If you go on a reduction or other special type of diet, be sure it supplies some butter or oleomargarine. Children still need their butter or oleomargarine (and quite probably a medically-prescribed vitamin supplement up to age six).

juice contains no vitamin C at all. Stewed tomatoes lose part of their vitamin C content while they are being heated, although fortunately their acid nature inhibits vitamin destruction. On the other hand, canning does not particularly decrease vitamin C content, since heat is applied after the food is sealed off from the air and very little oxygen is present inside the container.

One nutrient which is frequently lacking in foodstuffs grown in the United States is iodine. You can add this substance to your food very conveniently and substantially reduce the risk of unsightly thyroid gland enlargement by using iodized salt.

Improve Nutrition Without Spending More Money

"How can I get meat and vegetables a couple of times a day?" students often ask. "I can't afford that kind of meals at a restaurant, and I don't have time to cook them myself."

If you face this problem, three simple principles usually will keep your diet good enough to preserve your full level of energy and resistance:

1. Order food mixtures frequently. Food mixtures afford one means of having a varied diet without the expense or effort of preparing several dishes for each meal. One coed generally has vegetable or split pea soup, whole wheat bread, milk and fruit at supper, for instance. Her husky boy friend prefers stew or meat pie instead of soup. These choices combine some meat with several vegetables. At relatively little cost, they meet several nutritional needs.

2. Choose snacks to round out nutrition. One advantage of the count 4-5-5 plan for rounding out your diet is that it allows you to fit your snacks into your over-all program. If you drop by for a snack in the middle of the afternoon, think back to your previous meal. If you had ham sandwiches, pop, and cake, which met only your need for grain-derived foods and meat, you might order an apple and a glass of milk for your snack. This would add fruit and dairy products, bringing your count up to four. If you had jelly sandwiches, apple pie, and milk, which left you short of meat and vegetables, you might order tuna fish salad or a hamburger with lettuce, onion, and tomato. Snacks picked to round out your pattern cost no more and taste as good as ones which duplicate the nutritional values of your last meal.

3. Use inexpensive foods to meet nutritional needs. Frequent use of inexpensive foods in each group often helps mealtime economy without sacrificing nutritional quality. Liver or heart meets your body's protein needs just as well as sirloin steak. Whole wheat bread is as good as breakfast cereal. Canned or dehydrated milk is as good as fresh milk, and is a good substitute for cream in coffee or tea. Peas or carrots are as good as asparagus. Canned or dried fruits can replace expensive out-of-season fresh ones.

Benefits from Big Breakfasts

When a college student's diet fails to supply his full nutritional needs, the problem almost always turns out to be an inadequate breakfast. Breakfasts are especially important to students who live away from home because it is hard for them to adjust the size of their protein and fruit servings at other meals to make up for any morning servings they might miss. Eliminating the nonbreakfaster's late morning efficiency lag (an average of 25 per cent decrease in efficiency during the last morning hour as compared with the first hour after lunch) [2] can help a collegian, whose schedule concentrates this handicap on a single course.

Most students who skip breakfast have one of three problems: trouble getting up in the morning, lack of appetite on first arising, or dislike for standard breakfast fare. Revised rest patterns often make it easier to get out of bed (see Chapter 7). A small, priming-type feeding when you first wake up—a few crackers or a glass of juice—may help start your body processes so that you will have an appetite for breakfast by the time you have washed and dressed, or a small breakfast followed by a heartier midmorning snack may be the answer. Some students replace the standard breakfast items with soup, hash, or sandwiches if they have a profound dislike for cereal and eggs.

Vitamin Capsules and Nutritional Supplements

If your diet does not meet your nutritional needs entirely, vitamin capsules or nutritional substitutes will not fulfil your needs. Occasionally your doctor will prescribe these preparations to combat certain specific diseases or conditions. However, no supplement can replace proper choice and preparation of natural foodstuffs. Your body requires some specific substances which either have not yet been identified, cannot be manufactured, would be prohibitively expensive, or would make the supplement too bulky and unpalatable to be practical. The mainstay of good nutrition is properly selected natural foodstuffs, which beat the supplements hands down both in effectiveness and in economy.

Students who take vitamin capsules as a tonic or nutritional supplement in spite of the fact that their money might better be spent on fruit or dairy products should observe three cautions: *First,* they should not depend on the supplement to replace sound food choice, and should still do their best to

[2] Howard W. Haggard, M.D. and Leon A. Greenberg, Ph.D., *Diet and Physical Efficiency,* New Haven, Yale University Press, 1935.

fulfil their nutritional needs with natural foodstuffs. *Second,* they should select a balanced vitamin formula produced by a reputable drug firm, since formulas providing heavy dosage of the cheaper vitamins with small amounts of necessary companion substances may do more harm than good. *Third,* they should stick to compounds containing not over two to four times the minimum daily requirement for each vitamin, avoiding the heavy dosage "therapeutic formula" preparations.

HOW TO CONTROL YOUR WEIGHT

You look better, feel more energetic, and live longer with less illness and disability when you keep your weight within the recommended range. Weight control often requires continual effort, but the results are thoroughly worthwhile.

How Much Should You Weigh?

You can find your recommended approximate weight level from Table 1. These weights are not average levels: they are levels at which you can expect the best all-around efficiency, health, and survival. Weigh and measure yourself ordinarily dressed for comparison with this chart.

TABLE 1*

DESIRABLE WEIGHTS FOR MEN OF AGES 25 AND OVER

Weight in Pounds According to Frame (In Indoor Clothing)

HEIGHT (with shoes on) 1-inch heels Feet	Inches	SMALL FRAME	MEDIUM FRAME	LARGE FRAME
5	2	112–120	118–129	126–141
5	3	115–123	121–133	129–144
5	4	118–126	124–136	132–148
5	5	121–129	127–139	135–152
5	6	124–133	130–143	138–156
5	7	128–137	134–147	142–161
5	8	132–141	138–152	147–166
5	9	136–145	142–156	151–170
5	10	140–150	146–160	155–174
5	11	144–154	150–165	159–179
6	0	148–158	154–170	164–184
6	1	152–162	158–175	168–189
6	2	156–167	162–180	173–194
6	3	160–171	167–185	178–199
6	4	164–175	172–190	182–204

* *Courtesy Metropolitan Life Insurance Company.*

Table 1 (*continued*)

DESIRABLE WEIGHTS FOR WOMEN OF AGES 25 AND OVER

Weight in Pounds According to Frame (In Indoor Clothing)

HEIGHT (with shoes on) 2-inch heels		SMALL FRAME	MEDIUM FRAME	LARGE FRAME
Feet	Inches			
4	10	92– 98	96–107	104–119
4	11	94–101	98–110	106–122
5	0	96–104	101–113	109–125
5	1	99–107	104–116	112–128
5	2	102–110	107–119	115–131
5	3	105–113	110–122	118–134
5	4	108–116	113–126	121–138
5	5	111–119	116–130	125–142
5	6	114–123	120–135	129–146
5	7	118–127	124–139	133–150
5	8	122–131	128–143	137–154
5	9	126–135	132–147	141–158
5	10	130–140	136–151	145–163
5	11	134–144	140–155	149–168
6	0	138–148	144–159	153–173

For girls between 18 and 25, subtract 1 pound for each year under 25.

Overweight

Overweight usually results from a defect in the body's hunger control system rather than a defect in fuel use or storage. Ungoverned food cravings continue to affect people with a tendency to overweight after they have eaten enough to meet their actual needs. Either physical or emotional factors may be at fault. An overweight person does not turn food to fat more easily than anyone else. He simply eats more compared to what he burns. Even if he feels that he eats no more than his slim comrades, a careful account always proves that he supplies more fuel than his body would burn at normal weight. The basic facts of nutritional arithmetic apply to everyone.

Less fuel, fewer pounds

You will lose one pound a week for each 900 calories deficit between fuel supplied by food and fuel burned by bodily activity.[3] Since most college students burn at least 3,500 calories by virtue of their lively body processes and relatively intensive physical activity, a satisfactory rate of reduction

[3] 500 calories fuel from the fat per day, plus 400 which would have been required to digest food to yield this energy.

usually follows rigid adherence to a program providing 1,200 calories or more. Such a program (which you can get from your doctor or from the college health service) provides surprisingly large servings of widely varied foods. One day's menu on a 1,200 calorie diet might look like this:

Breakfast:

½ cup orange juice
¾ cup dry cereal with 1 cup milk
1 soft boiled egg
coffee or tea as desired (artificial sweetening)

Lunch:

2 frankfurters
sauerkraut (all you want)
¾ cup mashed potatoes
1 cup berries with 2 oz. light cream
1 cup skimmed milk

Dinner:

⅛ lb. chopped sirloin
¾ cup lima beans with 1 tsp. butter
cauliflower (all you want)
lettuce and tomatoes (vinegar and lemon juice dressing)
½ cup applesauce
coffee, tea, lemonade (artificial sweetening)

A reduction program allows substantially larger quantities to tall men (because of higher suggested weight) and to physically active people. Many overweight people who start such a program find that the diet allows much more than they usually eat, but proper methods of preparation and suitable selection of foods makes the actual fuel value sufficiently low for rapid results.

A nutritionally adequate reduction diet

You can lose from one to three pounds a week on a well-designed dietary program without risking undue fatigue, extra colds, or other physical problems stemming from poor nutrition. A sound reduction program meets every one of your nutritional needs through servings of meat, vegetables, fruit, milk, and whole grain just as a normal diet would. The only difference is that foods are chosen and prepared to keep down their total fuel value. Since your body can readily meet the need for extra fuel by mobilizing the reserve supplies it has laid up as fat, your essential body functions continue exactly as if you were on a normal diet.

Note that some reduction programs which work are not really suitable. You can lose weight on cranberry juice and dill pickles, or any other fad you might want to try. The only trouble is that you might lose your good health along with the excess poundage. Fad diets which do not provide for all your nutritional needs can definitely impair your strength and cut down your capacity to resist infectious disease, besides actually producing hospital-grade nutritional deficiency in some cases. Be sure that any dietary program you adopt has sound medical or dietetic backing if you want to lose weight without adverse health effects.

Exercise and weight loss

Most people feel somewhat better if they get a moderate amount of exercise. You should certainly continue the activity level which you have found suitable. However, the extra self-discipline required for a deliberate calorie-burning exercise program seldom proves worthwhile. This is true even though exercise speeds weight loss under experimental conditions. The experimental subject's will power is reinforced by solemn desire not to let the research team down, to serve humanity, and to stick to his word. He can stand up under appetite-increasing pressures that would make an ordinary man slip in an extra sandwich or two. Under ordinary circumstances, you lose weight faster by concentrating your mental energies on changes in eating patterns than by simultaneously undertaking the burdens of unaccustomed calorie-burning physical activity and of rigorous diet.

Contributing to this conclusion is the fact that your body is a very efficient machine. You can walk miles on the fuel derived from a single pound of fat. Although you may lose several pounds during an afternoon's exercise, most of this loss is fluid instead of permanent body substance. The amount of time and effort required to achieve any considerable, lasting weight reduction through exercise is much greater than that required to achieve the same amount of reduction through diet.

Physical, social, and psychological measures

People get fat when their food craving or hunger continues after their food needs are completely met. Several physical, social, and psychological factors which you can readily combat increase food craving or hunger. Among these are variations in the way your body uses sugar, exaggeration of food gratifications as living aims or as vicarious emotional supports, and undue stress upon food as a medium for improving friendships.

Frequent meals

If you have a tendency toward overweight, food cravings and exaggerated hunger from wide blood sugar fluctuations may be a factor. You can combat these problems in several ways:

1. You can eat slowly, allowing sugars from your first few bites to reach the blood stream and the brain before you have already consumed large additional amounts of food.

2. You can spread your food intake among at least three meals to prevent the rebound hunger, slow blood sugar rise at mealtime, and ravenous, rapid eating which frequently follow concentration of food intake into one or two meals.

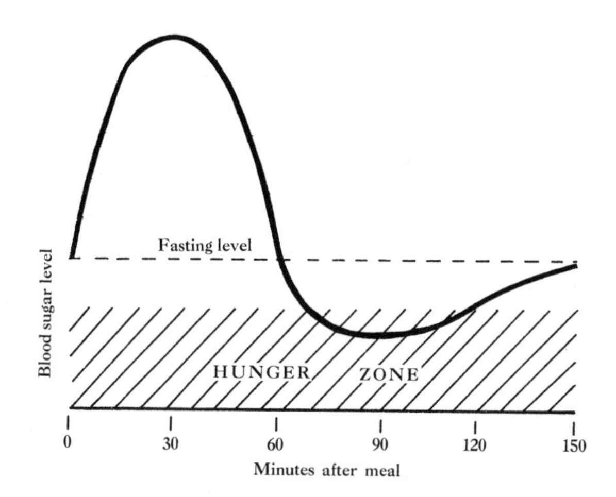

Figure 56. Effect of heavy carbohydrates feeding on blood sugar. Note "rebound hunger" about ninety minutes after meal.

3. You can use small, appetite-spoiling snacks if necessary. Slow sugar absorption, which leaves the brain signaling for more food long after an adequate quantity has actually been consumed, seems occasionally to be a factor in a tendency toward overweight. A piece of fruit or a glass of milk about thirty minutes before mealtime (with its caloric value subtracted from the meal itself) often solves this problem. The sugar from the snack boosts the blood sugar level up to or nearly up to the appetite-controlling level. As soon as sugars from the first few bites of the meal add their effect, low-sugar-spurred appetite ceases to be a problem.

Nonfattening gratifications

If the pleasures of the table are important enough to a person, and especially if he has developed few other sources of gratification, he will be strongly lured toward overweight. You can control this pressure in two ways:

1. You can get eating pleasure with less risk of overweight by emphasizing seasoning, variety, and atmosphere instead of richness and quantity. You can train yourself to enjoy a smoked oyster as much as a hamburger, a sip of liqueur as much as a swill of beer, a serving of Zucchini squash as much

as a heap of french fries. If you explore the possibilities of pleasurable eating without richness or gluttony, you will find the horizons to be broad.

2. You can develop other sources of gratification to take the pressure off your eating. Hobbies, sports, and social interests may meet the personal needs you have been assuaging at table.

Deliberate pampering

The food craving which drives people toward overweight often stems from the continual association of eating situations with personal security in our culture. From the time when you nursed at your mother's breast through the childhood days when candy was a frequently used reward and refreshments were the high spot of every date or party, food has accompanied your most loved, most secure, most pleasant moments. Even now, meals or snacks are frequently your only quiet occasions among friends and loved ones. No wonder that a need to feel loved and secure often throws this association into reverse gear!

You can help assuage or avoid these pressures in several ways:

1. You will do better with a reduction program if you undertake it during a period of relative freedom from stress.

2. Firm scheduling helps tremendously. Security depends on certainty about the future. If you know what you will be doing at 2:00 P.M. tomorrow, you are more secure than if you do not. A schedule helps give you that security. Overweight people who want to reduce, or people with a tendency toward overweight who want to keep their weight down, usually do much better if they keep to a written weekly schedule that covers at least their mealtime, bedtime, and work hours. Weekends and holidays are much less prone to wreck the program if they are completely planned at least a day or two in advance: the insecurity, boredom, and indecision of do-what-your-fancy-tells-you periods create tremendous food cravings for people who are prone to overweight.

3. If you pamper yourself and induce your friends and loved ones to pamper you during a reduction program, you do much better. An overweight person usually associates gifts of food strongly with affection: if his mother cuts two pieces of cake and gives him the smaller one, he feels distinctly hurt. He knows she is doing it for his own good, but he still feels distinctly hurt. Other gifts and attentions help control this element of stress: flowers instead of candy, extra time together, and expressions of affection in words and gestures help sustain morale during reduction and weight control.

4. Regular visits with a doctor, dietitian, or other interested people may help. If someone who is interested in you and your progress stands behind

you during a weight control program, you find the emotional pressures toward overeating easier to bear.

Weight maintenance

Most people who tend to become overweight find that perpetual dietary control wears out their will power. Nobody can count calories accurately enough to keep his weight exactly right for life. You can maintain your

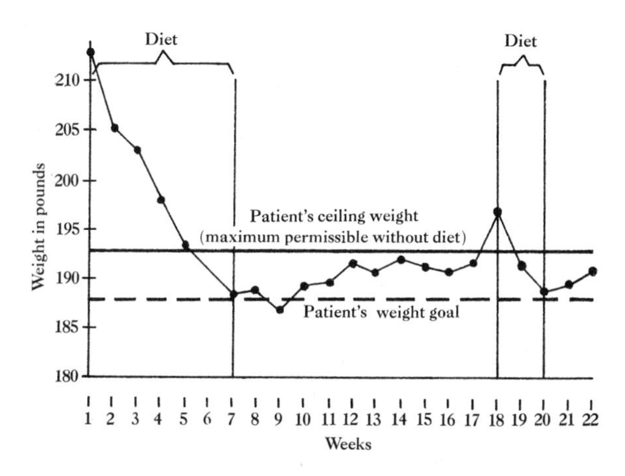

Figure 57. A weight reduction and control record, showing how brief periods on a rigid diet can control overweight's tendency to recur.

weight more easily by a two-stage program. First, set an ideal weight goal, reach it by an intensive reduction program, and then stop the diet altogether at that point. Weigh at least twice a week and go back on the full-scale reduction program the minute you go five pounds over your ideal. A written record or chart helps to reinforce this resolution. Most of my patients keep a graph with a double red line at the crucial when-I-hit-this-I-have-to-diet level. They find this graph makes them automatically adjust their food intake when weight gain threatens to put them back on the diet list. Almost everyone with a tendency toward overweight needs to follow a dietary program at least once a year, so a breakthrough to the red line need not be regarded as a drastic failure.

Underweight

Only very great degrees of constitutional underweight—at least 15 per cent below the recommended range—involve any risk in terms of either mortal or disabling disease. Moderate underweight decreases risk from heart disease, high blood pressure and diabetes more than it increases risk from tuberculosis and the like. Abrupt weight loss is something else again, and should not be confused with long-standing underweight. Many serious disorders which early treatment would greatly benefit first manifest their presence through abrupt weight loss. Any one who loses ten pounds or more within a period of six months is likely to profit from a complete medical examination.

You can enjoy a long life and good health without attempting a weight gain program if you have always been moderately underweight. However, these special precautions are worthwhile as long as your weight is low:

1. Get an annual checkup for tuberculosis, either through skin testing or x-ray. Ten per cent or more underweight makes you 2½ times as likely to get tuberculosis. Prompt detection and care greatly shorten the course and reduce the danger of this disease.

2. Pay particular attention to properly varied food choices. Underweight itself is not a sign that you are failing to meet all your body's food needs. However, it shows that you eat less food (in terms of total fuel value) than most people, and therefore must be particularly careful to eat enough from each important food group every day.

A weight gain program for underweight individuals

Although underweight involves no real health risks, many thin people want to gain a few pounds either for the sake of appearance or because they have found that extra fat reserves makes them feel better. A food program to correct underweight is quite practical, although it is just as difficult to follow as a reduction diet. Most people do best with gradual food adjustment. This calorie-building program often helps:

Record your food intake accurately for three to five days, checking fuel values with a complete calorie table. Be sure to take into account all butter or oleomargarine added to vegetables, syrup consumed with canned fruits, and sweetened or nutritious beverages. Continue to keep close track of all food intake the following week, but try to consume one hundred calories more per day than in the base period. Build up the diet by another hundred calories the next week, and continue until a satisfactory rate of weight gain occurs. High carbohydrate snacks an hour and a half or more before meals and bedtime snacks usually interfere the least with appetite. Higher calorie food choices at mealtime are also practical.

CHAPTER 15

Better Digestion

HAVE YOU SUFFERED A TEMPORARY STOMACH UPSET OR A SPELL OF HEARTBURN, diarrhea, gas pains, or constipation recently? What about more serious digestive problems like ulcers, hemorrhoids, or colitis? Victims of these disorders stream through my office every day. Yet most digestive disorders can be readily avoided. You can aid normal digestion and elimination in many ways, often preventing considerable misery and disability.

DIGESTIVE DUTIES

At both ends of the intestinal tract, you carry out essential functions deliberately rather than automatically. The frequency and rate at which you eat, the adequacy of chewing, and the promptness and regularity of evacuation greatly affect the workings of your digestive plant.

Chewing

When you chew your food, you accomplish three crucial processes: you break up food particles mechanically, you mix in saliva, and you stimulate your stomach to produce its digestive juices. The number of times you have o chew a bite in order to enjoy these effects depends upon the nature of he food. Any bite which you have to wash down or which scratches your hroat has not been chewed enough. Starchy foods require complete mastication even if their consistency is soft, because saliva plays a crucial part in digesting them. The old injunction to chew each bite ten times or more may erve to break the habit of bolting food, although it need not be followed trictly after you have established leisurely eating habits.

Frequency of Feedings

When you eat, your stomach acts as a reservoir to prevent overloading of your intestine, and also as a food-liquefying organ. Some food remains in your stomach for about ninety minutes after each meal. During this time, stomach acids and juices help to break down solid foods into smaller, more digestible fragments. A steady trickle of liquefied food substance passes

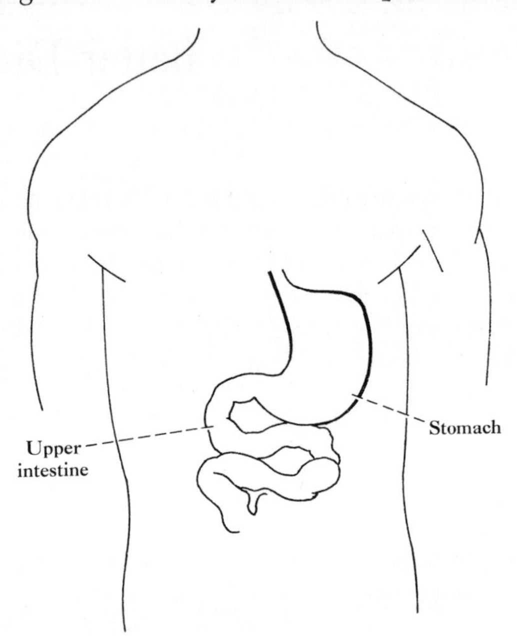

Figure 58. Stomach and upper intestine.

through into your intestine. Very few substances get into your system through your stomach wall, but the mixing, softening, and preliminary chemical treatment of foodstuffs in the stomach is an important part of digestion.

Your stomach can perform its functions easily on substantial volumes of food. However, if you load it beyond normal capacity, you may belch, feel uncomfortably full, get cramping discomfort or suffer heartburn. To avoid the necessity for overloading your stomach, it is generally wise to eat at least three times each day.

Eating speed

The rate at which food is consumed also affects the efficiency of your stomach. An attractive meal consumed with slow savoring of each bite stimulates the flow of gastric juice. An adequate period of time at table allows that stimulated flow to produce an ideal quantity of gastric juice. Constipation, feeling of fullness and gas pains sometimes seem related to rushed meals with inadequate gastric digestion.

Elimination

You can ordinarily forget about the food you swallow until its solid residues are ready for elimination. The urge to defecate arises when material moves into the last six or eight inches of the intestine. You can easily restrain this urge, but if you do so frequently and for long the nerve endings in the rectum may become quite insensitive. Normal urges then become barely noticeable or nonexistent. Such rectal insensitivity is one important cause of constipation.

The best way to avoid rectal constipation is probably by promptly heeding the calls of nature. In our organized, tightly scheduled society, however, you may also find it worthwhile to encourage those calls at a constant time. This is not only a convenience, but also a means of supplementing normal regularity through conditioned reflexes. To establish a habit time, select the most convenient period when natural urges often arise, and arrange to spend ten or fifteen minutes encouraging bowel action at that hour each day. At first, movements will rarely occur during this period. However, most people ultimately reach a point where prompt evacuation frequently occurs during their scheduled toileting, and urges at other times of the day become rare.

Constipation often stems from attempts to force the bowel into movements every day or two with habit-forming laxatives. Whether you develop a habit time or not, you should judge the efficiency of your bowel rhythm by the consistency of the stool and your freedom from complaints. Sausage-shaped, easily passed stools and freedom from constipation-caused cramps, nausea, or appetite disturbance indicate normal bowel rhythm, whether you have one movement a week or several each day.

OTHER HABITS AFFECTING DIGESTION AND ELIMINATION

The liquefied food mixture which pours into your small intestine from your stomach is only partially prepared for your body's use. Throughout the small intestine, other body-made chemicals are churned into the mixture. The liver and pancreas add secretions which liberate and chemically alter food substances. The intestine walls absorb nutrients and dispense them *via* the blood stream to other parts of the body for storage or use. The residues pass on into the large intestine where much of the water previously added with the digestive juices is reclaimed.

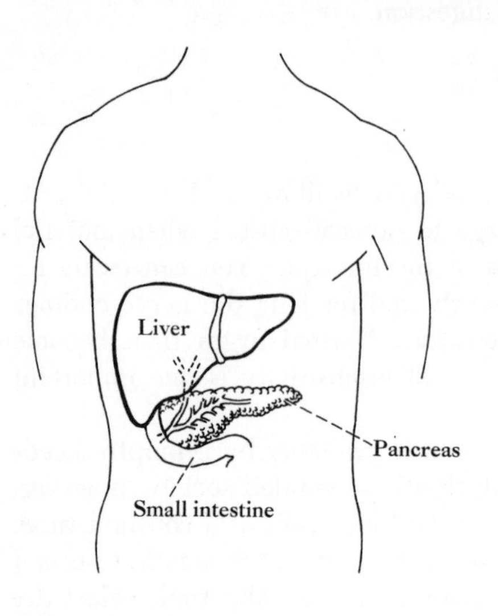

Figure 59. Liver and pancreas, showing their connection with the first loop of small intestine.

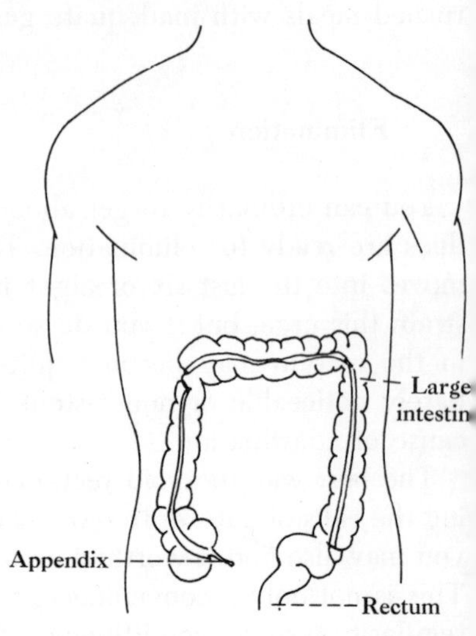

Figure 60. Large intestine. Material enters near blind end from the small intestine (not shown).

Moist-Bulk Foods

Unless the muscular tube of your large intestine moves material along promptly, excessive amounts of moisture soak up into your system out of the forming stool. The resulting lack of moisture, not lack of undigested fiber or bulk, is the most important single factor in constipation. Dry bulk material like bran may actually do harm instead of good.[1] Irritating laxatives increase the tightness in colon musculature, and ultimately make constipation worse.

What you need for preventing constipation and for curing mild tightness is extra moist bulk. Fruit is the most important moist-bulk food group. Never-irritating fruits, which almost everyone can eat with perfect safety, include stewed prunes, cantaloupe or honey dew melon, raisins, currants, applesauce, plums, cherries, and berries. Apples, figs, and dates are often

[1] Such materials have sometimes been recommended for "atonic constipation," a condition in which lax intestinal musculature supposedly slowed passage. Recent studies suggest that no such condition actually exists, with stretched intestinal walls actually the result rather than the cause of the problem. Certainly, if "atonic constipation" does occur it is a disorder of older people rather than collegians.

helpful, but should be eaten with caution at first, since they occasionally cause cramps or indigestion.

If you temporarily require more moist bulk than diet alone can provide, medicinal concentrates may be worthwhile. Check with your doctor or college health service to select a product which has no irritant laxative compounds in it. The mainstays contain substances like agar, psyllium seed, or methyl cellulose which take up a great deal of water inside the intestine to form a soft, nonirritating gel.

Water

If you fail to drink enough water, your body may reclaim enough extra moisture from the colon to aggravate constipation. The amount of water you need varies too much with activity and climate to permit a fixed standard. If you have a tendency to constipation, though, you may find it worthwhile to serve water with each meal and to make a point of drinking whenever you are thirsty. You might also increase your water intake when fever, hot weather, or exertion spurs extra moisture loss.

Exercise

When you walk or move, the alternate contraction and relaxation of your abdominal muscles gently massage your intestine. Good tone in your abdominal muscles helps support the inner organs in their proper position. Although the importance of these effects is hard to establish scientifically, most people with mild constipation get some help from a few minutes' walk or some other form of mild exercise.

Serious Forms of Intestinal Blockage

Intestinal obstruction, with complete stoppage of flow through either the large or the small intestine, causes serious or deadly illness and should not be confused with ordinary constipation. Abdominal cramps, bloating, and vomiting may mean intestinal obstruction even if feces passes during the attack (since intestinal contents beyond the obstruction remain free to move). Medical diagnosis and care usually relieve obstruction, but haste is essential since even a few hours' delay may lead to serious results. Obstruction usually results from scar tissue bands left by previous operation, from tumor, hernia or other serious disorder. It is *not* simply an advanced stage of constipation.

EMOTIONS AFFECT DIGESTION

Digestion is a complex, assembly line operation involving coordination of dozens of independent organs. This coordination is achieved through the autonomic nervous system, a web of nerve fibers and centers which is also very much involved in your emotions. Actual, visible, and measurable changes occur in almost every part of the digestive tract with strong emotion: gentle churning and orderly movement may be replaced by tight immobility or by backward and forward rushes. Acids and various other digestive juices may vastly increase or dry up. Shrunken or engorged blood vessels make the working surface of the digestive passages pale or engorged.

These physical changes lead to a variety of complaints. Emotional stress can lead to diarrhea or constipation, to loss of appetite, heartburn, nausea, vomiting or cramps, and to feeling of fullness or belching. Many perfectly normal college students develop one or more of these complaints during examination period, for instance.

Emotional factors contribute to many digestive diseases. Smoldering, unrecognized stress is more frequently responsible than frankly recognized upheaval. You deal intellectually with most acknowledged emotional upsets: either you steer clear of the cause, resolve the issue, or consciously and deliberately accept the situation. The conflicts which rankle are those you cannot quite bring yourself to face consciously and those involving obscure or symbolic emotional associations. For this reason, people who sincerely believe that they have no important emotional problems frequently suffer emotion-induced digestive distress or disease.

Pleasant Mealtime Aids Digestion

Relaxed, enjoyable companionship during meals definitely contributes to good digestion. Three assets besides the proper selection of an eating place (discussed in Chapter 2) prove helpful in this regard:

1. A store of timely topics of interest to fellow-diners helps to stimulate pleasant conversation and turn the conversation away from emotion-charged or hazardous areas. One technique for acquiring such a store: scan the morning paper or a weekly news magazine for items of interest to your usual companions.

2. A few minutes' leisure before, during, and after mealtime encourages pleasant social exchange. This need deserves some thought when you arrange your schedule.

3. Unfailing exclusion of business affairs and issues involving true personal conflict from table conversation avoids many unnecessary emotional strains. College students frequently enjoy heated discussion of politics, religion, and so on, and can detach themselves from the issues sufficiently to debate without anger. However, a dispute in which true acrimony is involved, or the controlled but intense stress of settling important family and business issues frequently causes distress when undertaken at table. Most people do better by setting a pleasant, cooperative tone, then broaching disputed issues afterward.

Stomach-Soothing During Emotional Upheavals

During periods of acknowledged emotional strain or upheaval, people with a tendency toward nervous indigestion can often avoid distress by following a stomach-soothing dietary program. Milk between meals and at bedtime is very helpful, since it neutralizes excess stomach acids before they have a chance to do any harm. Small meals of bland foods like creamed chicken on toast, poached eggs, cooked cereal, or soups place no burden on your digestion.

Dependency Conflicts and Digestive Distress

A great deal of digestive upset, ranging from occasional heartburn to continual ulcer pain, originates in conflict over dependency. Almost all of us want simultaneously to become self-sufficient and to enjoy the shelter and support of close ties with others. These ambitions come strongly into conflict when loving interest takes the form of material aid or correction of the other's missteps. The businessman whose daughter gets tossed out of college might buy her a new convertible with which to console herself (which pushes her toward his own living pattern), or use his influence to get her into another school (which he usually selects without asking her preference). He can rarely give her the feeling that he accepts her, faults and all, that he will stand behind her lovingly no matter what kind of life she makes for herself. The materialistic or dominating approach to dependency makes for inevitable conflict: when a person caught in this framework needs emotional support, he cannot reach out for it without surrendering independence and self-esteem. Smoldering emotional insecurity results, with indigestion or ulcer not far behind.

You can avoid this conflict while still meeting your own and your associates' dependency needs by making compassionate interest and emotional support the mainstays of your close interpersonal relationships. Compassionate interest does not sap independence. Emotional support does not threaten its recipient's feeling of worth. (Further discussion of means by which relationships can be placed on this plane appears in Chapters 3 and 4.)

Resentment and Indigestion

Drs. Wolf and Wolfe performed many experiments upon a man named Tom, who had an opening directly into his stomach from outside his body. To keep him readily available, they arranged to have him work as a janitor in the hospital. One day Tom showed up for an experiment with the inside of his stomach partly beet-red, its protective mucous coat completely gone and acid levels exceedingly high. Recognizing the changes as typical precursors of severe indigestion or ulcer formation, the doctors made careful inquiry into possible causes. They found that Tom had just taken a bawling out from his superior—not too unusual in itself, and no worse than a dozen other rebukes which had not harmed his stomach. But there was one difference: this bawling out was undeserved. This bawling out spurred intense feelings of resentment.

Many sufferers find that measures aimed at decreasing or handling resentment control digestive distress more easily than medicines or measures to soothe the consequent stomach irritation. Chapter 4 gives further details.

HOW TO WARD OFF OR MANAGE COMMON DIGESTIVE DISEASES

You get considerable benefit from prompt attention for ulcers, appendicitis, hernia, and hemorrhoids. You should know how to recognize your need for attention quickly when such disorders strike, how to meet the situation calmly, and how to prevent or slow the development of these diseases whenever possible.

Peptic Ulcer

In peptic ulcer, stomach acids and protein-digesting substances eat part way through the wall of the stomach or intestine. Although emotional factors probably underlie every case, an ulcer is a tangible, physical disease which calls for prompt medical or surgical control.

Your chance of having an ulcer justifies a visit to your doctor whenever you have frequent attacks of gnawing hunger-like or burning pain in the pit of the stomach. Ulcer pain usually begins an hour to an hour and a half after meals and is usually relieved very promptly by milk, baking soda, or antacid preparations. A few ulcer victims get their first warning from bleeding rather than pain: this shows up in the form of dead-black, somewhat bulky, soft stools associated at times with dizziness, fainting, or weakness from blood loss.

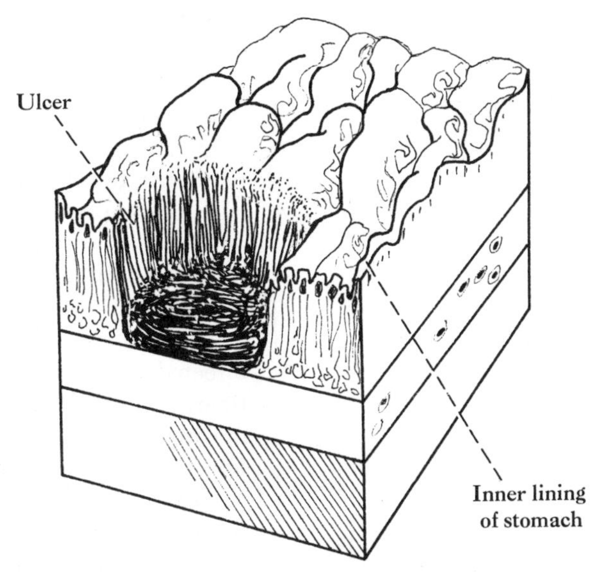

Figure 61. An ulcer penetrates part way through the stomach wall.

Revised living habits or psychologic guidance may help to prevent the initial attack or later recurrences, although such measures do not replace the need for medical or surgical treatment for the disease when complaints suggest that it is active.

Appendicitis

Although only one person in five has his appendix removed, almost everyone has one or more attacks of abdominal pain which make him wonder whether appendicitis is likely. The appendix is a narrow, blind pouch to the right of the colon which apparently serves no function. Infection in the appendix is dangerous mainly because the organ hangs free in the abdominal cavity, where germ-laden pus can discharge in a way that causes hazardous spread of infection under certain circumstances.

Appendicitis might underlie any attack of abdominal pain. In most cases, appendiceal pain starts in the pit of the stomach. It moves to the lower right portion of the abdomen inside four hours. The pain typically consists of cramps every two or three minutes, with mild to moderate soreness persisting between. However, many cases of appendicitis are far from typical. I have seen appendicitis cause pain on the left, steady pain rather than cramps, sudden fainting followed by mild abdominal pain. The only way to avoid the risks of inadequately treated appendicitis is by getting advice from your doctor whenever you have abdominal pain of any sort which persists for more than four hours, even if it occurs coincident with menstruation, diarrhea, constipation, or other manifestations which seem to explain it.

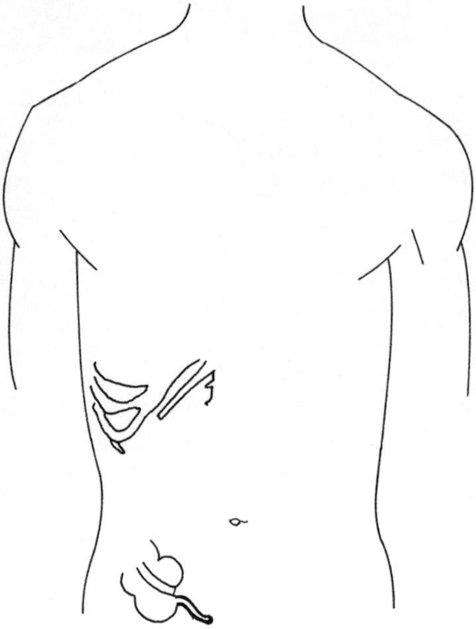

Figure 62. Appendix in relation to rib margin and umbilicus.

The risk involved in leaving an infected appendix alone is many times greater than the risk of removing an uninfected appendix. For this reason, your doctor has to play the odds: if he cannot be sure that your trouble lies elsewhere, he takes out your appendix. You actually cut your chance of having an unnecessary appendectomy by going to your doctor promptly, so that he has time to follow your progress for an hour or two before deciding whether to operate. Even so, perfectly sound medical judgment may sometimes call for removal of an appendix which at operation proves to be free of disease.

Hernia

When organs or membranes can slide out of their proper body compartment, a hernia or rupture is present. Hernia strikes most commonly in the groin, where a slight gap in the muscle layers of the abdomen often occurs around the blood vessels which supply the testicle. Hernia seldom causes pain. A sliding sensation when straining at stool, and perhaps muscular aching or stiffness in the area after strenuous lifting or exercise sometimes signal hernia. A bulge in one of the usual hernia sites merits your doctor's attention even though it appears only when straining, coughing, or lifting.

You can decrease your chance of suffering a hernia somewhat by following three steps, all aimed at minimizing episodes of increased pressure inside the abdomen:

1. Control constipation. Try adequate exercise, take extra fruit and fluid, and ask your doctor what further steps you should take if these methods fail.
2. Control cough. Get proper medical care for any severe, sustained cough.
3. Learn to lift with your back upright instead of by bending forward, and learn to breathe freely while lifting rather than holding your breath or straining.

Hemorrhoids

Hemorrhoids are dilated veins in the vicinity of the rectal opening. Bleeding, itching, and mild but continual discomfort frequently plague the victim. An irritating clot sometimes forms inside a hemorrhoid, causing pain and tenderness for several weeks.

Some of the rectal veins connect with large abdominal veins, which then break up into smaller channels again within the liver. Other rectal veins connect with large veins which run directly to the heart. Increased abdominal pressure, such as occurs during straining at stool or lifting, sends heavy flow of blood under high pressure from one system to the other through the rectal veins. Like heavy truck traffic over a dirt road detour, this heavy blood flow sometimes damages the delicate rectal vessels. Other disorders within the abdomen, such as rectal tumors or liver disease, can also force heavy detouring of blood through the rectal veins with similar results.

Every patient with bleeding from the rectum, even if hemorrhoids are obviously present, should have thorough medical study. About one case in fifty stems from some serious underlying disease, such as tumor or cirrhosis. Early treatment for these ailments makes a tremendous difference to your chance of permanent and life-long cure. Surgical cure of the hemorrhoids themselves is reasonably comfortable, safe, and effective, if the trouble they cause justifies it.

The same measures advised for prevention of hernia should prove helpful in keeping hemorrhoid formation to a minimum.

CHAPTER 16

Your Body in Action

PHYSICAL FITNESS AND ATHLETIC PARTICIPATION ARE EXCEEDINGLY WORTH-while, so long as they remain within the limitations imposed by health defects and pressing long-range needs. Let's examine both the benefits and the limitations of physical fitness programs and athletic participation.

BENEFITS OF REGULAR EXERCISE

Improved muscle tone and other effects of exercise offer five definite advantages other than recreational value:

Improved appearance

Regular exercise often improves body contours. Good tone in the abdominal muscles makes for a flatter abdomen. Firm hip and thigh muscles may make these parts measure two inches or more less than they do in a flabby state, even although no actual weight loss has occurred. Most people regard well-developed arm and shoulder muscles as masculine assets, and admire the robust skin tone athletic participation imparts.

Prestige and social values

Many elements in our society place heavy value upon athletic achievement and physical prowess. Coeds seem less likely to turn down a request for a date from a football star than from an honor student, for instance.

Through such social acceptance, athletes often acquire self-confidence and an assured manner which stands them in good stead.

The capacity to participate in sports is also an important social asset. How many of your friendships first warmed during or after sports activity? What percentage of close contacts with your best friends take their occasion from the world of sports, including noncompetitive activities like hiking, picnicking, and social swimming? Enough skill to participate in sports gives real satisfaction and help, even if you never excel.

Extra durability for your heart and circulation

Regular, mild exercise through the years helps open and maintain alternative small blood vessels within the heart muscle. Stoppage of all vessels to any one bit of muscle causes a coronary heart attack, one of the commonest forms of heart disease in this country. People doing physical work have many less coronary heart attacks than people doing desk work, and their attacks tend to be much less severe. You can accomplish similar results

Figure 63. One advantage of fitness. *Ewing Galloway.*

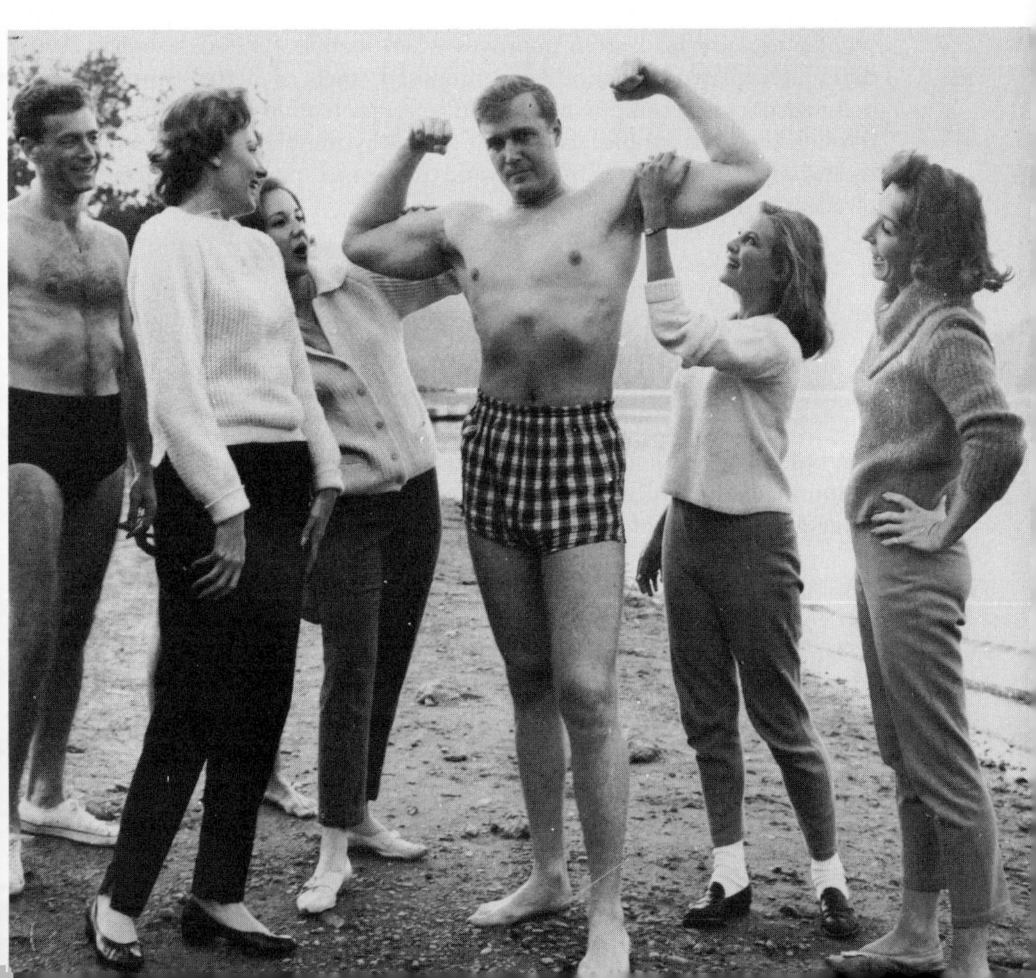

with recreational exercise, deliberate fitness-promoting routines like a twenty-minute walk to work each day, or calisthenics.

Less backache

Better muscle tone helps brace your spinal column and protects it from wrenching strains. I talked recently with a physician from an area of Europe where people usually walk or ride a bicycle, do their washing by hand, and generally perform enough physical work to maintain fitness. "We practically never see a patient with backache unless he has disease we can detect by x-ray or blood study," he told me.

In this country, about half the patients who complain of "nagging backache" have normal x-rays and blood studies. Postural strains and ligamentous stretching aggravated by muscular weakness seem to be at fault. Properly maintained muscle tone would presumably prevent the bulk of this distress.

Improved bowel function

Constipation seems to occur less frequently among people who take regular exercise, and often improves when victims take up exercise. Many different explanations have been proposed, such as better support of abdominal organs by improved muscle tone, promotion of intestinal function through the massage-like movement of nearby muscles, improved morale by recreational sports participation, and release of pent-up feelings through physical activity.

UNDUE EMPHASIS ON PHYSICAL FITNESS AND ATHLETIC PARTICIPATION

People who cannot achieve the ideal of total physical fitness for one reason or another often find their problems magnified tremendously by an exaggerated notion of its importance. Let me give two examples:

1. A college freshman learned that his vision tested 20/30 in each eye, one notch below average normal vision of 20/20.

"Isn't there something I can do?" he asked, his hands trembling from anxiety. "Can't you operate or something to get me back to normal?"

2. A young diabetic attempted suicide with sleeping pills.

"Why did you do it?" I asked him later.

"Because of the diabetes," he said.

"But it's no real handicap to you. You do everything you want to do, and you can keep the disease completely in check for the rest of your life."

"Sure. But it's always there. Every meal I eat is like a red flag waving in front of me—you're diseased, you're diseased, you're diseased. The other fellows order milkshakes, and I've got to stop and count up carbohydrates to see whether I can take a coke. It keeps beating in on me all the time, the fact that I'll never be normal again."

These people are victims of the "sound mind in a sound body" doctrine. They are perfectly fit for everything society actually expects of them. Yet the notion that freedom from disease or defect is essential to human worth turns minor physical inconveniences into major emotional roadblocks. The same phenomenon adds tremendously to the burden imposed by the smoldering diseases or defects almost all of us suffer in later life. It makes the normal adjustments of middle and old age into highly discomfitting miseries.

What are the actual facts? Only one person in fifty is physically fit for every conceivable type of employment. For practical purposes, physical fitness means fully developed physical capacities with which to meet the duties and responsibilities you yourself should carry. It is, or should be, an elastic standard which changes with your health, age, schedule, and occupation. A physically fit executive might drop from exhaustion after two hours in the mines. A physically fit octogenarian might be incapable of walking more than a few blocks without pausing to rest.

Athletic achievements also need to be kept in perspective. Athletics give satisfaction. Athletic achievement opens many doors for social and business development. But with the exception of a few professional performers, an athletic career ends in the twenties. Unless an athlete gives proper emphasis to more lasting skills and achievements, he faces the virtual certainty of becoming a has-been before the age of thirty. The wise athlete usually can make the most of his gifts without obstructing his permanent career development, but only by giving constant consideration to that necessity.

PROMOTING PHYSICAL FITNESS AND ATHLETIC SKILLS

The physical education department of your college probably offers a wide variety of assistance for developing physical fitness and athletic skills. Which among their offerings will offer the greatest long range health benefit for you? Perhaps these general principles will help you to make sound selections.

Pick at least two carry-over sports

After you get out of college, you will probably have very little opportunity to play team sports or sports involving special equipment and formal competition. Where will you find a working man's football team or pole vaulting competition, for instance? More ordinary, individual, or partnership sports frequently help you enjoy physical recreations through the years. You can play golf, tennis, badminton, squash, or handball for decades. You can bowl, fish, or hunt. When you develop athletic interests and skills which will fit in throughout your later life, you help yourself toward physical fitness and enhanced living satisfaction through the years.

Sports with social values

Shared activity helps build friendships. Sports you can pursue with your associates, either on a team or an individual basis, promote your social development. If you have difficulty meeting people or mixing with them, properly chosen sports participation may help you right now. If you plan a career in which personal contacts are relatively few—like scientific research or any form of writing, for instance—sports which let you get out with other people may help you throughout your future years.

Sports for emotional release

Leisure-time interests which meet repressed emotional needs serve a valuable health function. In our society, for example, expression of hatred or resentment is seldom given free rein. What would people think of you if you instantly struck the next person who offended you? You would not even feel comfortable about it yourself! Yet the emotional pressures which act whenever you are hurt or threatened are not prevented by civilized training. They are only turned inward before they lead to manifest actions or words. Result: continued smoldering stress.

Over the centuries, civilized man has found that he feels better after taking advantage of acceptable outlets for such feelings—games or sports through which he can carry out the pattern of violence without unpleasant consequences in society or in his own conscience. The civilized husband adds thirty yards to his drive by walloping the golf ball while his subcon-

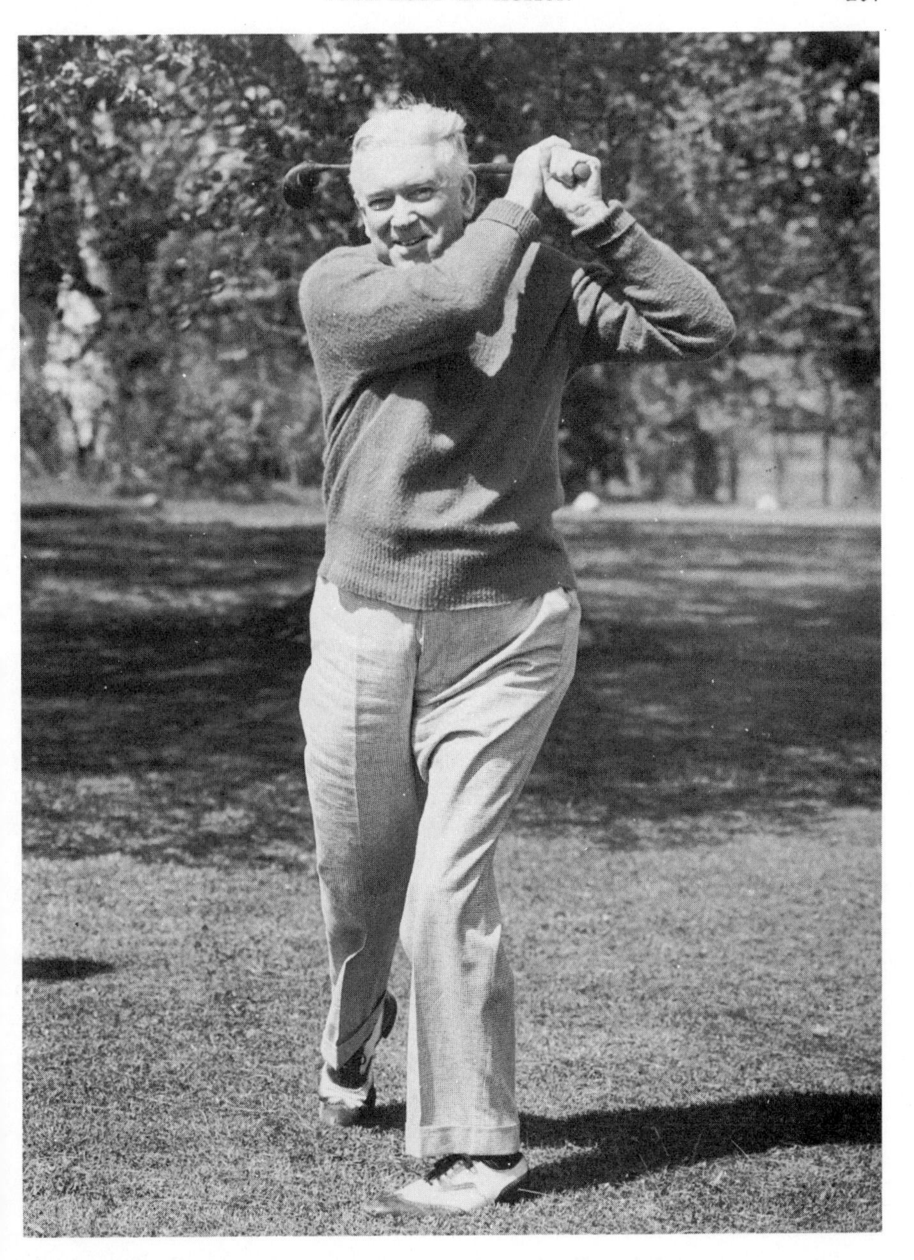

Figure 64. Thirty years out of college, and still enjoying golf. *Ewing Galloway.*

scious mind dwells upon his mother-in-law's head. The civilized student shoots an innocent rabbit: as the red gore trickles down upon the white snow, he feels release of the tension which stems from hatred for the college professor who flunked him. Even the civilized housewife takes vicarious joy in the blows landed by her pet wrestler, and bears up better under the refractoriness of her children as a result.

Foolish as such gestures might sound, sporting activity which gives release through hitting, shooting, chopping, killing, or otherwise abusing some acceptable target (or watching a figure with whom you identify perform such abuse) is very sound mental hygiene. It is particularly useful to people who must treat other people with emotional restraint, like the waitress who smiles at everybody, the psychiatrist who is blandly noncritical no matter how mean his patients act toward him, and the school principal who is the essence of sweet reasonableness to a steady parade of people who make highly unreasonable demands. If your work will involve intensive self-control in frequent contacts with other people, it is important that at least one of your sports interests involves some pattern of violence.

Transportation exercise or regular calisthenics

There are two ways to keep physically fit without taking much time for exercise. Probably best, because it is very regular and because you are more likely to keep it up through the years, is the custom of making your way to and from school or work in a way involving muscular activity. A brisk walk or bicycle ride involves much more exercise than an automobile trip, but may not take any more time than fighting traffic, parking, and getting where you want to go, for instance.

The other way of maintaining fitness with minimum time expenditure is through calisthenics. A well-designed daily workout can keep you fit if you continue the custom through the years.

BODILY POISE

You can expect several long-range benefits from improved bodily poise. Bodily poise conserves your energies for useful tasks and prevents undue fatigue; improves your appearance and promotes graceful movement; decreases muscular and joint strain, which helps to preserve your physical comfort through the years; and cuts your chance of injury through backstrain and through falls.

The Energy Drain of Upright Posture

Did you ever stand on your head? If so, you remember how tight you had to hold the muscles of your trunk and legs and how many sudden movements it took to keep yourself in balance. Your body is a collapsible sack of bones which remains upright only by virtue of continuous muscle bracing and continual efforts at balance. When you are standing or sitting, you accomplish these tasks automatically, thanks to the training of a lifetime plus your inbred balancing reflexes. But the need for muscular action to maintain posture is no less than when you are standing on your head: it is only more familiar. A substantial proportion of the work your muscles do is devoted to the task of keeping your body upright. A considerable share of the additional energy required by most tasks you undertake is consumed in maintaining and changing your own body's position: if you pick up and roll a sixteen-pound bowling ball, for instance, the bulk of the effort you expend is in rebalancing the fifty or more pounds of your own upper body, moving your entire body weight fifteen or twenty feet during your approach, and supporting your body in an abnormal and somewhat strained position during and after delivery. Postural efficiency both when stationary and in action definitely helps you enjoy greater energy and suffer less muscular fatigue and discomfort through the years.

Rating Your Own Posture

The most mechanically efficient positions and ways of moving seldom come about naturally. At least 75 per cent of American youth could gain substantial improvement in efficiency and appearance through postural training. Although most of the worst postural problems have had attention by college age, further improvement in posture is almost always possible. If you can get expert evaluation of your posture and body mechanics through the Physical Education Department of your school, by all means do so. Posture and body mechanics involve many individual variations which no self-administered test can take into account. If professional evaluation seems impractical, this group of screening procedures (which your teacher may want you to perform in class) will help you judge how much you might be able to improve your own posture:

The front wall test

Assume your usual standing posture with the tips of your toes barely touching the bottom of a smooth wall. Your chest should barely touch the wall. The tip of your nose should be approximately one inch away from the wall. The front of your thighs should be just far enough from the wall to let you slide your hands into the breach.

The back wall test

Stand with your heels, hips, and head against a smooth wall. Try to slide your hand between your low back and the wall. If the hollow of your back admits your hand, you should check with an expert in posture to see whether changed alignment might yield extra muscular efficiency, protection from injury, and a decreased rate of wear and tear on the joints of your spine.

The footprint alignment test

Walk across a stretch of soft ground or sand, or walk with wet feet across dry pavement. Draw a straight line along the center of your track. The inside margins of your heels should barely touch the line marking your body's course. Your toes should generally point straight ahead (although not always). If the toes point markedly inward or outward, appraisal of your body mechanics by a trained posture expert seems wise.

Appraisal of sitting posture

Feet flat on the floor, chest high, and back part of the top of the head stretched toward the ceiling make for ideal sitting posture. Your seat should be low enough to allow firm planting of the feet, your chair back should give support just above the rim of the pelvis, and surfaces on which you work should be more than four inches above the level of your knees.

Posture Correction

If medical examinations have never revealed any serious underlying disorder, postural defects usually result mainly from faulty habits and may respond to a few weeks' intensive retraining. Most people need to remind themselves continually of any new postural patterns they are trying to establish. These methods of self-correction have proved of considerable value:

Walking away from a wall

Stand with your heels four inches away from a wall. Flatten your back against the wall by rolling your pelvis forward on your hips, contracting your gluteal muscles and those of the lower abdomen. Try to leave the upper abdomen loose and tighten only the muscles from the umbilicus

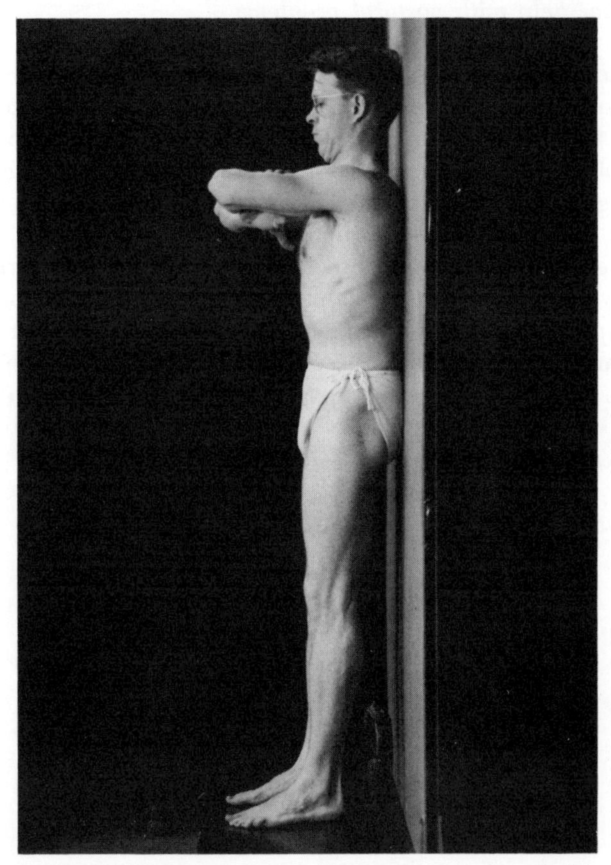

Figure 65. How to flatten your back against a wall. *From* Physical Medicine, *Frank H. Krusen, Copyright 1941. W. B. Saunders Co. Philadelphia.*

down. While learning this action, take several deep breaths to see whether the upper abdomen moves freely. Stretch the back of the top of your head toward the ceiling and raise your chest up. Rock forward away from the wall without changing the position of your trunk or head, and go about your daily activities.

Check sitting posture

Several times during the day, see if you are sitting tall with feet flat on the floor.

Further help with postural problems

If you do not make much progress in improving your posture with home measures, or if your posture problem is severe, you may want to get further help with it. A complete medical and orthopedic examination is a good starting point. If no disease or deformity seems at fault, the instructors in your college's physical education department may be able to give you substantial help. Gymnasium equipment, full-length mirrors, and various specific exercising and training techniques often let you correct posture problems which you have been unable to solve by yourself. In many colleges, posture improvement courses are offered as electives. In other institutions, you can enroll in special physical education classes to get individual attention. These courses give you an opportunity to spend twenty to thirty hours in guided postural training, which is often enough to establish lifelong improvement in bodily poise.

CHAPTER 17

Proper Care for Eyes, Ears, Nose, and Sinuses

By the time you reach college, your medical adviser usually depends on you to let him know if you have eye troubles. Unfortunately, visual problems sometimes take forms you may not instantly recognize. People who can read the fine print on the vision testing chart still suffer from eyestrain at times. If you want to keep feeling your best and working at peak, you need to recognize eye problems whenever they arise so that you can either correct or get help for them.

WHEN TO SUSPECT EYESTRAIN

Eyestrain may be troubling you whenever prolonged reading and close work or prolonged eye use at a distance (e.g., watching TV) leads to headache, inability to concentrate, irritability, or nausea.

Headache

Eyestrain headaches are usually steady rather than throbbing. Most victims describe them as dull discomfort over the eyes or at the back of the head. Discomfort usually starts in the late afternoon or evening, generally responds to aspirin, and always subsides during a night's rest.

Inability to concentrate

With or without headache, many people who have eyestrain suffer an impaired ability to concentrate. Many students who eliminate eyestrain of which they had previously been unaware (for instance, students who get glasses after visual defects are detected in routine examinations) report improved capacity for prolonged intellectual work.

Irritability, tension, and fatigue

Many people react emotionally to eyestrain. A dull, depressed feeling often results. Irritability, tension, and fatigue also occur.

Nausea or loss of appetite

Among preschool and school-aged children, vomiting is very frequently the principal complaint caused by eyestrain. By college age, stomach disturbances from eyestrain are somewhat less severe. Nausea and loss of appetite occasionally occur from eyestrain at any age, though.

HOW TO CONTROL EYESTRAIN

You get exactly the same complaints whether you do close work in dim light, allow the light-sensitive layer of your eye to be overstimulated, overwork the focusing and light-adjusting muscles, or overburden the muscles which turn your eyes. The extra brain work of interpreting the blurred images of poor vision causes eyestrain symptoms, too. Well-chosen home measures or proper professional care can conquer every one of these problems.

Work and rest

Your eyes can stand intensive use for a brief period. However, the level of strain you can tolerate for thirty minutes may cause headaches or fuzzy thinking after an hour or two. One way to keep this from happening is to arrange your work so that tasks involving less intense use of vision alternate with periods of very close work. Brief rest intervals help considerably, too. The custom of closing your eyes for a few seconds at the first good stopping point after turning each page helps keep you fresh. You may also find you are more efficient in doing close eye work at the start of each study period than later.

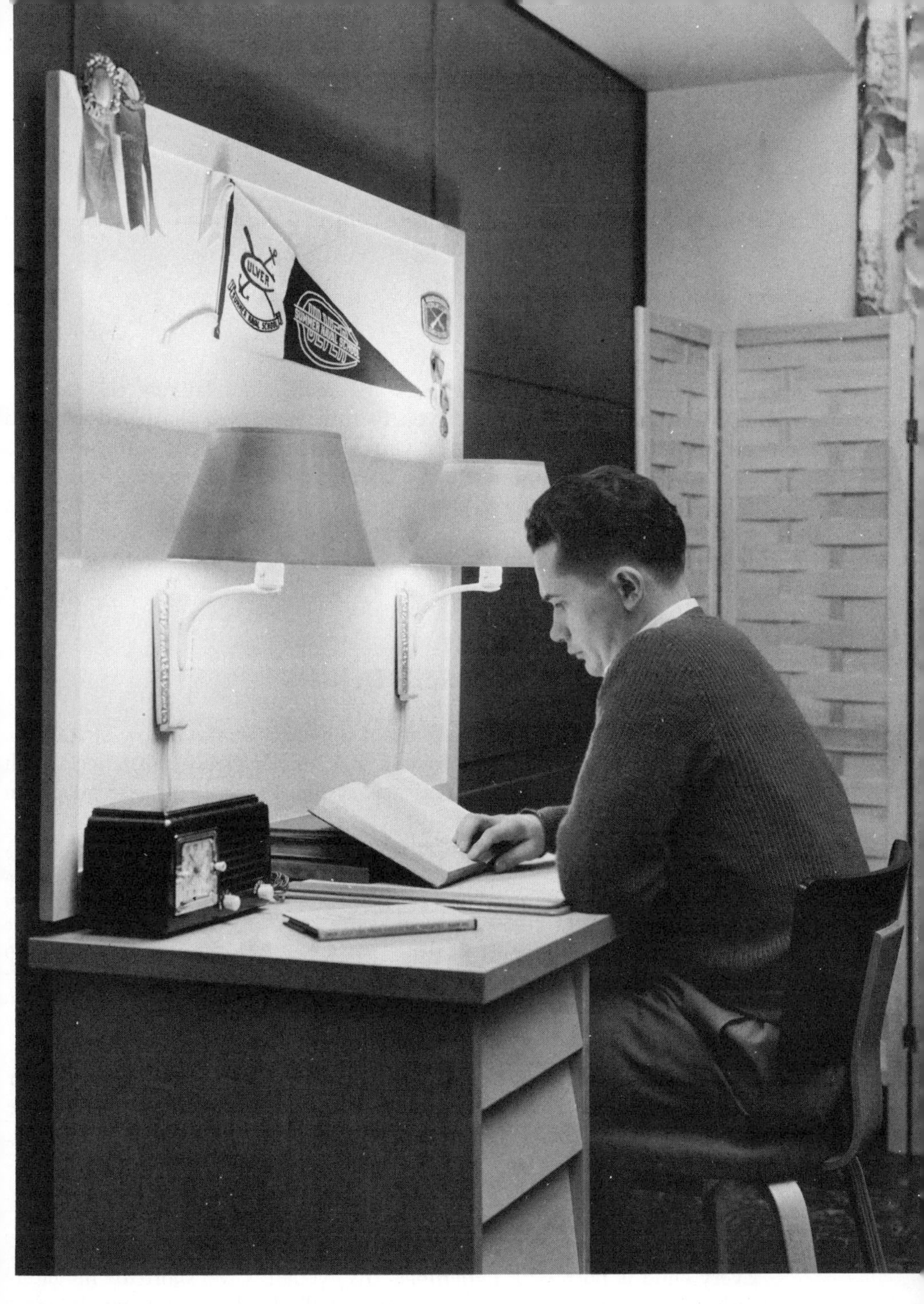

Figure 66. Good reading posture. *From* Studies of Lighting and Seeing for the Student at Home, *Mary E. Webber, Illuminating Engineering Vol. XLIV, No. 5, May 1949.*

Lighting

Follow the suggestions for adequate subject lighting and adequate gloom and glare free background lighting in Chapter 2.

Posture during eye use

The muscles which turn your eyes are small and relatively easy to tire. A study posture which requires you to turn your eyes sharply downward while reading, such as a lying or very slouched sitting posture, places a great deal of extra strain on the eye-turning muscles. This strain results in exactly the same complaints of eye fatigue and eyestrain which lighting defects would produce. An upright study posture with the book directly in front of your face and at the proper distance from it definitely helps prevent eye-induced fatigue.

Optical Defects

Your eye has a lens system made up of the clear front window of the eye, a watery substance, a highly refractile lens, and a glassy substance which fills the interior of the eyeball. This lens system focuses a precise image on

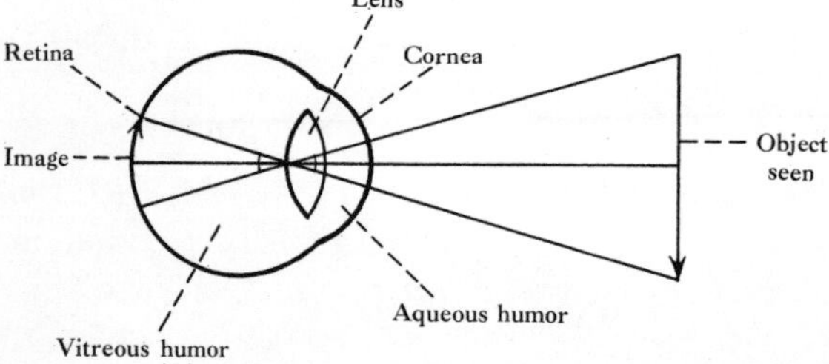

Figure 67. The normal eye focusses images precisely on the retina. *Adapted from* Parson's Diseases of the Eye *by Sir Stewart Duke-Elder, 13th Ed. (1959) with permission of J. & A. Churchill, Ltd., London.*

the sheet of light sensitive nerve cells at the back of your eyeball. Your vision is impaired if this lens system fails to focus light accurately on the retina. Four defects are very common:

Hyperopia or farsightedness

Every child is born with hyperopia. His eyeball is too short for his light-focusing lens system. As he grows, his eyeball slowly catches up. In most cases, the size of the eyeball matches the focusing plane of the eye's lens system at about age eight. If the eyeball grows too slowly to fit the particular lens system with which it must work, the individual remains hyperopic.

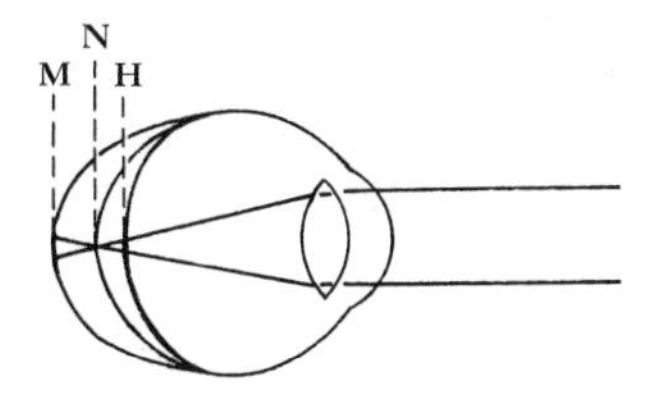

Figure 68. A lens system which focusses perfectly in a normal eyeball (N) gives a fuzzy image in hyperopia's short eyeball (H) or in myopia's long one (M). *Adapted from* Parson's Diseases of the Eye *by Sir Stewart Duke-Elder, 13th Ed. (1959) with permission of J. & A. Churchill, Ltd., London.*

In mild cases, he can rightly be called farsighted: by unconscious focusing effort similar to what a person with normal vision uses to look at close objects, he changes the shape of his eye's lens to get a clear image of distant objects. He is unable to bring close objects into focus, just as a normal person cannot see clearly within two or three inches of his eye. In severe hyperopia, distant vision is also impaired.

Hyperopia causes three important complaints. Most victims have headaches and other eyestrain symptoms brought on by continual tightness of the focusing muscles in their eyes. A few victims complain of blurred vision, although lack of a standard of comparison keeps most of them from recognizing this problem until after the defect has been corrected. The fact that clear images cannot be obtained from both eyes at once, plus natural reflexes which associate focusing effort with eye convergence, produce crossed eyes in many hyperopic infants and children.

Myopia or nearsightedness

If your eyeball grows or stretches until the retina is farther back than the focal distance of your eye's lens system, myopia results. This condition usually becomes evident in the later elementary- or high-school years and becomes steadily worse until about age twenty-five. The victim can focus on objects held close to his face, but sees distant objects as blurs. You should suspect myopia if the most comfortable position for reading a book brings the pages closer than ten inches to your eyes, if you have difficulty recognizing acquaintances across the street, if you get headaches from watching movies, or if you find yourself sitting much closer to the television set than other members of your family.

Astigmatism

Astigmatism, the most common cause of defective vision, is the least likely to result in severe visual impairment or other complaints. The optical curves in an astigmatic eye are slightly assymetrical, so that the curves in different planes (horizontal, vertical, etc.) focus light at different distances. When your eye is focused as perfectly as possible on either a near or a distant object, the imperfect focus of a portion of the light reaching the eye still makes things look fuzzy.

Astigmatism very often occurs in conjunction with either hyperopia or myopia.

Presbyopia

You focus your eyes at different distances by changing the shape of your crystalline lenses. After about age forty, this lens slowly becomes inelastic. Vision may be quite sharp for either distant or nearby objects, but not for both. Reading glasses or bifocals ultimately become necessary.

GLASSES

Properly fitted glasses can bring light into perfect focus on your retina whether you have hyperopia, myopia, astigmatism, presbyopia, or any combination of these visual defects. Although your eye doctor determines the

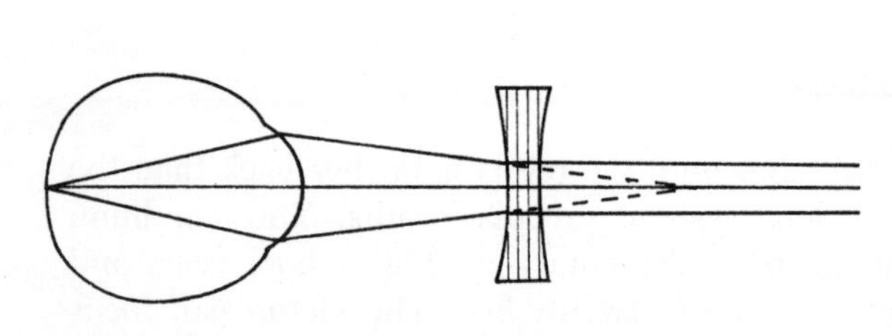

Figure 69. Myopic eye will not focus unaided on objects more than a few inches away. Glasses bend light to bring distant objects into focus. *Adapted from* Parson's Diseases of the Eye *by Sir Stewart Duke-Elder, 13th Ed. (1959) with permission of J. & A. Churchill, Ltd. London.*

exact shape of lenses required, he usually leaves the selection of frames and glass type to you. Here are several points which you may want to keep in mind:

1. The size of your lenses determines the breadth of your field of keen vision. If you have myopia or severe astigmatism and plan to drive a car, a fairly large lens surface is wise.

2. Generally speaking, glasses which follow or accent nearby facial contours look best. However, glasses can be used deliberately to provide

vertical, diagonal, or horizontal lines. A brief review of the principles involved in choosing makeup[1] is often helpful in selecting attractive frames to fit your face.

3. Ordinary lenses are not shatterproof. If you plan to wear glasses while you play athletic games or are otherwise exposed to falls or injury, hardened lenses are worthwhile.

College students often wonder about contact lenses. Contact lenses are mainly useful for moderate or severe myopia. They provide a very broad field of vision, are safe to wear even during contact sports, never fog up, and are virtually invisible. However, many people need glasses because of visual defects other than myopia and cannot use contact lenses. Contact lenses are expensive to buy and keep insured against breakage and loss. Discomfort from having something always in your eye ranges from occasional awareness to perpetual and unbearable annoyance: about one-third of the people who try contact lenses never get so that they can wear them; another third wear them for limited periods only.

OTHER EYE TROUBLES

Impaired vision, eye discomfort, and headaches related to eye use are often due to other eye disorders rather than to imperfect conformity of the eye's focusing system with its size or shape. If these other eye problems are present either alone or in conjunction with light-focusing difficulties, prompt identification and countermeasures are very worthwhile. In some instances, prompt treatment with medicines or prompt surgical operation will save or restore eye function which would otherwise be permanently lost. In others, the eye condition may reflect a serious disease state such as diabetes or high blood pressure, for which prompt care might be salutory. In the remaining cases, glasses and other such measures will prove ineffective, while more appropriate measures will often bring relief. Here are the most important eye disorders other than refractive error, arranged approximately according to the age at which they usually appear:

Muscle Imbalance

Crossed eyes and other eye muscle disorders lead to three separate problems: they are unsightly, they frequently cause impaired vision or blind-

[1] Check with your college librarian for a good book on grooming or cosmetology.

ness in one eye, and they interfere with depth perception, which is quite vital in this age of fast-moving automobiles and planes.

All infants have in-co-ordinated eye movements for several weeks or months after birth. Consistent crossing or divergence deserves attention even in the very young infant, but occasional, independent eye movement can be ignored. By six months, however, an infant should have good eye co-ordination. Any tendency toward crossed or divergent eyes beyond that age calls for a doctor's care even if it occurs only when the child is fatigued.

With prompt attention, eye specialists can cure most cross-eyed children without the need for surgery. Most cases are due to hyperopia, often hyperopia which is worse in one eye than in the other. If this condition is corrected with glasses before the child's brain learns to ignore nerve signals from the less useful eye, the child can often be taught co-ordinated eye motions.

Glaucoma

Glaucoma, an increased pressure within the eyeball, is the most common cause of blindness in the United States. When it strikes a child or a young adult, pain in the eyes and a dusky red band on the white of the eye surrounding the iris usually result. Medical care within the first few hours is essential if vision is to remain unimpaired.

A more gradual, subtle onset marks the commoner form of the disease, which usually strikes in the forties or fifties. On a dark night, the street lights often seem surrounded by rainbow-hued halos. Restriction of the field of vision may also be notable: the victim can see objects which he looks at directly, but has difficulty driving in traffic and has to look down at his feet when he walks to keep from tripping. A rapid change in focusing distance is also notable: some patients feel the need for new glasses only a few months after having a new pair fitted. Any of these signs deserves a doctor's attention. Prompt care usually saves vision and often averts the need for an operation.

Diseases of the Retina

Bleeding, infection, or other changes involving the light sensitive sheet at the back of your eye commonly cause visual problems. Large and persistent spots in front of the eyes or impairment of vision in one or several parts of the visual field point toward this sort of trouble.

An eye doctor frequently detects diseases ranging from diabetes or high blood pressure to tuberculosis or brain tumor through changes he can see in your retina. Even if these conditions are not themselves responsible for visual difficulties, the prompt care you get for them through an ophthalmologist's guidance may be very helpful.

Cataract

A cataract is a defect in the crystalline lens of the eye which renders it opaque or hazy. A few babies are born with cataracts; some young people get cataract through injury. However, the vast bulk of cataracts occur after

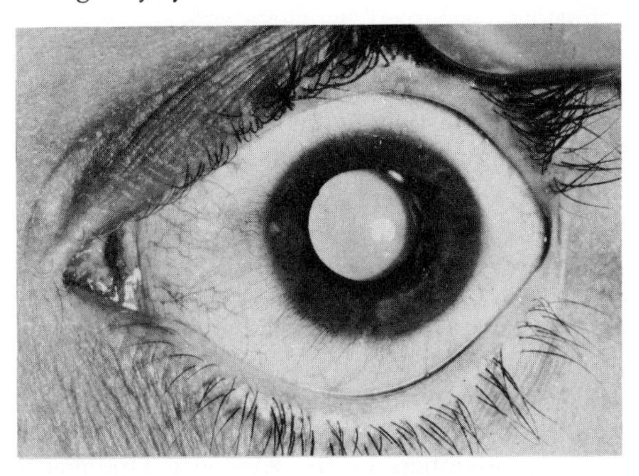

Figure 70. Cataract. *From* Parson's Diseases of the Eye *By Sir Stewart Duke-Elder, 13th Ed. (1959). With permission of J. & A. Churchill, Ltd., London.*

age fifty. The condition reveals itself as a whitish coloration of the pupil, and causes impaired vision. Treatment is by removal of the crystalline lens. Glasses bring light in to adequate focus on the retina after the light-obstructing cataract has been removed.

Scars of the Cornea

Congenital defects, injury or disease sometimes leave the eye's clear window permanently shaded with white scar. This portion of the eye gets its nutrition without direct blood supply, from oxygen and other substances floated to it across the underlying watery pool. The responses which ordinarily lead to rejection of parts grafted from one person's body to another's are mediated by blood vessels, and do not always occur in the cornea. Doctors can often restore vision to people blinded by a scarred cornea if some other individual will permit use of his own eye tissue (which is generally removed shortly after death). If you should wish to make such a donation, the Society for Prevention of Blindness in your state or area will be glad to help you with the necessary arrangements, or you can write to the Eye Bank for Sight Restoration, New York, N. Y.

SOURCES OF EYE CARE

Most students are confused about the qualifications and functions of the three main professions concerned with eye care.

An *ophthalmologist* or *oculist* is a physician specializing in eye care. His training includes college work, four years of medical school, and three to five years' further training in distinguishing and managing eye disorders. He supports himself by charging fees for examining or treating your eyes rather than by making a profit on the sale of glasses.

An *optometrist* is not trained in medical methods of diagnosis and care. However, he has received considerable professional training in improving vision by optical means, with emphasis on the fitting of glasses. His training includes considerable material on recognition of eye disorders, but very little on medical diagnosis and care of eye disorders. Many practicing optometrists received only four years of training after high-school graduation, although present-day graduates receive five years' training and further increase seems likely. Members of the American Optometric Association have pledged themselves to support-by-fees like that practiced by eye physicians, but a large proportion of optometrists still practice on an "eyes examined—glasses fitted" basis which ties their income to your purchase of new lenses or frames.

An *optician* supplies lenses according to the recommendations of your ophthalmologist or optometrist, installs them in frames, and adjusts or adapts the frames to assure comfort and efficiency.

Ophthalmologist *vs.* Optometrist

When you or some other member of your family needs eye care, you have to choose between a medically trained eye doctor and an optometrist. Here are several points which you should keep in mind:

1. Only the ophthalmologist or oculist can use drops. It is impossible to fit glasses accurately for victims of hyperopia so long as they can change the shape of their eye's own lens by involuntary focusing effort. The medically trained eye doctor paralyzes the focusing muscles of the eye completely with drops, assuring visual correction with the eye's focusing muscle at omplete rest. The optometrist attempts to achieve similar ends by relaxing he eye muscles for twenty minutes or so. However, prolonged tightness of he eye's focusing muscle, which almost always accompanies uncorrected yperopia, leads to long-sustained spasm of the muscle: up to three days, ccording to one authority. This would seem to give the medically trained ye doctor a marked advantage in accurately fitting glasses for hyperopic ndividuals (at least until the lens loses its elasticity in middle age).

2. *The ophthalmologist or oculist treats eye diseases involving more than ision.* Redness or irritation of the eyes, pain in the eyes, spots in front of he eyes, patches of impaired vision, or other signs of eye disease rather han purely optical disparities deserve medical attention, which makes an phthalmologist your best bet. Even if complaints are mainly of poor vision, he chance of a disorder which calls for medical treatment increases sharply rom age forty-five on. This would appear to give the ophthalmologist or culist an advantage over the optometrist after this age.

3. *A payment plan which ties the examiner's income to your purchase of lasses encourages abuse.* While some optometrists who work in close lliance with opticians are undoubtedly honest, others seem to have sucumbed to the temptation to sell more glasses than their patients can use. oth the American Optometric Association and the ophthalmologists' groups trongly oppose the "eyes examined—glasses fitted" pattern of payment. Having seen several cases which seem hard to explain on any other basis, feel sure that abuse is a real risk in "eyes examined—glasses fitted" estabishments, and advise my own clients to pay a fee for an examination rather han to take a chance on getting stuck for several times as high an expendiure for lenses which they do not need.

HOW TO CONSERVE HEARING AND EAR COMFORT

One of the most common problems for which college students seek medical advice is accumulation of wax in the ears. Hearing loss is frequent by college age, too, and becomes steadily more so as the years go by. You can take several practical steps to control these problems now and in the future.

Ear Wax

Everybody's ears form wax. Chewing and speech impart slight motions to the outer ear canal, which usually milk the wax out. In some people, either the shape of the ear canal or the consistency of the wax hampers this action. Wax accumulates in a thick, dry plug. Itching, impaired hearing, and ear discomfort frequently result.

Removal of ear wax

Any attempt to dig out ear wax with a hairpin or other small object is very likely to damage the eardrum and delicate middle ear structures. If you have a tendency to accumulate ear wax, best let your doctor remove the heavy plug and advise measures to prevent reaccumulation.

Hearing Tests

Mild or moderate hearing loss muffles or distorts sound without blanking it out. Gradual onset or long duration give many victims no clear standard for comparison. A great many people therefore have hearing defects of which they are unaware. If these people learn of their difficulty through a hearing test, they can often cure or stop the progress of the underlying disorder, make hearing loss less of a handicap through ear training or use of an aid, and arrange classroom seating and the like to suit their special perceptual needs.

Doctors or trained technicians can test hearing very accurately with a pure tone audiometer. This instrument produces a sound of designated pitch and loudness so that the precise level of loudness detectable at various pitches can be determined. Results are reported in units of hearing *loss*, so that high plus readings show poor hearing and minus readings show extraordinarily good hearing. Because the difference between good and poor hearing may be a thousand or a millionfold, an ordinary unit of measurement would make reports arithmetically clumsy, and an exponential unit has been chosen as standard. The decibel doubles about every five units, so that a 20 decibel loss is four times and a 40 decibel loss in 64 times as great as a 10 decibel loss.

As a poor second best when audiometry is not available, the whisper test is sometimes used. The tester practices whispering just loud enough that several people with presumably normal hearing can barely distinguish numbers or words at fifteen feet distance. A person who cannot hear at this distance then moves closer until sounds become plain. Inability to distinguish numbers or words with either ear from ten feet or more distance justifies more accurate testing and professional appraisal.

Middle Ear Infection

Earache, fever and pus or matter draining from the ear result when the middle ear cavity becomes infected. Scarring may lead to persistent hearing loss unless treatment clears up the process promptly. The germ-laden back portions of your nasal passage connect through a small tube with the normally germ free middle ear cavities. Germs move through this passage

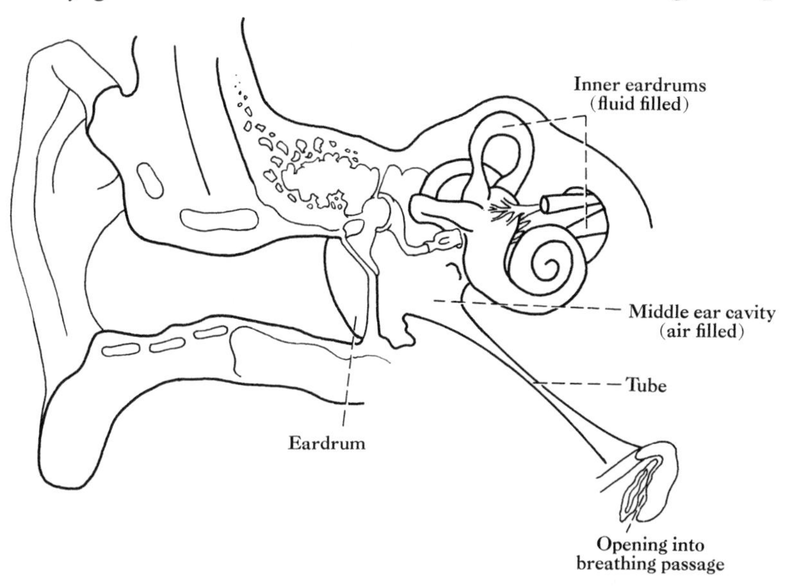

Figure 71. The ear. Air moves through tube connecting middle ear cavity and breathing passage with change of altitude, nose blowing, and other pressure alterations. Eardrum is normally air-tight.

mainly with bursts of air generated by nose-blowing, sneezes, and coughs. Severe infection can destroy part of the eardrum, making another possible portal for infection to enter. Smoldering or repeated infection can leave scar tissue which binds down the delicate moving parts inside the middle ear cavity. Poor hearing results, with especially severe loss in the high-frequency ranges through which you achieve most distinctions required to understand human speech.

How to avoid smoldering or repeated middle ear infections

You can usually avoid smoldering or repeated middle ear infections, and thus help to conserve your hearing. These steps seem both practical and efficient:

1. Blow your nose gently, or not at all. Although it may sometimes be socially inept, the most hygienic way to dispose of nasal secretions is to sniff them back and either spit them out or swallow them. Your normal stomach acids destroy the germs, and no bursts of air carry infection into either your ears or your sinuses. Second best: blow gently with both nostrils open. Absolutely worst: blowing hard with the more open nostril deliberately held closed.

2. *Try not to encourage use of antibiotics for your colds.* The "ounce of prevention" approach does not work in keeping ear infections from arising in the course of ordinary colds. Ear infections are just as frequent and last longer when penicillin is used for colds. Probable explanation: when all the germs which penicillin can affect are killed, other germ families take advantage of the lack of bacterial competition to multiply prodigiously. These germ families cause infections which do not respond to ordinary treatment measures, as infections with the original germ families would have done. Patients who use up old supplies of antibiotic, pressure their doctors for strong medicines, or otherwise encourage use of antibiotics for colds actually do themselves more harm than good.

3. *Arrange care promptly for middle ear infection.* Many middle ear infections today do not drive you to a doctor with severe pain. Milder earache, uncomfortable fullness in the ear, slight evening fever, and mushiness of hearing make up a pattern of smoldering infection which, because it is frequently neglected, leads to more hearing loss than abrupt, severely painful ear infections. If you see your doctor promptly for such complaints, he can usually clear up the situation quickly and inexpensively.

Ear Injury from Noise

Loud sounds can cause permanent hearing impairment. In avoiding this hazard, you will want to keep several points in mind:

1. Sound intensity varies as the square of the distance from the source. A farm tractor which causes no hearing damage when you are sitting in the driver's seat will still damage your ears if you put your head close to the motor.

2. High pitched sounds seem less loud than they are. Your ears receive sounds of different pitches with different rates of efficiency. Since ear damage from noise strikes an octave or so below the pitch of the offending sound, a high pitched whine can still cause serious ear damage even if it does not seem terribly loud and falls well outside the speech frequencies.

3. Continual exposure to noise levels which do not instantly damage your ears can ultimately cause permanent harm. Industrial noise, farm machinery, airplane engine noise, and so on are as dangerous as shotgun blasts when you work around them for weeks or months.

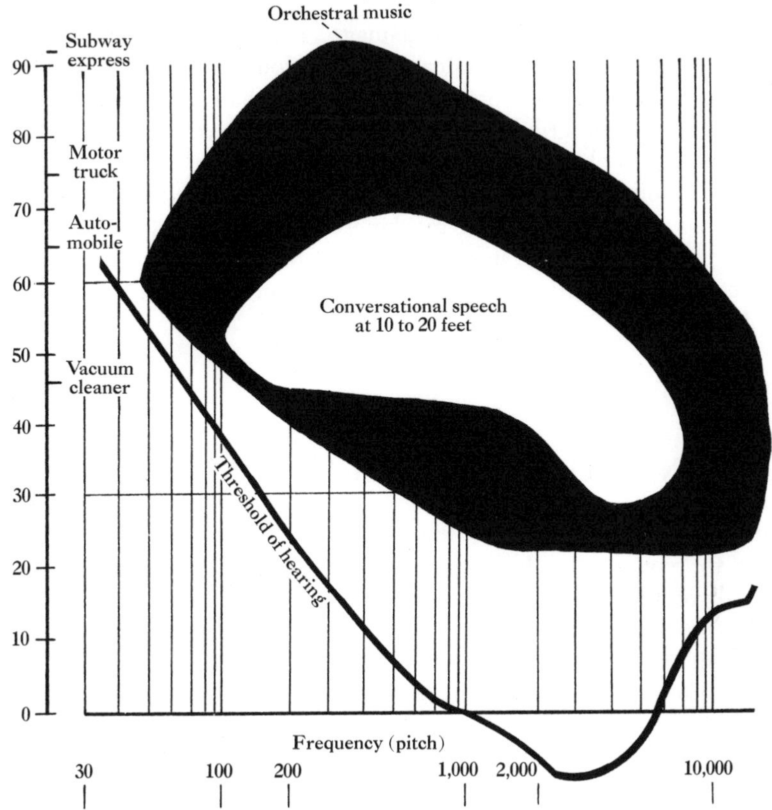

Figure 72. Threshold of hearing (softest sounds audible to the average ear) varies considerably for sounds of different pitch. Threshold levels are shown here in relationship with commonly perceived sounds. Note that proper hearing of music and speech requires greater keenness of perception in the upper than in the lower frequency ranges and that the margin between the usual thresholds and important-to-perceive sound levels is quite narrow in the upper ranges. *Adapted from* Radio Today *by courtesy of Maico Electronics, Inc.*

How to protect your ears against noise damage

Several practical steps help you to avoid noise-induced hearing loss.

1. Approach known noise hazards gradually. Too many people walk right up to a screaming jet or fire off a magnum load in a twelve gauge shotgun without first making any effort to find out whether their ears are noise sensitive. If these people would try their ears out at greater distance, fire a few rounds of smaller shells, or use well-fitted earplugs during their earlier exposures, many of them would get warning complaints on time to avoid permanent hearing loss.

2. Stay alert for signs of noise damage. Pain in the ears during noise exposure, ringing in the ears after hearing a loud noise, or impairment of hearing quality commonly precede permanent changes. Impaired hearing quality usually is described as "a tin ear" or "everything sounds like it's coming through a cheap radio with bad speaker crack."

3. Have careful tests of hearing during early months of exposure to loud noise. If you work around noisy machinery at any stage of your career, get a hearing test before you start and after a few weeks of exposure. Tests often detect slight hearing loss months before permanent or severe changes take place.

NASAL AND SINUS COMFORT

Your nose not only gives you the sense of smell, but also acts as air conditioner for your entire breathing passage. It filters out and disposes of almost all of the germs you breathe in and warms and humidifies each breath. These functions subject your nose lining to hazards and strains which frequently cause considerable discomfort or disease. A few simple measures often help your nose to bear its burdens without difficulty.

How Your Nose Handles Germs

Your nose traps the vast bulk of the germs you inhale upon its inside surface. Three mechanisms help keep it free from infection in spite of its constantly germ-laden state:

1. A sticky mucus blanket covers the entire inside surface of your nose. Normally, this is exceedingly thin and virtually invisible. However, myriad germs stick to it. Tiny sweeper cells in the nose lining sweep the mucus blanket continuously back toward the throat. Every six to seven minutes, the entire nasal passage gets a fresh coating of mucus, and the old layer with its millions of ensnared germs goes down into the stomach.

2. Your nose has a delicate but highly effective germ-combating sheet of lining tissue.

3. Your nasal lining has a tremendous network of tiny blood vessels through which extra circulation can be brought in to heat up or moisturize the air, fight infection, and repair tissue. There are so many vessels which are normally not needed that the nose lining can swell to many times its usual thickness by opening up reserve vessels.

How Your Nose Handles Dryness

Your nose wafts each breath past crinkled fins which project from its interior. The vast surface which these fins provide allows moisture and heat quickly to permeate each fresh breath.

Although the ideal moisture level in the air you breathe is approximately 70 per cent, a normal nose can moisturize air down to 25 per cent or less without difficulty. At lower moisture levels, the stream of dry air hitting

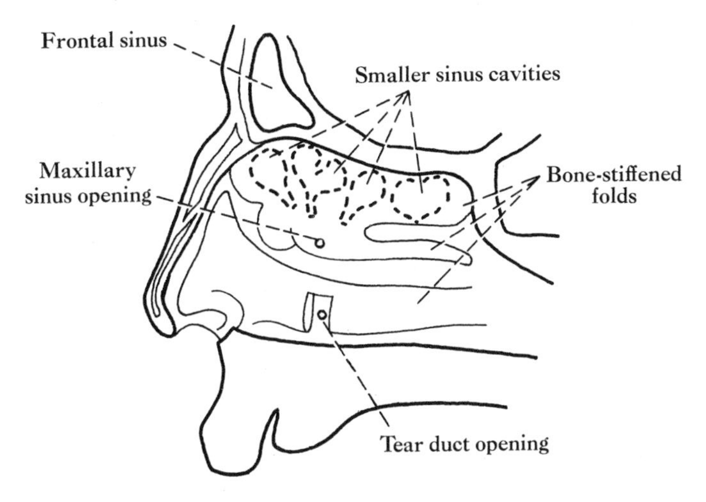

Figure 73. Bone-stiffened corrugations jut into nasal passage, partially covering sinus and tear-duct openings. *Adapted with permission from* Developmental Anatomy, *Leslie Brainerd Arey, 6th edition (1959) W. B. Saunders Company, Philadelphia.*

just within the nose dries the mucus blanket into irritating crusts. Further drying action damages the lining layer of the nose, and this sometimes allows germs which would otherwise be excluded to cause infections. It sometimes allows tiny splits to form with resulting discomfort and nosebleeds.

Practical Steps for Nasal Comfort and Protection

You probably can eliminate considerable nagging discomfort and prevent a substantial number of colds or other infections by measures aimed at protecting your nasal lining. These steps frequently have value:

1. Push down that thermostat. Nasal drying stems from low relative humidity. Relative humidity is determined by the relationship of the moisture content of the air with the total amount of moisture that air could hold at the prevailing temperature. The total amount of moisture air can hold approximately doubles every five degrees as you warm it. Nice, moist air at 20° becomes quite dry by the time you heat it to 68°, and crackling, desiccating dry at 80° or 85°. The simplest and most practical way to raise the relative humidity of the air you breathe is to lower its temperature. Sixty-eight degrees seems the most healthful daytime level. Nighttime settings can be five to ten degrees lower. Adequate clothing and covering for personal comfort is a necessary part of this program, of course.

2. *Humidify your surroundings if possible.* A humidifier in the warm air hood of an air circulation furnace or a shallow pan on ordinary radiators contributes worthwhile moisture. Substantial increases in relative humidity often result. However, you usually cannot evaporate enough water to reach ideal humidity levels in this way.

3. *Lanolin or pure petroleum jelly.* If crusting or dryness-induced nosebleeds continue after taking the above steps, lanolin or unmedicated petroleum jelly applied just inside the nasal orifice provide considerable protection.

Direct moisturization

In many cases, either nasal drying or nasal irritation due to rapid fluctuations in relative humidity at the change of seasons causes crusting, drainage back into the throat, and other unpleasant symptoms. You can combat moisture-deficiency effects by spraying or snuffling plain water, mild salt water (one teaspoonful to the pint), or a special solution your doctor can prescribe.

What about Sinus Trouble?

Your paranasal sinuses are air-filled hollows in the bones near the nasal cavity. They open into the nasal cavity through small orifices. Your sinuses normally keep themselves free of germs and irritants by sweeping a mucus blanket through into the nose continuously. If infection or irritation gets a start in one of your sinuses, however, the resulting swelling of the sinus lining often stops up the sinus opening and interferes with this mechanism. Infections in the nose often cause so much engorgement of the nose lining that it bulges into or down upon the sinus opening, causing blockage, irritation, or infection.

Probably most victims of sinus discomfort do not actually have sinus infection. Whenever a sinus gets stopped up, the moving mucus blanket which normally clears irritants from the sinus can no longer carry out its function. The sinus becomes irritated and painful whether germs are present or not. While medical measures often prove very helpful, sinus irritation does not involve the major health threats which make prompt care urgent for true sinus infection. Throbbing pain, fever, and general aches and pains in conjunction with sinus discomfort point toward actual bacterial infection, which could spread to the bones of the skull or into the brain cage if unchecked. Prompt and intensive medical care is always worthwhile.

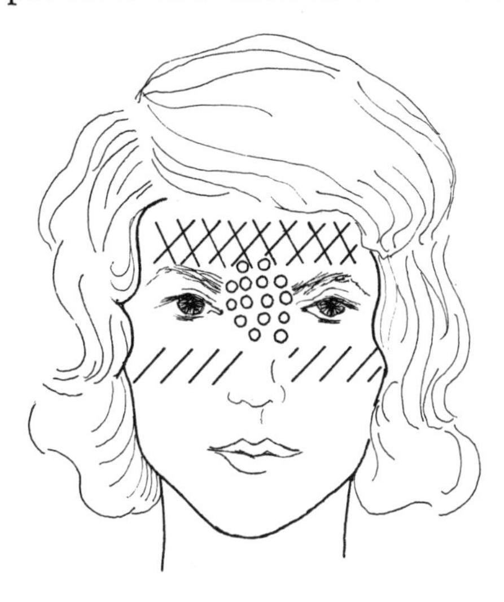

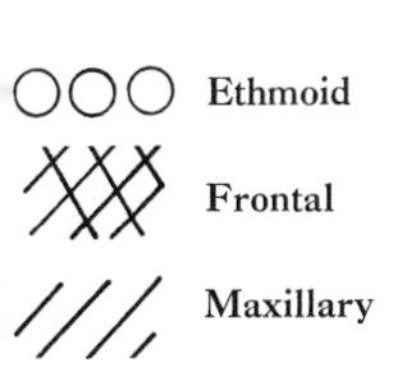

Figure 74. Sites where discomfort might be due to sinus trouble.

If you are subject to sinus discomfort or infection, certain preventive measure may help you to avoid some future attacks:

1. *Avoid extreme pressure changes.* A rapid descent in air or water raises the pressure inside the nose and drives germ laden material into the sinuses. Main practical application: sinus sufferers should enter the water by wading or with a shallow racing dive and avoid deep diving or underwater activity. Nose plugs are of no help because air pressures change inside the lungs and breathing passages on descent into the water whether the nose is open or not. The whole chest acts like a gigantic bellows to build pressure in the closed-off nose.

2. *Control nasal air blasts.* Sneezes, coughs, and violent nose-blowing drive germ laden material into the sinuses. Cold and cough remedies containing codeine and similar prescription-only drugs are the only readily available medicines effective enough against coughing and sneezing to prevent this effect. You can rid yourself of nasal secretions without blowing violently either by sniffing or by blowing gently with both nostrils open.

3. *Prevent sinus blockage.* As long as mucus can move out of a sinus freely, infection is unlikely. Your doctor can correct many conditions which

cause continual or repeated episodes of sinus blockage, such as a crooked wall between the two sides of the nose, hay fever, or other allergy causing swelling of the nasal lining.

4. Avoid prolonged or frequent use of nose drops. Many doctors advise drops or spray for two or three days during each cold to shrink the nose lining, which is generally safe. However, the drops themselves often cause severe congestion beginning an hour or two after you use them if you continue them for too long. When you take more drops to relieve that congestion, you perpetuate your problem.

CHAPTER 18

How You Avoid or Resist Germs

INFECTIONS, WHICH ARE DISORDERS CAUSED BY GERMS, CREATE A GREAT DEAL of suffering, disability, and expense. Most infections occur only when a substantial number of germs from one infection-causing family simultaneously attack one individual. If you can either cut down the number of disease-causing germs you encounter or build your resistance against them either by individual or by community action you will avoid a substantial burden of illness, disability, and death.

THE INFECTIVE DOSE

Infectious disease is always the result of an accumulation of germs sufficient to overcome your body's resistance. The number of germs required to set off infection may vary sharply between different individuals and in the same individual at different times, but a certain number of germs from the same family must attack your body simultaneously to cause disease.

The fact that a substantial number of these germs must pass from the infected person to a potential victim before he becomes ill refutes the common argument that "we've already been exposed to Mary's cold [or measles, or whatever it might be], so there's no sense trying to do anything about it now." If you or the community stop further exposure you will avoid illness completely even if you have acquired all but one single microorganism of the number necessary to start an infection. If you or your community keep further germs from reaching your tissues, you will not acquire a given infection even if the number of germs already passed has brought you to the very brink.

So far as your personal health precautions are concerned, the notion of the infective dose puts emphasis on close or continual contacts and associations. Casual contact with strangers seldom permits passage of infection. Even if the people you talk to over the counter or brush against in a bus were exuding infectious organisms at a fabulous rate, the odds are very much against your acquring an infective dose in a matter of a few seconds. On the other hand, the people with whom you share meals and quarters can give you an infective number of germs even if they are exuding relatively few organisms per hour. Those with whom you talk for any length of time in the course of your business and social affairs or with whom you share a classroom can easily deliver an infective number of germs also. You must, therefore, emphasize arrangements and behavior in your home and social and ordinary business or school life in your efforts to avoid germs. A furniture arrangement which keeps people six feet instead of four feet apart in your living room makes more difference than accommodations to reduce crowding on your commuter bus, for instance.

The notion of the infective dose puts heart and soul into community measures to halt spread of disease. If Johnny gets mumps while at school, some already-exposed classmates will be saved from infection if the boy is excluded promptly. If Mr. Smith's x-rays show tuberculosis, prompt follow-up and control measures (if studies establish the need for them) may save many of the victim's associates from contracting the disease. Since a definite number of germs must pass to a given individual before the infection will develop, there is often time for preventive action after the threat becomes known.

Limited Germ Spread Helps Everybody

If you can keep an infection from spreading from Mr. Jones to Mr. Smith, you not only protect Mr. Smith himself but also all of the people to whom he would have given the disease and those to whom the people he infected would have passed it along, and so forth. Measures which limit the spread of disease thus benefit the entire community, not just the individuals directly concerned. For example, suppose that a disease would normally spread to two new victims from each person afflicted and would show up in exactly one week. Each case today would cause two cases next week, four a week afterward and sixteen the following week. Now suppose that community measures such as immunizing injections, prompt withdrawal of infected individuals from contact with all others, and improved sanitation or housing protected half of the people formerly destined to become diseased. Each case this week would lead to one case next week, one the week afterward, and one the following week. Any slight further control effort would lead to a break in the chain and total protection for all the remaining uninfected people. Moreover, natural or seasonal elements often interrupt further spread of the disease, leaving uninfected people free of further risk.

Basic Methods for Limiting Microbial Spread

Both individual and community programs to limit the spread of infectious disease generally use one of three basic approaches.

1. Quick cure or suppression. If you cure a disease before its victim has a chance to pass his germs along, further spread does not occur. It is cheaper to cure a person of syphilis than it is to keep him from spreading his disease or to find and warn everyone to whom he gives it. An operation to remove the tubercular portion of a person's lung costs less than the sanitarium care he would otherwise require for months or years to keep him from spreading his infection. Treatment for scarlet fever kills the germs within twelve hours, relieving the need for prolonged confinement.

Treatment early enough to prevent spread usually costs no more in money, effort, or misery than treatment undertaken solely for the current disease victim's sake. In a sense, the prevention of further disease spread by prompt cure is virtually free, which makes it preferable to other methods whenever it can be applied. However, quick detection and cure can never do the whole job. Infected persons can seldom be found before they are capable of spreading their disease. The period of communicability, which is the period when sufficient numbers of germs are being spread to make delivery of an infective dose to another person possible, usually starts before illness begins. Spread may occur during an infection which is so mild that the disease is not identified or even one which the victim does not recognize as an illness at all. Moreover, curative measures are not available for many communicable diseases.

2. Increase specific or nonspecific resistance. Measures that increase the number of organisms that must reach a potential victim before infection occurs limit the spread of disease. Immunization, better nutrition, and general health improvement fall into this category. The next section discusses these measures in detail.

3. Block the pathways by which microorganisms spread. You can greatly improve your own chance of escaping communicable disease by trying to obstruct each of the common pathways by which organisms leave one infected person's body and reach another potential victim. Community measures to ensure sanitation even among people who seem in good health also help. The more stringent control measures are only worthwhile when serious infection threatens, as specifically discussed in the next chapter. The less stringent living customs and sanitary practices may prove worthwhile every hour of every day.

Respiratory Spread of Infection

The most common pathway by which disease spreads is the respiratory route. Every time you breathe out through your nose or throat, you expel thousands of germ-laden droplets into the air in front of your face. When you speak, sneeze, or cough, clouds of such droplets spray forth. Although most of the germs contained are harmless, the causative agents of many diseases are spread in this way.

Germ-laden droplets move from person to person in several ways. Mostly, they move in the form of heavy mist sucked into the recipient's breathing passages before even the heavy globules can settle to the earth. Six feet of space effectively protects you from this type of germ transfer. A small percentage of germ-laden mouth moisture sprays forth in very tiny droplets which dry into particles so light that they continue to waft about in the air for twenty-four hours or more. This mechanism results in disease mainly when the infective dose is very small, either because of the low resistance of the potential victim (e.g., in a nursery for newborn infants), or because of access to tissue of low resistance (e.g., in a surgical operating room, where germs from the air may settle into an open wound).

Shared drinking glasses, toys on which several children chew or blow, and inadequately sanitized dishes are other possible ways of transferring germ-laden mouth moisture. The kiss also deserves mention, if only to add a little thrill of danger to an impregnable custom.

Space and isolation

Space is one of your most important weapons against respiratory spread of disease. Most germ-laden droplets fall to earth within six feet even during conversation or after a cough or sneeze. You definitely can decrease potential disease spread by arranging your class seating, your home, or your office in a way that encourages people to sit six feet or more apart. Proper spacing is especially important when people stay together for long periods and when they talk a good deal. For instance, passive listeners in a lecture hall do not need as much space to insulate them against each other's germs as members of a seminar in which everyone takes his turn at talking.

Isolation uses the distance barrier to keep an infected person from spreading germs to new victims. Isolation means keeping the infected person in a separate room from people who might contract his infection. Whoever takes care of the sick person usually takes precautions against carrying disease germs outside of the sickroom on hands, clothing, linens, dishes, or sickroom utensils, and against contracting the sickness himself.

Quarantine is a much more stringent technique for limiting the spread of communicable disease. After an infective dose of germs gets to your body, they multiply and spread without causing fever or other complaints for several days or weeks. Toward the end of this period, considerable numbers of germs may appear in body secretions. Communicability thus often begins some days before actual illness commences. Quarantine takes this fact into account by isolating everyone who might possibly have become infected until after they would have become ill. Quarantine is usually applied only to control very serious disease outbreaks such as smallpox and plague.

Sanitary measures

Although most Americans are quite conscious of the risks involved in exchanging saliva, a few inconsistencies frequently mar our sanitary practices. Each member of the family always has his own toothbrush, but all frequently use the same bathroom glass to rinse their mouth. Mother pounces with horror when the youngsters take turns licking a sucker, but sits back calmly while they pass the harmonica back and forth. Sis passes up the remnants of little Joe's dessert because he touched it with his fork, then chews on the pencil he just took out of his mouth while she does her homework. Without making a fetish of sanitation, you can probably eliminate several such hazards in your own home. Simply walk through the house asking yourself what articles in each room are placed in the mouth or used in a way that smears them with mouth moisture. Then arrange that each such item be reserved for one person, or thoroughly cleaned immediately after each use.

The Fecal-Oral Route

The next most common pathway by which germs spread is the fecal-oral route. In many diseases, infectious material leaves one person's body with the intestinal discharges. Faulty sewage disposal may release this infectious material in potentially dangerous ways, or microscopic quantities of infectious material may get into circulation by way of the original victim's hands. Both of these pathways lead to other individuals by way of water, food, direct transfer, or indirect transfer. The recipients swallow infectious material in quantities or under conditions which prevent the stomach acids from destroying it.

Adequate sewage disposal and water supply

For personal health purposes, you can usually assume that any approved municipal system for disposal of sewage or for purifying water is adequate. Sewage and water problems usually fall directly on your own shoulders when you move into a suburb, visit a summer resort, or buy a farm. Here you are very likely to supply your own sewage disposal system through a septic tank and cesspool or through a privy, and secure your own water through a well.

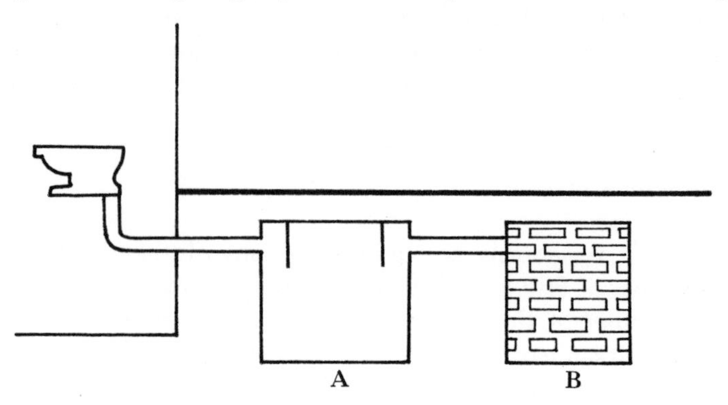

Figure 75. Individual disposal system. Sewage moves first into septic tank (A) where bacteria liquefy solid wastes. The liquid effluvient passes on to a cesspool (B) whose walls are laid in such a way that numerous chinks and channels let liquid material seep into the surrounding ground.

The biggest single problem arising out of septic tanks and cesspools is poor drainage. All water you use in your home has to sink into the ground immediately surrounding your cesspool. Unless this is located in sandy or loose soil and unless the elevation is such that the water table never floods out your system, sewage will ultimately back up.

Adequate space between draining sewage and wells is another absolute essential. A septic tank does not purify sewage: it only allows bacterial decomposition of solid wastes. Germ-laden fluids still flow through to the cesspool and into the ground. Feedlots (with concentrated animal droppings) and privies create similar hazards. A well should be at least fifty feet, and preferably a hundred feet, away from any such germ source and should be definitely uphill from it. If many germ sources are concentrated in a small area, as in a typical suburban housing development, even more spacing may be needed. Rock and limestone bases require greater spacing, too. They contain fissures in which water often flows rapidly and contrary to the surface contour of the ground.

Well construction deserves considerable attention. A good many wells in current use on farms and in summer camps do not provide the six foot concrete apron and other design features needed to keep rain or reflux from washing germs back down the inside of the well. Figures on well depth are often deceptive, too: what determines water purity is how far down the water goes through filtering dirt before a single drop of it can enter the well, not how far down the well extends in order to obtain adequate flow. A hundred-foot well with a twenty-foot casing is only twenty feet deep for purposes of purity. Twenty-five feet is usually a safe depth in sand or loam, but seventy-five feet may be required in other soils.

Body wastes and germ-soiled hands

Cleansing of the rectal area after bowel movements is fraught with sanitary hazards. Bacteriologically speaking, toilet paper is a snare and a delusion. Hordes of infectious germs readily penetrate it. Only thorough washing of your hands after bowel movements gets all of the intestinal bacteria down the sewer, where they belong.

Soilage of the hands with material from the intestinal tract also frequently occurs as a result of rectal itching, especially in young children. Pinworm infestation, which can only spread when eggs from the rectal area get into someone's mouth, is one of the commonest childhood disorders in America. Best single protection: thorough hand-washing after naps, on arising in the morning, and before meals. Frequently trimmed fingernails also help.

Food as a germ-spreading agent

Bacteria can multiply in food. A single infectious organism of certain families may grow into millions or billions within a matter of hours. Moreover, food is sometimes handled or prepared in such a way that infectious organisms can spread themselves through hundreds of different portions. One breach in a restaurant or dormitory's sanitary technique may lead to an epidemic.

Some foods are notorious for disease-spreading potential, and are distributed mainly under government supervision for that reason. Government standards are imposed on milk and dairy products through grading and labeling. If you want dairy products of the best sanitary quality, you should get only grade A products. Look for the word "pasteurized" on the label, too. Pasteurization gives substantial extra protection against milk-borne disease without appreciable extra cost or impairment of flavor. Watch the label with special care when you buy farmer's or gourmet varieties of cheese, which often reach the market without pasteurization.

In the case of meat products, government sanitary standards are imposed separately from grading standards. If the meat you buy has official "inspected and approved" stamps on it, proper precautions have been observed regardless of grade. Utility beef is just as sanitary as prime, the difference being mainly in fat content and other qualities affecting taste and texture.

The way food is stored and prepared is very important, too. Proper refrigeration, sanitary handling, and service without prolonged maintenance at lukewarm temperatures are key points.

Insects and Ticks as Carriers of Disease

Insects sometimes convey disease agents mechanically from feces or other infected material to a person's food or to his skin. "The fly who does not wipe his feet" feeds alternately on filth and foodstuffs, unless insect-tight outdoor toilets, screened windows, and properly covered food supplies frustrate him. Insects and ticks also act as vectors for certain diseases, which means that the disease-causing organism actually goes through part of its life cycle within the insect's body, then remains for a time ready to invade the human body. The commonest insect- or tick-spread disease in this country is Rocky Mountain spotted fever, which fortunately involves only a few, none-too-populous areas. Prompt search for ticks after possible exposure and their removal within eight hours usually prevents infection. Mosquitoes probably play some part in spread of certain forms of encephalitis. Flea-conveyed plague has spread widely among certain American animals, but human epidemics have not resulted. On the world health scene, insect-carried diseases such as malaria, yellow fever, epidemic, and murine typhus, and a variety of tropical diseases create many problems. The best way to control these disorders is usually to eliminate breeding of the insect vector. Insecticides, screening or netting to avoid bites, and medicine to suppress infection are also widely used. Whenever you visit countries in which insect-borne diseases occur, you should inform yourself about the necessary precautions.

Direct and Indirect Contact

Infections of the skin frequently spread from person to person by direct personal contact, or by indirect contact through infectious material deposited on towels, combs and brushes, or furniture. Infections such as impetigo and ringworm of the scalp often spread in this way. Individuals who have such conditions should take precautions against spreading them. However, the disease-spreading potential of such objects as doorknobs, money, and so on has been greatly exaggerated in the past. Such objects practically never play a part in the passage of disease.

Transmission of disease by blood transfusion, during drug injections, and in other bizarre ways are too infrequent to call for any special action on your part. Spread by sexual contact is discussed in Chapter 20.

RESISTANCE

You come into contact with disease-causing germs every single day. Only your resistance to those germs keeps you from being perpetually ill. By building and maintaining your resistance, you can avoid many infections which would otherwise make trouble for you.

General Resistance

General resistance is a capacity to respond quickly and efficiently to threats from microbes. Like any form of physical vigor, general resistance is partly inborn and partly the product of good morale, good nutrition, and adequate rest.

How much can you accomplish by building up your general resistance? At Trudeau Sanitarium, the doctors and nurses worked continually with tuberculosis patients, but masks and other measures to decrease passage of germs were almost unknown. By omitting masks, the superintendent felt that the importance of maintaining resistance was emphasized. The staff dining room provided a variety of excellent food, house rules required ten hours in bed at night, and excellent recreational and social facilities helped maintain morale. Result: a superb record regarding tuberculous infection among staff members.

You can probably cut your risk of various infections, from tuberculosis to the common cold, by following these principles:

1. Determine and fulfil your own basic rest requirements.
2. Follow the counting plan outlined in Chapter 14 for ideal nutrition.
3. Give recreational and social needs a definite place in your schedule.
4. Shift these patterns instead of abandoning them during periods of heavy work load, such as examination time. By using rest breaks instead of extra nighttime sleep, interspersing brief play periods with study sessions, and so on, you can maintain your efficiency much better than by plain, undiluted drive.
5. Give special emphasis to rest, nutrition, and morale when exposed to

unusual communicable disease hazards. Why not spend a little extra time in bed during epidemics of influenza or after one of your close associates comes down with a communicable disease? An extra hour in bed each day for a week might save you several days of illness by building your resistance before the germs take hold.

Tissue Immunity

Certain body tissues resist thoroughly many of the germ families to which they have previously been exposed. For instance, tissue immunity from an attack of mumps may keep the previously involved gland healthy even though general body mechanisms fail to protect the salivary glands not previously involved.

Perhaps the most important function of tissue immunity is to fight off the myriads of germs to which certain of your body parts are constantly exposed. Your nose lining, your mouth, and the inside of your intestine are constantly bathed in germs which would cause deadly infection in other parts of your system. Your skin glands continually harbor germs which cause raging infection when they get into deeper tissue.

Tissue immunity has one harmful indirect effect: it often makes people overconfident about the innocuous nature of saliva and surface dirt, and that overconfidence often leads to serious infection. Your mouth is second only to your rectum in bacteriologic filthiness. The immunity you have developed to its germs affects only the immediate vicinity. If you allow mouth germs to get into a wound by sucking it, for instance, serious infection may result.

Specific Immunity

An important factor in your resistance to infections is specific immunity. Every germ family has certain distinctive chemical compounds on its surface or makes certain distinctive poisons. When you have specific immunity against a given germ family, your blood and tissue fluids contain antibodies against one or more such chemical compound. Antibodies are biological substances your body makes specifically to combine with certain presumably harmful chemicals. When a germ family to which you have specific immunity starts to invade your body, antibodies quickly combine with the germs or with the poisons they make. Germs are killed or immobilized and poisons neutralized. Specific immunity does not make you completely immune in the sense that infection is impossible. However, it greatly improves your resistance against the affected germ families.

Once your body learns to make a given type of antibody, it can make large quantities very quickly. Perhaps three weeks are required to bring your antibody level to its infection-fighting peak when you first make contact with a given germ family or presumably harmful substance. If you have another contact with the same germ or substance years later, that same peak level will be reached in twenty-four hours. Moreover, your body increases its supply of every kind of antibodies which it has ever made whenever its production of any antibody is stimulated. This effect helps you fight off other germs when illness lowers your general resistance.

Naturally Acquired Immunity

Naturally acquired immunity is specific immunity which results from antibodies formed through direct contact with the germ family concerned. Natural immunity is produced in the course of most infectious illnesses. It also may be produced by repeated contact with small numbers of germs, even though these never succeed in causing infection.

Your past history of disease often affects decisions you must make in protecting yourself against further episodes. You usually can depend on naturally acquired immunity to keep you protected for life after an attack of measles or chicken pox. A slightly less reliable degree of lifelong immunity follows German measles, mumps, and whooping cough. Past attacks should not greatly influence you in deciding what precautions to take against other diseases.

Naturally acquired immunity probably plays a considerable part in protecting you against many minor disorders and in making those disorders mild. Foreign students in American colleges and Americans in foreign colleges suffer some extra frequency and severity of disease which seems at least partially due to their lack of previous exposure to the locally prevalent infectious ailments.

Active Immunization

Active immunization is a form of artificial immunization which stimulates the subject's body to produce its own antibodies against a certain disease. Active immunization produces prolonged immunity, but takes several weeks to be effective. Active immunity, therefore, is used mainly for long-term protection instead of being given after exposure to disease is known to have occurred. Active immunity is usually produced in three ways:

1. Inoculation with killed or detoxified material. Most of the material used for producing active immunization contains no living matter and causes absolutely no infection. The inoculated substance may be a suspension of killed organisms or a neutralized poison. The portion of the germ or poison to which antibodies form remains unaltered, while either death or chemical alteration makes the material innocuous.

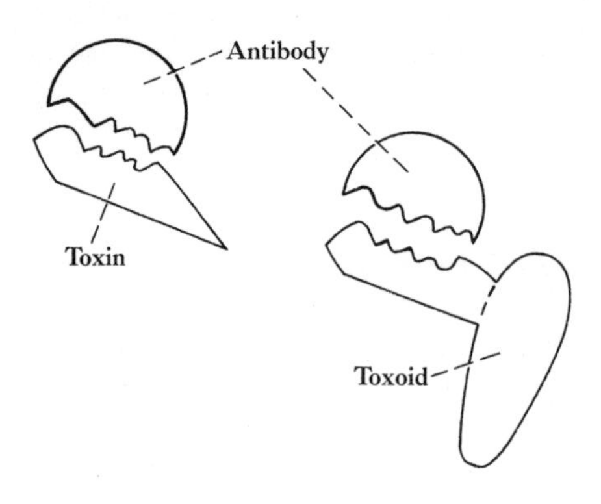

Figure 76. Diagrammatic representation of how a toxoid retains intact the portion of the toxin molecule to which antibodies form in spite of chemical changes which render it harmless.

2. *Inoculation with living material other than the disease agent.* Infection with an organism slightly different from that which causes a serious disease sometimes gives immunity against the serious disease itself. The mild infection may be naturally occurring, as in immunization against smallpox: this vaccination is really deliberate infection with cowpox, a very mild disease originally found mainly in milkmaids. The mild infection may be the result of change in the causative organism of the more serious disease through laboratory manipulation, as is true of yellow fever vaccine. In either case, a very mild infection yields effective protection against a dangerous disease.

3. *Inoculation with actual disease-causing organisms.* Live virus polio vaccines use unaltered disease organisms. These are selected for low capacity to invade the nervous system, but set up a definite, transmissible infection. Since our aim is to prevent paralysis, not polio virus infections *per se*, this approach seems valid.

Live organisms are also commonly used in veterinary practice to immunize young calves against infectious abortion. It is not used in humans at present.

Passive Immunization

Passive immunization supplements your own store of antibodies against a given disease with antibodies made by another person or animal. A mother gives her unborn child passive immunity lasting several months through antibodies passing into his blood stream from her own. Artificial passive immunizing agents give protection for several weeks, which is very helpful when exposure to infectious disease occurs.

The material used in conveying passive immunity against tetanus, diphtheria, and several other diseases is derived from animals. The animal (usually a horse) builds a high antibody level in response to active immunization and repeated booster doses. Immunizing antiserum consists of that portion of his blood in which the antibodies are most concentrated.

The material used to convey passive immunity against measles and hepatitis is derived from human blood donations. Blood from a hundred or so adult donors is pooled, so that blood from a number of persons who have been exposed to measles and hepatitis inevitably will be included in each batch. The portion of the blood which contains antibodies, namely the immune serum globulin, is separated from the rest and used for immunizing injections.

Your Immunization Needs

Although many of the diseases you can readily avoid through immunization have become rather rare in the United States, the potentiality of severe outbreak frequently remains. Every infant gets worthwhile benefits from active immunization against smallpox, diphtheria, tetanus, whooping cough, and poliomyelitis. Although different doctors advise slightly different schedules, the following general principles usually hold:

Smallpox

Vaccination in infancy and revaccination at approximately five-year intervals will maintain reasonably good levels of immunity. You seldom get fever, swelling, and soreness after your first vaccination with this program, because immunity from previous vaccinations usually reduces your response.

Diphtheria

Diphtheria immunization in early infancy followed by booster shots or tests of immune status every six years usually gives excellent protection.

Tetanus

Active immunization for tetanus has several advantages over taking antitoxin after injuries. It gives better protection when typical tetanus-inducing wounds occur. It causes many less unpleasant or dangerous allergic reactions. It gives a considerable degree of protection against the many cases of tetanus which arise out of mild scrapes or cuts, out of small children's injuries (of which responsible adults may be unaware), and out of infection which outlasts antitoxin-conveyed protection. After initial immunization, a booster every four years maintains good protection. A prompt booster after injury restores immunity quickly enough to avoid tetanus for up to ten years after the last previous inoculation.

Whooping cough

Whooping cough is very dangerous to infants, who therefore deserve inoculation within their first six months. One booster is advised at school age. Further boosters are worthwhile in the event of known exposure.

Poliomyelitis

At this writing, the recommended program for poliomyelitis prevention involves two injections one month apart, another after seven months, and annual boosters thereafter to age forty. Live virus vaccines give promise of longer lasting immunity but are still experimental.

School and Community Immunization Programs

Immunization helps everyone in the vicinity as well as the person immunized. When immunity keeps you from becoming ill, it usually also keeps you from passing disease along to other people, who in turn would pass it further still. An immunization program benefits the entire public rather than the immunized individuals alone.

Most health departments offer free immunization through well-baby clinics, school immunization programs and other free or low-cost agencies. Such programs try to reach all people, rich and poor alike, on the theory that immunization of any individual helps everybody. They should be clearly distinguished from welfare services, which are intended only for people unable to help themselves. You can take full advantage of public and school immunization programs without in any sense feeling that you are placing an undue burden on your fellow citizens.

Immunization in the Face of Special Hazards

Whenever you plan foreign travel, you should write to the State Department for up-to-date advice regarding immunizations; since uncomfortable reaction to these immunizations is usually less severe if they are spaced a week or more apart, an early start helps. Revaccination for smallpox is almost always necessary. If typhus, cholera, yellow fever, or any of several other diseases are occurring in the areas you will visit, immunization is wise.

CHAPTER 19

What To Do about Common Infections

PERHAPS NO OTHER HEALTH PROBLEM PLACES A GREATER BURDEN OF PERSONAL decision on you than infection. Early medical care of appropriate preventive measures make a tremendous difference, yet you must decide for yourself (and sometimes for your family) when such measures should be initiated. Well-chosen hygienic precautions and first aid measures can keep many very mild illnesses (for which you will not usually see a doctor) from leading to worse troubles. Even when you call your doctor immediately, you make many of the health decisions and carry out many of the procedures considered in this chapter.

INFECTIONS YOU CAN ATTACK IMMEDIATELY AFTER EXPOSURE

A few years from now, the chances are that you will get a printed card or a telephone call to the effect that your youngster has just been exposed to a certain childhood disease at school. In many cases, that card or call will give you an opportunity to ease a really serious health burden for your child. Here are the facts with which you can determine whether disease may be imminent and steps available to prevent or modify it.

Measles

A child who has not had the measles benefits greatly from protective measures applied after known exposure. Such exposure can be presumed to have taken place during classroom or other indoor association any time after the original victim develops sniffles and sore throat, which is usually about three days before the rash commences. Your doctor probably will suggest immune serum globulin in such an instance and try to make the disease milder instead of to prevent it altogether unless the exposed child is already ill with some other serious disease or is very young. By permitting a mild attack, your doctor lets you achieve a lasting immunity which no available artificial immunizing agent will convey.[1]

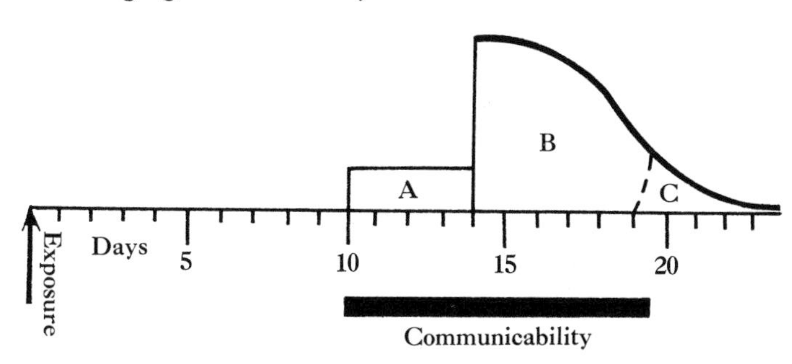

Figure 77. Course of measles. (A) Premonitory phase with mild to moderate fever, runny nose, aches and pains. (B) Active phase with red rash, fever, cough, watering, uncomfortable eyes. (C) Convalescent phase: rash turns brownish, skin peels slightly or flakes, disease no longer communicable.

Whooping Cough

If you have had inoculation against whooping cough in infancy, a booster dose after exposure frequently gives protection. If a very small child is exposed to whooping cough without having had inoculation, his doctor will probably urge passive immunization.

Streptococcal Sore Throat and Scarlet Fever

Sore throats caused by streptococcal infection frequently cause serious consequences. Streptococcal sore throat, scarlet fever, and so-called "scarlatina" involve identical risks of spread or complications and need not be distinguished from each other. Streptococcal infection often extends itself from the throat to the sinuses, ears, or bronchial tubes. Streptococci also set off mechanisms which frequently lead to rheumatic fever or to serious kidney disease. Once an attack of rheumatic fever has occurred, future streptococcal infections very often bring on recurrences.

Moderate doses of penicillin or other such medicines often will ward off

[1] Preparations now being tested seem promising, but are available only for experimental use.

or quickly cure streptococcal infection. These principles give some guidance to preventive use:

1. If you have definitely had rheumatic fever, your doctor probably will advise penicillin or similar preventive care.
2. If you may have had rheumatic fever, your doctor probably will recommend penicillin or similar treatment for every sore throat and preventive treatment whenever any close associate develops a streptococcal sore throat.
3. If you sustain family or household contact with streptococcal sore throat your doctor probably will advise penicillin or similar preventive care even if you have never had rheumatic fever or nephritis.
4. If you have a sore throat accompanied by fever of over 100° or by shaking chills, your doctor probably will want to examine you promptly to see whether penicillin treatment seems worthwhile.

Tetanus

The germs which cause tetanus thrive in certain types of wounds. Puncture wounds (e.g., from stepping on a nail) very often cause trouble. So do severe injuries from gunshot or from automobile accidents. Tetanus can result from almost any injury, however.

Tetanus is particularly frequent in rural communities. A great many animals harbor tetanus germs in their intestinal tract. These germs can live for several months in sand or soil. By that time, they have been tracked from the feedlot to every nook and cranny of a farm area.

If you have renewed your active immunization against tetanus recently, you probably have adequate protection against tetanus from minor scrapes and burns. You still require a booster with puncture wounds and serious injuries. If you do not have current active immunity, you should probably check with your doctor whenever an injury penetrates, breaks, or blisters your skin.

Rabies

If rabies virus is present in an animal's saliva, he has very little time left to live. When you must decide whether a bite or lick might have exposed you to rabies, the animal should be penned or tied for ten days. If he is still alive and well thereafter, you have no cause for concern. If he dies, his head should be packed in ice and sent special delivery to your state health department laboratory.

You should make every effort to identify and confine the animal which bites you or a member of your family, since this step often helps you to avoid the many injections and considerable risk involved in rabies vaccination. The animal should be penned or on a leash, not merely observed. Complaints produced by rabies may otherwise make him wander off, leaving the issue unsettled. The animal should not be shot unless already manifestly sick, and should not be shot through the head in any case (because definite tests for the presence of rabies cannot be done if the brain is destroyed). Bites by an animal which cannot be identified or penned should always lead to consultation with a doctor.

Other Serious Infectious Diseases

When you have family or household contact with hepatitis, diphtheria, or poliomyelitis, steps to give protection or boost preexisting protection are in order.[2] Suspect hepatitis if fever, nausea, or loss of appetite and dark colored urine or yellowish skin coloration occur. Suspect diphtheria if mild sore throat causes intense prostration. Suspect poliomyelitis if headache and backache follow three or four days of mild sore throat. Check these suspicions with your doctor, who will make the necessary arrangements for immunization and assistance if your fears prove justified.

INFECTIONS YOU CAN LIMIT BY PROMPT IDENTIFICATION

Several infections are often very mild when they first appear in the family group but ultimately spread to members of the family who become severely ill. If you suspect these processes and check with your doctor, serious health problems often can be avoided.

Impetigo

Impetigo is ordinarily a mild skin disorder of school children and adults, but it is a very serious, sometimes deadly disease in infants. Impetigo spreads easily from person to person, either by direct contact or by shared use of towels and linens. You should learn to recognize it (or at least suspect it) in order to protect your youngsters from exposure.

In its early stages, impetigo causes irregular-shaped blisters filled with

[2] Polio inoculation cannot be begun after exposure, but booster does help already-immunized individuals.

cloudy, yellowish fluid. Itching is intense, so the blisters are often broken by scratching before you spot the condition. A thick, crumbly, yellowish to dark brown scab forms over the sores. Sometimes new blisters appear nearby, where the germs have spread through scratching. Impetigo may start on the unbroken skin, but it also often starts in a healing scrape or wound. Your doctor can usually prescribe inexpensive measures which will give prompt cure.

German Measles

The unborn infant often sustains severe damage if his mother suffers an attack of German measles, especially during the early months of pregnancy. For this reason, you should try very hard to limit the spread of this disease even though its ordinary form is quite mild.

A German measles rash usually is easiest to spot on the trunk, and often comes out best after a hot tub or shower. You can often note slightly enlarged glands along the back of the neck either by running your fingers up and down the sides of the neck muscles or by shining a light tangentially on the area. Although your doctor cannot do much about German measles, you probably will want him to make a definite diagnosis and give advice on how to keep the condition from spreading.

Mumps

Many college students have never had mumps. Reinfections among people who already have had one attack are fairly common. The disease often involves the testicles in men of college age and above. While this very rarely leads to any impairment of fertility with modern care, it does make for a relatively long and uncomfortable illness.

You should suspect mumps if a swelling appears in the cheek and jowl. This swelling is usually very soft and ill-defined. It increases and becomes painful when the victim sucks on a lemon or eats a sour pickle. Mumps also can involve the salivary glands under the chin and beneath the tongue instead of in the cheek. In these locations, swelling may be quite firm. Sucking on a lemon or sour pickle causes discomfort, but usually no additional swelling.

Chicken Pox

Suspect chicken pox when tiny blisters, often surrounded by reddish margins, appear at the hairline and on the outside of the upper arms, spreading somewhat more thinly to other body areas. Some of the blisters have tiny dents in the center. A degree or so of fever is common, with itching, mild headache, and sometimes loss of appetite or slight aches and pains as accompanying complaints. Your doctor will suggest measures to control itching, since scratching of the blisters often leads to serious skin infection.

Most doctors today feel that the chicken pox virus also causes a somewhat more protracted and uncomfortable ailment known as shingles, which most commonly strikes middle aged or old people who have recently been exposed to chicken pox. Certainly, adults who have not had chicken pox or whose resistance might be expected to be low because of advanced age or smoldering disease should try to avoid close contact with chicken pox during its communicable stage (which lasts about five days after the rash appears).

Other Serious Infections

Severe headache, backache, aches and pains, fever, chilliness, sore throat, cough, or rash may signify serious infection. Among college students, severe and unexplained fatigue also deserves medical evaluation, frequently signaling infectious mononucleosis. Infectious mononucleosis is a virus infection which causes considerable changes in the white blood cells, lasts six to eight weeks, and virtually always responds to adequate amounts of bed rest. Most infectious disorders respond very quickly to prompt care, making medical evaluation of possibly infection-caused complaints especially worthwhile.

COMMUNITY AND SCHOOL PROGRAMS

Teachers and other school personnel often can detect evidence of communicable disease quite early in its course. They look closely at their charges many times during each day—more closely at times than parents, whose supervision becomes quite distant as the child's patterns of self-care and play become independent. Teachers watch children perform a great many different activities in which difficulties and abnormalities are revealed. They have considerable experience with children of similar ages, and have a group of normal youngsters always available for comparison. These points, plus the special health training they have had and the availability in most schools of a qualified nurse, often allow teachers and other school personnel to detect an illness of which even the parents have been unaware.

Most schools either return sick children to their homes or have the parents come for them. In order to protect other children from communicable disease, schools tend to send home any child under suspicion of having such an illness, even though they know their suspicions sometimes will prove unjustified. Some schools also notify parents of children who have been in classroom contact with communicable disease. This service helps in arranging protection against whooping cough or diphtheria. Such notices help make you alert for signs of disease when the risk is especially high, and help keep sick children who might spread infection further from coming to school. Rules concerning readmission after an absence also help keep youngsters whose disease is still infectious from reentering school as soon as they feel well enough to attend (or Mother feels that she has to get back to work).

Most communities take some action to keep victims of communicable disease from moving around freely and spreading their germs. For the usual childhood diseases, placarding generally suffices. A prominent notice states that chicken pox, measles, or whatever the case might be afflicts someone inside the home. This helps the neighbors keep susceptible youngsters out of contact with the victim. In more serious illnesses, community-imposed isolation sometimes seems necessary. The isolated victim must stay in until he no longer is capable of spreading disease, but his family can move in and out of the home freely. Only very stringent situations, such as a case of smallpox, call for quarantine, in which all possibly susceptible people in contact with the disease must remain confined until the danger that they will become ill has passed.

FIRST AID FOR MILD INFECTIONS

Although you will generally want to check with your doctor whenever you become ill, a common cold or a minor skin infection is not a medical emergency. So long as fever, extreme sore throat, prostration, or other signs do not suggest serious infection, first-aid type treatment usually suffices until the doctor's next regularly scheduled office period.

First Aid for Ordinary Colds

First aid and hygienic measures are very helpful for mild colds and scratchy throats. These measures will not conflict in any way with the program your doctor may ultimately suggest.

Rest

The best way yet discovered to build your powers of recuperation from minor illness is by rest. A brief rest break once or twice during the day is very valuable. Twenty to thirty minutes after lunch or before supper accomplishes more than an extra hour in bed at night. Ten hours of quiet relaxation at night help, too. Strenuous physical exertion probably slows your recovery and should be avoided.

You may be able to conserve considerable energy for disease-fighting purposes by changing your transportation arrangements temporarily during a cold. A high proportion of the physical energy you consume goes toward moving your entire body weight from place to place, lifting it up flights of stairs, and so on. Although you do not ordinarily think of these tasks as work, they may involve several times as much expenditure of muscular effort as hand-and-arm tasks to which you devote conscious attention. If you can ride more and walk less while ailing, you probably will recover more quickly.

Decreasing exposure to new germs

While you are suffering from a cold or throat irritation, your resistance to other germs is definitely impaired. Bacterial infections like sinusitis, tonsillitis, bronchitis, and pneumonia frequently complicate an ordinary cold. One of the best ways to avoid such secondary infections is to keep more or less to yourself. Whether you go to bed or not, you can often keep your distance from other people while you are ailing.

Controlled nose blowing

Violent nose blowing shoves germ laden material up into the sinuses and middle ear cavities. You can dispose of nasal secretions without these harmful results by sniffing and swallowing or by blowing gently with both nostrils open.

Hot gargles

Gargling serves two purposes: hot solutions soothe soreness, and the removal of germs from the area decreases secondary infection. Antiseptic gargles have no real advantage. Whether you wash germs away or kill them makes no difference. Half a teaspoonful of salt to a glass of hot water works quite well.

Aspirin

Aspirin is generally a safe home remedy, so long as you do not let the relative comfort it brings influence your decision as to whether you need medical aid. Aspirin decreases fever, headache, and other disease-produced miseries. You should be sure to base your judgment of the disorder's severity on your condition without aspirin rather than on the lowered temperature and lessened complaints achieved through this drug.

Nose drops

More harm than good comes from nose drops as generally used. Oil-base nose drops are definitely harmful. Prolonged use of any kind of nose drops often leads to a form of sensitivity which makes the nose become very stuffy an hour or two after the drops are used. When more drops are used for the resulting stuffiness, you get into a vicious circle that may last for years. Nose drops are also completely useless during the initial, runny-nose stage of a cold. Probably nose drops are best reserved for special instances of sinus blockage and the like, on a physician's recommendation only.

First aid for minor skin infections

Any signs of spreading infection from a scratch, scrape, or burn deserves immediate medical care. Watch especially for throbbing pain, swelling, redness, red streaks running toward the trunk, and fever. Milder infections still deserve attention, but can usually wait until scheduled office hours. These measures help until medical care can be arranged:

1. *Rest.* Motion spurs the flow of tissue juices from one part to another. If infection has a start, this extra flow of tissue juices may help it spread. You may be able simply to cut down on use of the affected part. You may require a bulky bandage to decrease movement. In a few instances, you may want to use a splint or sling.

2. *Elevation.* Infections throb less and heal faster if the blood goes downhill from the infected area to your heart. Whenever you get a chance, you should prop up the infected part. When you lie down, an infected foot or leg does best on two pillows arranged so that the lower leg is roughly parallel with the floor. You can raise an infected hand or arm on extra pillows or put it in a sling which keeps it on top of your chest.

3. *Heat.* Hot soaks or hot, wet cloths help most infections. If you have a candy or darkroom thermometer, adjust the heat to about 112°. You can go by feel, using water as hot as is comfortable for a part which has not been immersed. Remember that some body parts become so accustomed to heat

that you can burn them if you continually add as much hot water as they will tolerate. Hot applications should last at least twenty minutes for maximum benefit.

4. *Drainage.* Infections heal better if the pus and matter formed in them can drain away freely. One of your body's main ways of fighting infection is through white blood cells, which swarm to the scene, devour germs, then die and turn into pus. New hordes of white blood cells cannot get to the scene until the old ones are out of the way.

In many cases, hot soaks draw pus toward the surface. The gentle removal of the thin, stretched layer of dead skin cells at the infection's head or of drainage-blocking crusts or scabs will speed healing. Do not squeeze sores or pick at them until they bleed: once an opening is present, hot soaks will rapidly and safely draw out any remaining material.[3]

5. *Cleanliness.* Any draining infection pours millions of germs onto your skin surface. If these germs are capable of invading the unbroken or slightly scraped skin, further infections may result. You can usually prevent this difficulty by taking these steps:

a. Wash off the entire area with rubbing alcohol after each soak or compress.
b. Bandage draining sores if they will rub against your clothes and spread their germs.
c. Take a daily shower or sponge bath, preferably using mildly antiseptic surgical soap.

[3] Heat is not advised for acne pustules because it increases the activity of the underlying acne process. Gentle, straight-in pressure with a blackhead squeezer after opening may therefore be necessary, as noted above.

CHAPTER 20

Protecting Yourself from Tuberculosis and Venereal Disease

YOUR OWN BEST INTEREST AS WELL AS THE WELFARE OF YOUR FRIENDS AND neighbors demand periodic tests and prompt medical attention for tuberculosis and venereal disease. True, many facilities are provided primarily because detection and cure is the cheapest way to limit spread rather than because of an interest in your personal welfare: Nevertheless, these facilities do you nothing but good. People often think of tuberculosis sanitariums as pest holes set up exclusively to keep tuberculosis victims shut off from their friends and neighbors, and of VD contact investigators as sex-centered busybodies. The truth is that most enlightened state programs for control of tuberculosis depend on topnotch care rather than police power to enlist their patients' cooperation, and most VD investigators are personifications of tact.

TUBERCULOSIS

Tuberculosis is a form of infection which characteristically smolders along for a period of years before the victim gets well or dies. The causative organism can be positively identified under the microscope, can be grown in a test tube, and can be detected in small numbers by its ability to infect certain laboratory animals. Tuberculosis usually involves the lungs, but may also occur in the envelopes of the brain, in the kidneys, the skin, the lymph glands, and other body parts. Although x-ray changes may strongly suggest the presence of tuberculosis, the only way to positively identify the disease is to find the causative organism in material coughed up, in stomach washings, or in other body fluids or tissues.

Primary or Childhood-Type Tuberculosis

Your first infective encounter with tuberculosis germs usually leads to a very mild, often unrecognized infection. The germs do not cause violent bodily reaction at this point; you usually get no fever, no loss of appetite, no weakness, and no cough. After a few weeks, your body builds immunity against the tuberculosis germs and drives them back into a few centers, where they are walled off in tiny pockets of lime. The germs remain present

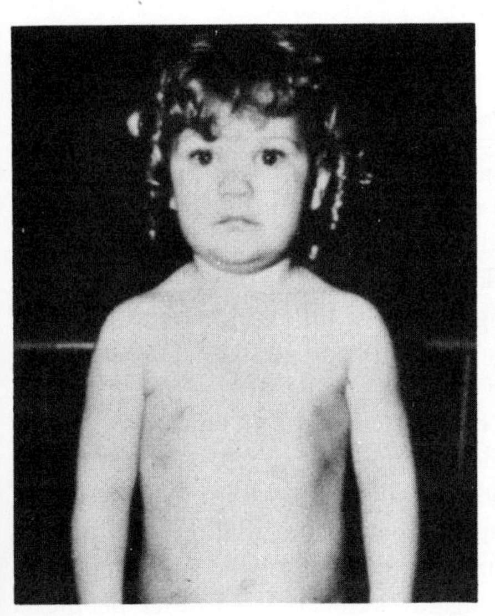

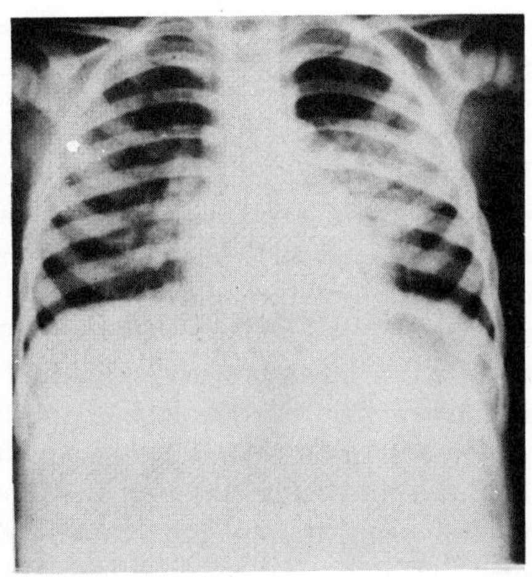

Figure 78. Childhood tuberculosis. (A) Victim apparently healthy and well nourished even though x-ray (B) shows definite disease (whitish clouding in middle third of left lung). *Courtesy Clay-Adams Medicrome.*

in these pockets for many years. Although they occasionally spread into nearby tissue if your resistance becomes very low, they generally cause no trouble.

A few people have trouble fighting off their first infective dose of tuberculosis germs. Further lung inflammation occurs, with cough, fever, and substantial x-ray changes. In rare cases, germs invade the bloodstream and set up scattered patches of infection in other parts of the body. These risks probably justify medical surveillance and a moderate amount of extra rest if your initial tuberculous involvement is detected. Sanitarium or hospital care is not needed unless complications actually occur.

What your Mantoux test means

A positive Mantoux test means that you have at some time encountered an infective dose of tuberculosis germs, but it does not tell whether you successfully resisted them. Shortly after your first encounter with an infective dose of tuberculosis germs, your skin becomes sensitive to small amounts of certain chemical substances normally associated with those germs. In doing the Mantoux test, your doctor injects a small amount of harmless material derived from tuberculosis germs into your skin. Swelling or redness at the site 48 hours later signifies effective exposure to tuberculosis germs at some time in the past.

Mantoux reaction and resistance

If you have a positive Mantoux reaction, your body can probably resist a larger number of tuberculosis germs than if you have a negative reaction. However, you are also carrying around a number of live tuberculosis germs in little lime pockets, which can break loose and cause trouble for you. If tuberculous infection becomes active again, either through breaking loose of old infection or through invasion by a new crop of germs, your body will react to that infection in self-destructive ways. The hazards of more serious disease if a breakthrough occurs and of internal germ residues are greater in this country than the lack of specific immunity.

These hazards are one reason for the prevailing opposition to widespread BCG vaccination in America. BCG vaccination, an inoculation with a relatively benign strain of tuberculosis germs, is often practiced in Europe and Asia. In these areas, the risk of acquiring tuberculosis from other people is very high. The extra resistance imparted by BCG, which turns the Mantoux reaction positive, frequently outweighs any risks and difficulties involved. If tuberculosis later occurs, though, it is of the more severe, secondary invasion type. BCG vaccination makes the Mantoux test completely useless in detecting tuberculosis. The vaccination itself leads to serious illness in an occasional individual. The disadvantages of BCG vaccination seem to outweigh its advantages for the average American, although some authorities recommend it for nurses in tuberculosis hospitals and other high-exposure occupations.

Calcifications

A chest x-ray often hows the flecks of lime in which tuberculosis germs are walled off after a primary infection. Similar calcifications also form as a result of infection with certain relatively innocuous organisms. Therefore, small calcifications with a positive Mantoux test mean exactly the same thing as the positive Mantoux test alone: effective exposure to tuberculosis germs in the past. Calcifications with a negative Mantoux test come from a healed nontuberculous infection which generally involves no significant threat.

Secondary Invasion or Adult-Type Tuberculosis

When tuberculosis germs break loose from their pockets of lime, or when a new tuberculous invasion occurs after your Mantoux test is positive, a more serious type of infection generally results. The lungs are almost always involved first, although other organs may become involved later. Early treatment usually brings about a complete, lifelong cure, but healing rarely if ever occurs without a prolonged and definite attack on the disease.

Advantages of early treatment

The earlier you get treatment, the better your chances of survival and the briefer your period of confinement. The vast majority of patients whose tuberculosis is detected by x-ray before they have complaints or symptoms are completely cured within six months. Patients who wait until physical com-

Figure 79. Time spent: one minute. Time saved: perhaps a year or more of sanitarium care. *Courtesy New York City Department of Health.*

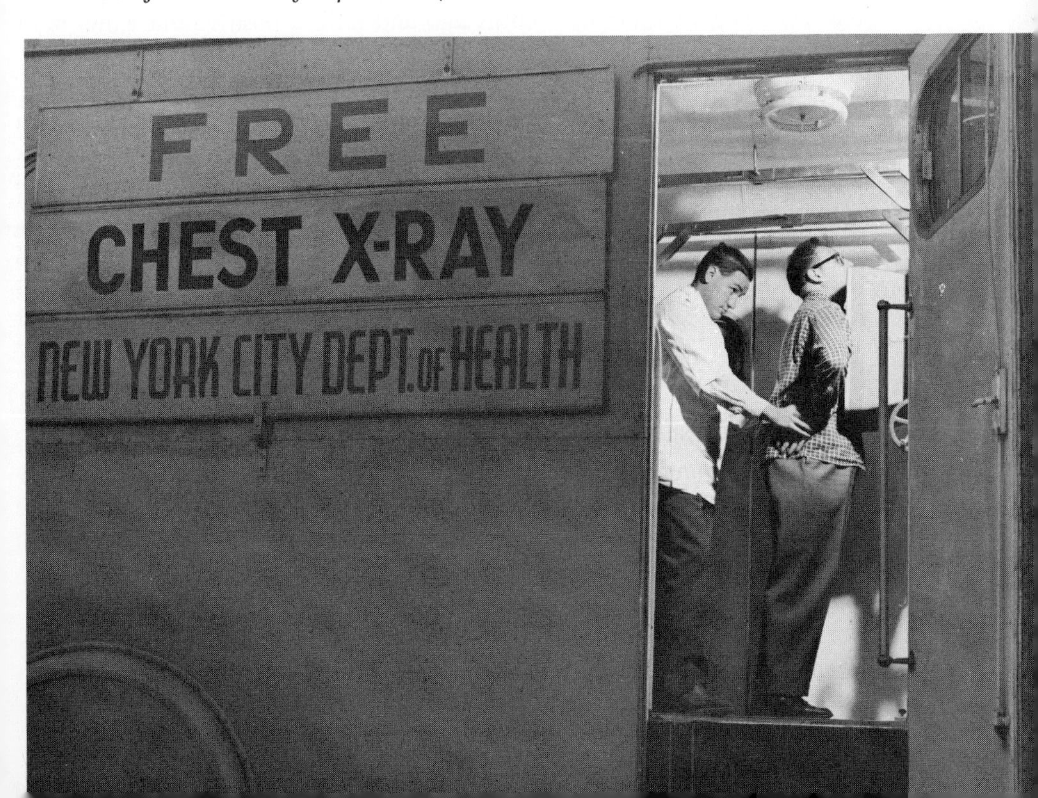

plaints drive them to medical care have already allowed their disease to progress for an extra 2½ years. Many of them will never achieve permanent cure, and those who do will generally have to undergo years of sanitarium or bed care. If you acquire a new tuberculous infection or suffer reactivation of a past primary infection, detecting your disease by routine tests instead of waiting until it causes complaints can save you many months in the hospital and greatly increase your chance for a cure. It can also protect your family and friends from acquiring your infection.

Your personal program for tuberculosis detection

In most communities, you can get periodic tests for tuberculosis at little or no cost: the public and voluntary health agencies make testing available as a means of combating spread of the disease. The basic program usually advised is this:

1. A Mantoux test at least every year as long as the test remains negative. People who have recently had contact with active tuberculosis, such as family members of a patient or nurses on a tuberculosis ward, should have a Mantoux test every three months. Medical students, nursing students, and similar high-exposure groups should have tests every three to six months.
2. A full-sized chest x-ray if your Mantoux test becomes positive, and at intervals thereafter. The once popular miniature x-rays have been replaced by full-sized films because they involved considerable extra radiation. If you know that the change in your Mantoux test is recent—for instance, if you had a negative test six months ago and have a positive one now—most authorities would advise you to have a chest x-ray every three months for a year, every six months for five years, and every year thereafter.
3. A testing program to find the source of infection if Mantoux conversion occurs while the number of close associates is still limited. If one of your children develops a positive Mantoux test during his elementary school years, for instance, the chances are that some adult whom he sees frequently has active tuberculosis. The infected individual can often be found among household members, school employees, relatives, or family friends, both to his benefit and to the benefit of other people whom he might infect. Note that the child himself and his classmates cannot spread the disease: primary infection does not involve enough germs to let its victims deliver an infective dose.
4. Awareness of possible tuberculosis symptoms, both in yourself and in your relatives and friends. Complaints deserve extra attention in older people, both because they are more prone to ignore them as "just old age" and because tuberculosis is much more common after midforties. Cough,

especially if it produces phlegm or blood-tinged material, may mean tuberculosis. Pain in the chest, weight loss, slight afternoon fever, and cold sweats at night are other suggestive signs.

Tuberculosis Treatment Today

False ideas about the care of tuberculosis often lead to ruinous delays in accepting treatment. In particular, the prospect of a long period of isolation from family, friends, and employment often proves hard to face. The actual facts are reassuring:

1. Doctors cure many tuberculosis patients through surgery. Lung operations today involve no more risk or discomfort than long-established procedures like gall bladder operations. The remaining healthy lung tissue usually expands to fill up the chest, restoring more reserve breathing capacity than natural healing (with lung-shrinking scar) usually provides.
2. Drug treatment often allows patients to leave the hospital very promptly. Many cases which would once have required months or years of bed rest are now going back to school or work promptly, thanks to drugs which suppress or kill the tuberculosis germ.
3. Sanitariums are active, relatively pleasant treatment centers nowadays. Even if prolonged bed care is necessary, interesting recreational activities are possible, and frequent visits by relatives and friends are perfectly safe.

Community programs

The main means by which tuberculosis spreads is through the breathing passages. Victims of the secondary invasion or adult-type often cough up germs in large numbers, but not in large enough numbers to infect anybody with just one cough. People who share the household or working place with a tuberculosis victim or who come into frequent contact with him accumulate an infective dose over a considerable period of time.

Whenever a person is found to have a contagious form of tuberculosis, public health nurses try to arrange Mantoux tests or chest x-rays for everyone who might have been infected, and follow those patients along. School employees and other people whose jobs bring them into close contact with a great many children are often required to have annual x-rays. Many communities arrange x-rays for everyone in a certain high-risk group such as patients being admitted to general hospitals (who have much more chance of having the disease than their healthier brethren) or workers in certain industrial plants. Wherever tuberculosis is found, prompt arrangements for isolation and for curative care quickly limit further spread of disease.

Tuberculosis can also be spread through milk. Smoldering tuberculosis infection of the cow's udder seeds every drop of the milk with infective numbers of germs. In this country, an intensive public health campaign has almost wiped out tuberculosis among cattle. The customary practice of pasteurization, supervised by community agencies, kills any tuberculosis germs which get through. Milk-borne tuberculosis is quite common in certain foreign countries, though.

VENEREAL DISEASES

Since venereal diseases spread almost entirely through sex contact, your only major danger of acquiring them is generally through sexual relations with a partner who has previously had contact with at least one other person (i.e., the source of his or her infection). The more promiscuous your partner is, the greater the chance that one or more previous contacts have conveyed infection. Highly promiscuous people, who have sexual contact during the same period of time with several partners each, fling connections for potential infection wide through the entire community. Less promiscuity thus means less venereal exposure. The number of sex partners, not the amount of sex contact, determines your VD risk. With no sex partner, you have no venereal risk: with a single, loyal partner you have relatively little venereal risk, while sexual activity shared among several partners who in turn are promiscuous involves very substantial hazard.

Venereal Disease without Promiscuity

Since the organisms which cause the common venereal infections all die rapidly when deprived of moisture and warmth, it is virtually impossible to acquire infection from a toilet seat or borrowed article of clothing. However, homosexual relationships and other forms of intimate body contact without sexual intercourse can spread various venereal infections. Syphilis causes infectious mouth sores at one stage, and, therefore, can be readily spread by kissing. In an occasional instance (e.g., an outbreak among Chicago school children traced to a street vendor who spit on his apples before polishing them) indirect contact through food or dishes seems at fault. Dentists and dental assistants occasionally acquire syphilis by placing their fingers against an unnoticed mouth sore.

Venereal diseases can also be acquired without any moral lapse by the unborn baby of a syphilitic mother, the infant being born to a victim of gonorrhea, and the loyal spouse of a promiscuous deceiver. All of these instances controvert the arch-moralist's idea that we should leave venereal diseases uncontrolled as just punishment for sinners.

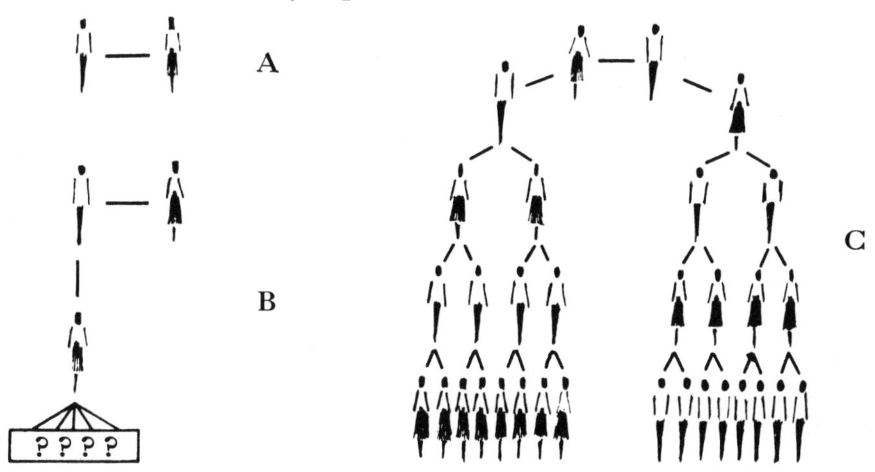

Figure 80. Effect of promiscuity on venereal risk. (A) Loyal couple: no risk. (B) Excursion by either partner opens possible channel of infection to both. (C) Promiscuous society (here assuming 3 contacts per person) spreads a network of possible infection-conveying contact throughout the community.

Personal Protection

Besides limiting promiscuity, several other measures give a degree of protection against venereal infection. Mechanical barriers such as condoms and sheaths lessen the degree of exposure during intercourse. When coupled with reasonably prompt and thorough soap and water scrubbing of the entire area from waist to knees, such precautions definitely reduce the likelihood of getting syphilis. Preventive drug therapy has proved reasonably effective if used within twelve hours after contact. Almost any doctor or hospital emergency room can administer such treatment. Prompt attention for suspicious symptoms is very worthwhile. Burning on urination a few days after sex contact, any sore or pimple-like bump on or near the genital area within eight weeks after contact, or any other complaints described below should lead to a physician's evaluation. Blood tests are worthwhile after every possible exposure. Tests six weeks, three months, six months, and one year after exposure usually identify syphilis promptly if it occurs. Long follow-up is especially worthwhile if penicillin or other antibiotics were used either as preventives or as treatment for some other illness during the first two months after exposure.

Community Action

Public agencies and voluntary health organizations have played an enormous part in reducing the scourge of venereal disease. Health departments provide free laboratory services to aid early diagnosis of venereal disease (and simultaneously to learn about each new case as soon as tests confirm its nature). In many states, examination for venereal disease before marriage encourages detection in people who might not otherwise have tests. Some health departments provide free treatment upon the precept that cure halts spread more effectively than any other approach. They trace possible sources and targets of infection in order to identify and cure individuals who might otherwise disseminate the disease further.

Other official agencies try to control prostitution, which has always proved to increase the spread of venereal disease even when legalized, inspected, and rigorously regulated. Voluntary agencies generally confine themselves to public education about venereal disease and to lobbying for better legislation.

VD as a Taxpayer's Burden

Venereal disease places a considerable burden on taxpayers, among whom you will shortly hold an honored place. The burden is large because some consequences of venereal disease caused prolonged disability. Take syphilis of the brain, for instance. With modern treatment, perhaps one-third of the victims recover. A few go rapidly downhill and die (as they all did before modern treatment was available). The rest remain sick enough to require hospital care, but live out their years—often twenty or thirty years, each of which costs the taxpayers several thousand dollars. Victims of syphilitic heart disease, spinal cord syphilis, and so on, also generally wind up on the welfare rolls, in the charity wards, or in public mental or chronic disease hospitals. Serious complications from gonorrhea call for drastic surgery or prolonged care in thousands of cases, too. The total cost is staggering.

By comparison, the cost of finding and curing venereal diseases early in their course is reasonable indeed. The cost of caring for one patient with brain syphilis for one year is enough to pay for detecting and curing several syphilis victims in the early stages of their disease. Each such early case also would probably spread his disorder directly or indirectly to many further victims if he were not found and cured. The cost of treating thousands of

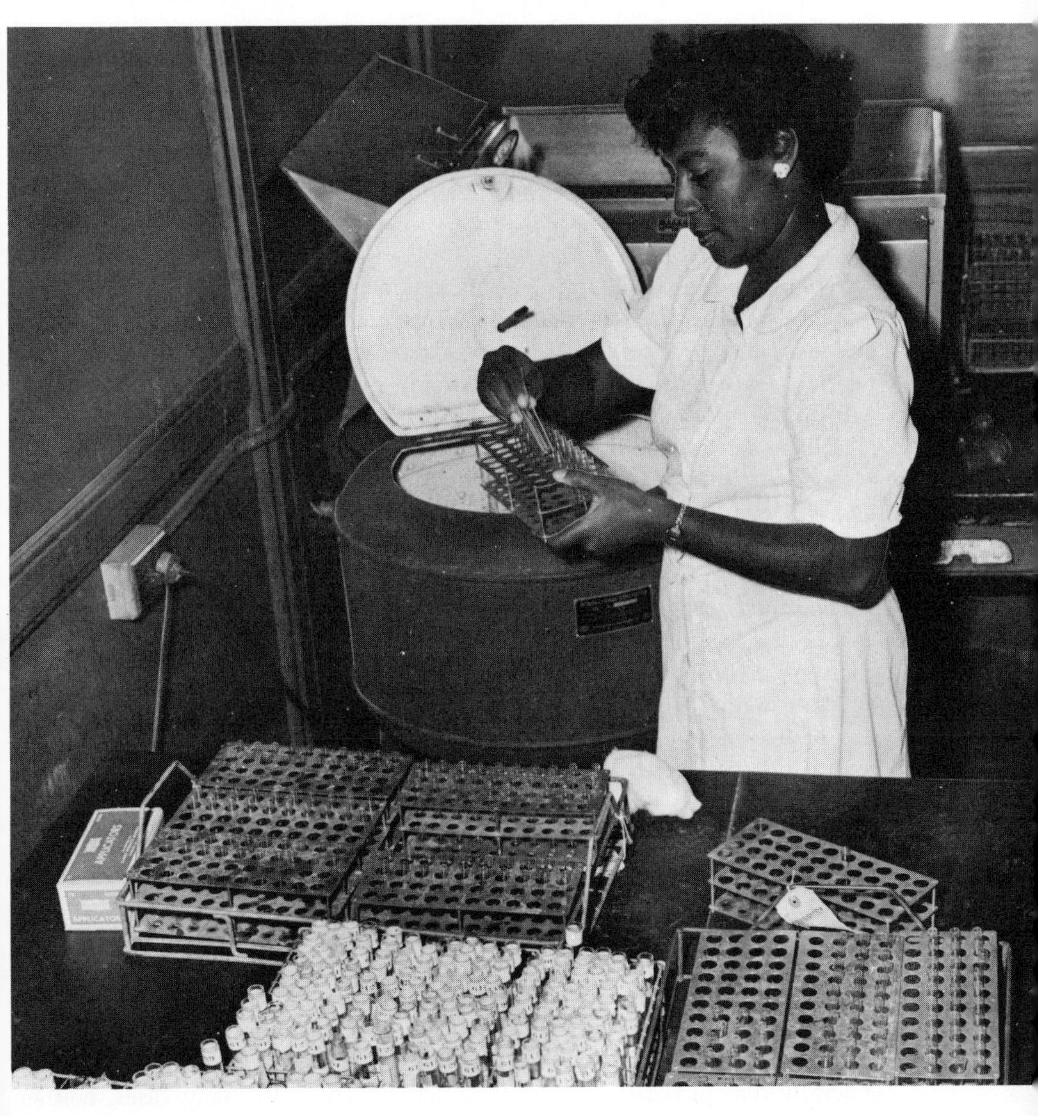

Figure 81. Laboratory tests being done at New York City Health Department. *Courtesy New York City Department of Health.*

newborn infants to prevent gonorrheal eye infection is less than the rehabilitation and public support which one blinded victim of the disease would require.

As a taxpayer, you will pay hundreds of dollars for care of venereal disease. Early detection and care is far cheaper than grudging, last-minute aid. You might sometimes wonder why your dollars should go to provide free care for venereal diseases when the ailments you suffer receive no such aid. In the long run, however, this policy has proved worthwhile.

THE NATURE AND COURSE OF VENEREAL DISEASES

Syphilis and gonorrhea are very common venereal diseases in the United States. Several other venereal conditions [1] cause slow-healing sores of the genitalia and occasional other complications. Since these conditions are relatively rare and will be readily distinguished only a physician (whom you will presumably consult for any possibly venereal sore anyway) you need take little account of these in your personal program of VD alertness.

Syphilis

The initial sore of syphilis occurs between three and six weeks after contact, and is located at the site where germs invade your body. This is generally on or near the genitalia. The sore is usually tense, firm and swollen, but only mildly tender or painful. It is generally somewhere between the size of a dime and a quarter, often with a punched-out or scab-covered central depression. Usually there is only one such sore, but in some cases two or three sores appear simultaneously. Women frequently do not notice any sore, presumably because of its internal location. The initial sore heals spontaneously in three weeks or so unless its course is shortened by treatment.

Several weeks later, a rash sometimes appears. This rash consists of red spots which are often widespread over the entire body, sometimes even involving the soles and palms. Patches of infection may form inside the mouth at this stage. The rash heals itself completely without treatment. Blood tests usually become positive within six weeks after infection, and generally remain positive for at least several years. In many cases, neither the sore nor the rash occur, and blood tests afford the sole clue to the presence of disease.

Syphilis can spread through sexual contact for about two years after its onset. Transmission to an unborn child can occur for five years after infection. The disease no longer spreads thereafter, even if it causes disabling or deadly disorder. A few days of treatment also makes it impossible for the disease to spread further, even though the cure is never completed.

Unrecognized or inadequately treated syphilis can lead to later involve-

[1] Lymphopathia venereum, granuloma inguinale, and chancroid.

ment of various body organs, such as the heart, liver, skin, or brain. These problems generally arise from ten to twenty years after the initial infection, long after the earlier manifestations have ceased to give any trouble.

Gonorrhea

In men, gonorrhea usually makes its presence known within nine days after sexual contact. The predominant complaints are of burning and stinging on urination and a discharge of pus or matter which either flows or can be easily milked from the penis. Prompt treatment at this stage usually brings the disease under control. Without treatment, extension to the prostate gland and other organs commonly leads to serious disabilities.

In women, gonorrhea has a more subtle, time-bomb effect. Many victims have no obvious sign of infection at first. Others note burning or stinging on urination or whitish vaginal discharge. If the disease is unchecked, menstrual periods may become somewhat heavier and somewhat more frequent. Attacks of lower abdominal cramps may occur from invasion of the tubes, which usually occurs shortly after menstruation. Further extension leads to widespread infection of the ovaries and tubes with intermittent discomfort. Scar formation or pus pockets often block the tubes, causing infertility. While prompt treatment usually prevents all this, the lack of definite complaints during the early, readily cured phase of the disease frequently leads to its neglect.

Gonorrhea victims can spread their infection from shortly before complaints develop until completely cured. The disease is sufficiently hard to detect in women that infection of babies' eyes during the process of birth was a major cause of blindness as long as doctors reserved treatment for children of women suspected of being gonorrheal. The law now requires that preventive measures against gonorrheal eye involvement be given to every newborn child. Difficulty with detection (plus the fact that an uninfected woman can harbor and spread germs from an infected sexual partner for many hours) has proved a major problem in areas with legalized prostitution.

CHAPTER 21

How To Keep a Sound Heart and Blood Vessels

IF YOU APPLY FOR A LIFE INSURANCE POLICY, THE MEDICAL EXAMINER CHECKS most thoroughly on your heart and blood vessels. Insurance companies pay tremendous attention to these organs and to conditions likely to lead to later trouble with them, because the condition of your heart and blood vessels has more to do with your continued life and health than that of all your other organs combined. Perhaps you should give your circulatory system similar emphasis in your own health program through the years.

HOW YOUR HEART AND BLOOD VESSELS WORK

Although you may have a clear understanding of how the heart and blood vessels work from high-school health courses, a quick review with emphasis on points most commonly confused may be worthwhile.

The Heart: A Double-Barreled, Positive-Pressure Pump

Your heart has two main pumping chambers, each of which is serviced by a smaller, priming chamber. The pumping chambers work completely independently of each other, one pumping blood into the lungs after it returns from the general circulation and the other pumping blood through the general circulation after it returns from the lungs.

The heart only forces blood out of its pumping chambers, and cannot suck blood into them. The priming chambers help to fill the pumping ones as quickly as the sluggish flow of blood returning through the veins permits: they fill while the pumping chambers are closed off for a heartbeat, and add their contents to blood currently returning through the veins when the pumping chambers relax. They do not speed return of blood through the veins, however. Your heart acts entirely as a positive-pressure pump, creating no suction whatever to speed flow through the veins.

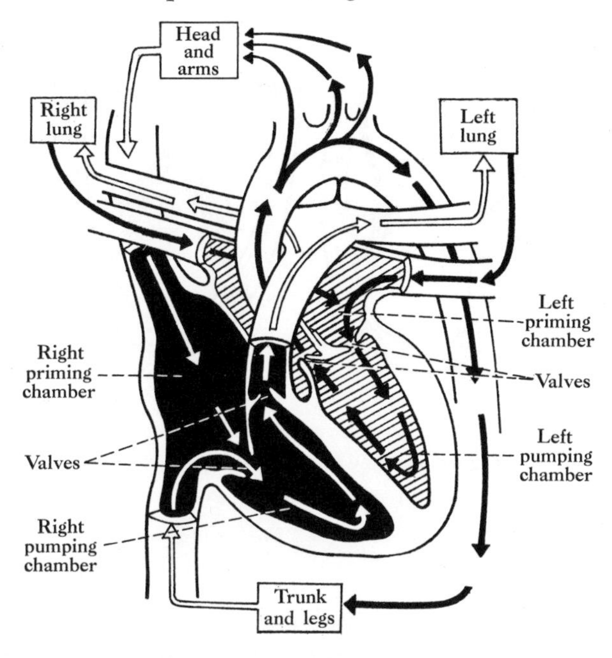

Figure 82. Heart and circulation. The right side of the heart pumps blood which returns from all other parts of the body through the lungs. The left side of the heart pumps blood which returns from the lungs to all other parts of the body. *Adapted with permission from an American Heart Association diagram.*

Heart valves

At each end of each pumping chamber, pliable, flap-type valves operate to keep the blood flowing in the right direction. The valves fold back out of the way when the blood is moving forward and billow out into the stream of blood when it starts to flow backward, sealing off the corresponding chamber opening.

The heart muscle

The lining of your heart's pumping chambers allows very little blood or nourishment to filter through. Most fuel and oxygen for its own use reaches your heart muscle through small vessels known as the *coronary* arteries, which branch off from the body's main blood vessel shortly after it leaves the heart. These arteries interconnect, permitting many detour pathways in the event that one of them gets stopped up.

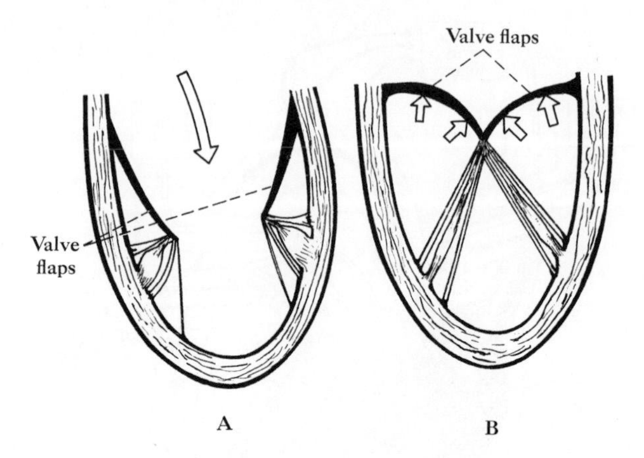

Figure 83. How the heart valves work.

The aorta

Your heart pumps blood in spurts, but your body needs smooth, continuous circulation. The aorta, your principal artery, smooths out blood flow by acting as an elastic-walled storage tank. Each heartbeat stretches it slightly, building a level of pressure inside which drives blood continuously through the smaller arteries and capillaries. Incidentally, your pulse does not signal the arrival of blood pumped by your most recent heartbeat: the pulse is a pressure wave, spreading like the ripples on a pool of water after a stone is thrown in. It moves eight times as fast as the blood itself.

Circulatory balance

When you stand up, blood vessels leading to your brain open up very substantially and blood vessels to your feet and legs partially close. If this adjustment does not occur instantly, too little blood flow reaches your brain and you become giddy or faint. Likewise, your circulation adjusts itself to heavy demands for circulation in your digestive organs after a meal and in your muscles during exertion. It sends more blood through your skin when you are warm and keeps more in the deeper layers when you are cold.

These adjustments are made mainly through nerve fibers in the sympathetic nervous system, which operates without conscious control. Small arteries can contract or dilate to decrease or increase the flow of blood through any one body part. Acting in concert, their contraction or dilation markedly affects the pressure your heart must work against in order to maintain blood flow.

Blood pressure

When your doctor takes your blood pressure, he applies measured degrees of pressure to your arm with a cuff and listens over your main arm artery as he adjusts the pressure to various levels. When the pressure in the instrument cuts off all blood flow, he hears nothing. When the pressure drops so that pressure within the artery is greater than that in the instrument during part of the pulse cycle, he hears the artery popping open and shut or the blood gurgling through the partially obstructed vessel. The highest pressure at which this occurs is the peak pressure during a pulse cycle, called your *systolic blood pressure.* When the pressure in the instrument no longer collapses the blood vessel wall at any phase, blood flow becomes smoothly continuous and silent. This point represents the pressure persisting in your arteries between heartbeats, or your *diastolic blood pressure.* Blood pressure is usually written as if it were a fraction, with the systolic pressure as the numerator and the diastolic pressure as the denominator. Normal levels vary considerably, but the upper limits of normal in adults are 150 systolic and 100 diastolic.

Venous return

Blood moves uphill in the veins mainly through the massaging action of nearby muscles. Inside most of the larger veins, small valves direct blood

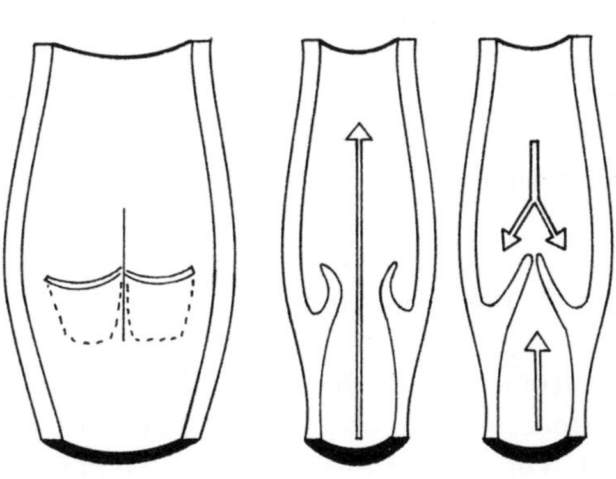

Figure 84. How vein valves work. *Adapted by permission from* Health and Safety for You, *by Diehl and Laton, Copyright 1954. McGraw-Hill Book Co., Inc.*

flow. These valves are like shirt pockets sewn to the inside of the veins. They flop out of the way when the blood flows in the proper direction and billow out to obstruct the passage when blood starts to flow backward.

In some areas, as in the lower leg, venous return is quite complex. Here, the large veins located between the calf muscles and the leg bones act more or less like bellows. When the leg muscles contract, they squeeze on these deep veins and force blood up through vessels in the thigh. When the leg muscles relax, valves prevent the blood from flowing back down into the deep veins, which fill instead from nearby surface and smaller veins. Other valves prevent the blood from flowing into the surface or smaller veins during the muscle contraction phase.

Unduly Frightening Circulatory Complaints

Undue concern about your heart can be just as disabling and uncomfortable as heart disease itself. Several complaints or findings which seldom if ever indicate the presence of significant disease frequently give rise to such upsets. Here are the six main sources of undue alarm in the order of their frequency.

1. Seemingly skipped beats

Nobody has a perfectly even, regular heartbeat throughout the day. If you made an electrical recording of your pulse and heartbeat, you would find fairly frequent breaks in the rhythm. On the record of your pulse, these breaks would seem to be skipped beats. Many people are conscious of them and report a sensation "like my heart turning over" or "as if my heart stopped for an instant, then gave a hard, sudden beat." What actually happens is a single, out-of-rhythm heartbeat which occurs soon after its predecessor. The heart's pumping chamber is still empty at this time, so no pulse wave is produced. The heart then pauses to get back on rhythm. The pumping chambers are overfilled by the time the next heartbeat is due, and send an extra-large spurt of blood forth into the aorta. This is a perfectly harmless and normal event.

2. Functional murmurs

At some time in their lives, about half the people in America have a heart murmur, which is an extra gurgling noise heard in association with the heartbeat. Very few of these people have any real heart disease. Murmurs due to real heart disease usually sound much different than the innocuous ones, and can also be distinguished by laboratory or other tests. The so-called functional murmurs are just extra noises which have absolutely no significance. They call for no limitation in strenuous exertion, require no additional watchfulness, and deserve to be ignored completely.

3. Left chest pains

College students very frequently visit a physician because of twinges of pain in the left chest. These pains may be like cramps underneath the nipple or may spread in a band of cramping or burning discomfort along one or more rib lines in the left side.

Such pains are virtually never due to heart trouble. As we will soon see, heart pain is usually in the middle of the chest and has a distinctive, crushing character. Left chest twinges and discomforts are usually due to gas in the stomach or to cramped study postures with resulting muscle spasm or nerve pressure. They deserve care like any other pain or complaint, but should not stir fear of heart disease.

4. Temporary elevation of the blood pressure

Young men and women frequently become inwardly upset during a physical examination, and get a temporary, emotionally-induced rise in blood pressure. Even after rechecks prove to be normal, the patients often feel that a serious threat is hanging over them. Actually, a transient rise in blood pressure means nothing. Your blood pressure probably soars to high levels many times during the year as part of normal emotional and physiologic phenomenon. A single high reading does not signify any disease whatever, as long as rechecks show that your blood pressure is normal when you are calm, rested, and accustomed to the procedure.

5. Lightheadedness, numbness, and tingling

Patients often report attacks of lightheadedness with numbness and tingling of the hands and feet and with some breathing difficulty or tightness in the chest. These attacks usually come at a time of extra emotional pressure or difficult living adjustment. The key problem is deep and rapid breathing on an emotional basis. Excessively heavy, deep breathing dissipates blood acids by blowing off carbon dioxide. A shift to the alkaline side results, causing lightheadedness, numbness, and tingling. Often the patient becomes further concerned about these complaints, becomes still more upset emotionally, and breathes all the deeper. A medical checkup usually proves reassuring.

6. Fainting spells

People with perfectly normal hearts and blood vessels faint under circumstances of emotional or physical stress. Fainting is due to changes in blood vessel caliber which temporarily deprive your brain of adequate circulation. This is a result of sympathetic nervous system response to stress or to emotion and does not signify circulatory weakness.

COMMON CIRCULATORY DISORDERS

You can take many effective steps to ward off common circulatory disorders. If one of these diseases strikes, you can probably make your doctor's treatment very much more effective by consulting him promptly, taking proper emergency measures, and keeping yourself free of misapprehension.

Personal Prevention of Heart and Blood Vessel Disease

You can take highly effective measures, either on your own or with your doctor's advice and help, to ward off several important diseases of the heart and blood vessels. Here are the main facts, arranged according to the age at which the disorder combated would otherwise strike:

Preventing rheumatic fever

Rheumatic fever, which strikes predominantly among children and young adults, is a disease caused by an unusual bodily response to certain strains of streptococci. Many victims of rheumatic fever do not get heart disease (especially with modern care), but enough of them are left with permanent heart damage to make rheumatic heart disease an important health problem. Once you have had an attack of rheumatic fever, you know that your body responds to streptococci in this highly undesirable way. Measures to prevent further streptococcal infections, perhaps including continuous treatment with penicillin or some other antibiotic (see Chapter 19) are very much worthwhile. You might discuss such measures with your physician.

Prompt treatment of streptococcal infection has also proved highly effective in warding off later rheumatic fever attacks even in individuals who have never had previous rheumatic difficulties. You can therefore help to ward off this disease for yourself and your family if you encourage prompt medical care for sore throat, especially when accompanied by high fever.

Varicose veins

If you prevent engorgement of normal veins, you defer or prevent the formation of varicose veins, which are enlarged, tortuous leg veins. The vein valves which direct blood flow from the surface to the deep leg veins are barely big enough to close the vein passages when the veins are at their normal size. The muscles in your legs do not rhythmically squeeze blood out of the deep veins when you stand still, as they do when you walk. Prolonged standing therefore leads to leg-vein congestion. Sitting causes a similar problem which is less intense only because the blood does not have to move as far uphill. After you stand or sit still for some time, the veins may become engorged until the valves are no longer effective. When these valves are not working, every contraction of the leg muscles squeezes some blood back into the delicate-walled surface veins instead of up through the main leg veins. The surface veins gradually balloon out into varicosities. The volume of blood eddying back and forth between surface and deep vessels increases as the surface veins enlarge, and the volume sent up toward the heart becomes very small. Varicose vein victims suffer considerable leg-weariness and calf cramps because of this interference with circulation. With continued neglect, skin eruption and slow-healing leg sores may result.

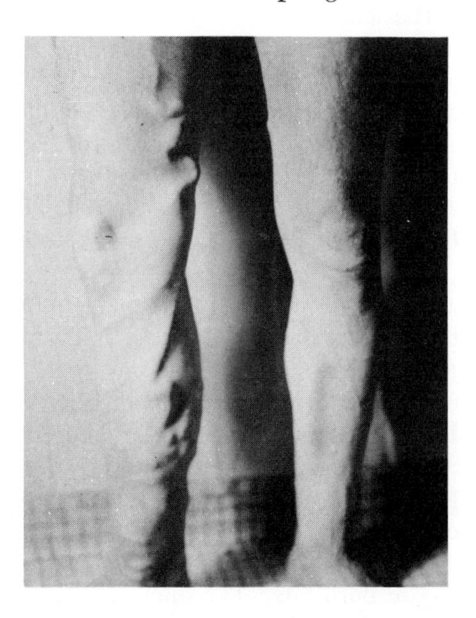

Figure 85. Varicose veins *Courtesy Annals of Surgery.*

If any blood vessel in your lower leg becomes as thick as a lead pencil or if you tend toward leg-weariness and cramps after prolonged standing, measures to prevent leg vein congestion may be worthwhile. Simply propping up your feet occasionally to let gravity aid your circulation may suffice. If discomfort makes more intensive leg drainage worthwhile, lie in the inverted bicycle position and jiggle your feet slightly with the foot and ankle muscles relaxed. Thirty seconds of such gravity-aided leg vein drainage for every two hours or so of standing gives considerable relief from leg-weariness and congestion. If frank varicose veins are present, ask your doctor about treatment. Ask further advice early in the course of any future pregnancy (when the pressing of the developing infant on veins from the legs adds to congestion).

Hardening of the arteries

Hardening of the arteries is a disease, not a part of the normal aging process. Complaints seldom appear until damage has accumulated over a period of forty to sixty years, but the hardening process itself actually starts in infancy, hits its peak in young adults, and slows down in old age.

Hardening of the arteries causes spotty thickening of the involved vessels' lining layer, which reduces or cuts off blood supply to various organs or areas. Such thickening is the principal cause of coronary heart attacks, high blood pressure, stroke, and several other disabling or deadly ailments.

A number of factors play a part in determining how rapidly your own arteries will harden. Heredity undoubtedly increases or decreases susceptibility to this process. Of more practical importance, since you can't pick your grandparents and you can pick your food, is the part played by diet. If you eat enough to keep your weight above the recommended range (see Chapter 14) you definitely speed hardening of the arteries and its various sequels. Studies of heart disease in areas with various dietary customs strongly suggest that consumption of excessive amounts of fat also does harm. Apparently the problem is mainly in your body's handling of certain substances, namely cholesterol and its chemical cousins, which form within your body as you burn fats.[1] The thickened spots of hard arteries are full of this substance. A number of studies have shown that blood cholesterol levels (and presumably deposit of cholesterol in your artery walls) increase when you eat chemically saturated fats (usually those solid at room temperature) as

[1] Certain foods, such as cream and eggs, contain large amounts of cholesterol. Dietary cholesterol has little influence on your blood cholesterol level, however. To quote Frederick Stare and his coworkers (Frederick J. Stare, M.D., Theodore B. Van Itallie, M.D., Mary B. MacCann, M.P.H. and Oscar W. Portman, M.D., "Nutritional Studies Relating to Serum Lipids and Atherosclerosis," *J.A.M.A.*, 164: 1920–1925, August 24, 1957): "No rigid control of dietary cholesterol seems necessary. It has been well shown that alteration of dietary cholesterol from as little as 200 mg. to as much as 1,000 mg. per day does not affect the level of cholesterol in the blood."

opposed to chemically unsaturated ones (usually liquid at room temperature).[2]

Although the exact role of saturated and unsaturated fats in the causation of hardened arteries has not been precisely defined at this writing, the evidence seems to justify such measures to avoid excess consumption of saturated fats as you can take without major inconvenience. Three general approaches deserve your consideration:

1. *Weight control.* Less total calories presumably mean less fats, which may or may not be the reason for the proved effectiveness of this measure in staving off arteriosclerosis.

2. *Decreased fat consumption.* Without any cuts whatever in your use of table fats like cream and butter, you can decrease fat consumption substantially by eating less fried food and rich pastry. Since Americans have tremendously increased their use of fats in the last generation, such a program involves no excursion into the unknown realms of nutritional experimentation, and frequently offers bonus benefits in decreasing acne and overweight problems.

3. *Replacing solid shortenings with unsaturated preparations whenever convenient.* Home economists and nutritionists see no advantage in artificially solidified shortenings over corn or cottonseed oil in most cooking uses. You can buy corn oil or cottonseed oil in any grocery store under several well-known trade names. "Old fashioned" peanut butter differs from chemically altered products only in consistency rather than in flavor or nutritional value. Even if you regard the hazard of excess saturated fats as unproved, what harm will you do by playing safe?

Coronary heart disease

In addition to measures helpful against hardening of the arteries, evidence is accumulating that a certain minimum of physical exercise helps to prevent or lessen the impact of coronary heart disease. Physically active workers suffer many less coronary heart attacks than sedentary workers, and the attacks they suffer tend to be considerably less severe. This is true even when occupations are paired off to eliminate possible social status factors (e.g., when mail carriers are paired off with letter sorters of identical civil service grade). Apparently the significant point is frequent, moderate exertion, not strenuous work or vigorous athletic indulgence: athletes and heavy workers have little or no extra advantage. A few minutes' walk to and from work or

[2] The terms "saturated" and "unsaturated" refer to the chemical formula of the individual fat molecules, which are considered fully saturated if they contain as much hydrogen as is chemically possible.

a bicycle ride each day would probably suffice to put most sedentary work ers in the lower-risk group.

The effect of smoking on your chance of getting coronary heart diseas seems definite and reversible (see Chapter 7). This effect rather than th more highly publicized cancer problem explains most of the doubled deat rate found in heavy smokers.

Muscular contraction of artery walls often results from emotion-induce nerve imbalance. Hard-driving, dynamic people seem especially prone t coronary disease. Heavy executive or professional responsibility definitel increases your chance of having this disease. Accumulated emotional pres sures often need release through one of the channels discussed in Chapte 4 or through measures specifically advised by your physician.

High blood pressure

Certain psychologic and social problems are commonly associated wit high blood pressure. Difficulty in self-assertion and in expressing hatred o other emotions seem related to hypertension in some cases. The meek littl man who prides himself on self-containment, but still fumes inwardly, ma be boosting his blood pressure toward the danger point. Chapter 4 dis cusses practical emotional outlets and describes sources for further psycho logic aid.

The relationship of high blood pressure to salt intake may or may not b significant. People who salt their food without tasting first are more pron to high blood pressure than people who salt to taste or never salt, bu nobody knows whether extra salt causes hypertension or salt craving is a early sign of hypertension-causing disease.

RECOGNIZING AND ARRANGING BETTER CARE FOR HEART DISEASE

Naturally, you will want to go to your physician immediately when yo suspect that you might have heart disease. Here are the changes whic should make you suspect these disorders, and the measures you should tak until the doctor comes.

Rheumatic fever

Most rheumatic fever victims have an easily recognized, abruptly begin ning illness with fever, joint pain, and medically detectable evidence o eart involvement. One or more joints become red, swollen, and painful: arge joints such as a shoulder or hip, elbow or knee, ankle or wrist are nost commonly involved. Each joint clears up completely inside two or hree days, but others simultaneously flare. Patients almost always survive vithout serious heart damage, partly because their dramatic illness virtually orces them into adequate care during the crucial early months.

Unfortunately, many rheumatic fever victims have smoldering rather than brupt and readily recognizable disease. In these patients, joint discomforts nay be mild and brief enough that they pass for "growing pains." Fever eldom calls the condition to your attention, but the afternoon temperature s often up one degree or so when you become suspicious enough to measure t. Frequent nosebleeds may occur for no apparent reason. Pallor is sometimes notable, and rheumatic children often lag considerably in growth. 'requent colds and sore throats may also indicate impaired vigor and reistance.

If three or more signs of rheumatic disease are present, special medical ests are certainly in order. Even two of these signs, if severe and typical n nature, justify a physician's attention.

Congestive heart failure

You should watch for congestive heart failure with special care in people who have had high blood pressure, rheumatic fever, or any form of heart isease. The signs by which you can recognize congestive failure and the mergency measures you can take for it are the same whatever the underying disorder. Swelling of the feet and ankles in the late afternoon and vening usually shows up first. This swelling is due to extra fluid in the ssues. It is soft, so that thirty seconds of firm pressure with the tip of your nger will leave a definite dent. Blueness or duskiness of the lips and tongue ometimes shows up at this stage, too. When the victim lies down at night, ne fluid shifts up into his lungs. In the middle of the night, he wakes p feeling as if the room is very stuffy. He gets up and sits by the window, nd the condition clears (not because of the fresh air, but because his upght position lets some of the excess fluid siphon out of his waterlogged ngs into his legs and feet). If he gets no medical care, he soon finds that ny extra exertion, such as walking up one or two flights of stairs, gets him ompletely out of breath. The amount of exertion required to make him lose is wind steadily decreases, until even ordinary tasks of living make him huff nd puff.

If congestive failure comes on slowly and you become suspicious when nly swelling of the ankles or a single, self-relieving nocturnal smothering oell has occurred, you can safely wait until morning to call your doctor.

More severe attacks require oxygen for relief of short-windedness. In mos
cases, the victim can be carried in a chair to an automobile, propped uprigh
so that he can breathe comfortably, and taken to a hospital where oxygen i
available. In rapidly developing or extreme cases, an oxygen-equipped am
bulance or rescue squad can give considerable relief. A doctor should b
summoned, but it is usually wiser to have him meet you at the hospital tha
to waste time on a home visit.

Coronary heart attacks

Most coronary heart attack victims have pain. The pain is crushing, "lik
a mountain sitting on my chest." It centers on the breastbone, but ofte
runs up to the neck, down the left arm, or down the right arm. The victim als
feels faint, dizzy, or weak. He looks very pale. His skin feels cold an
wet.

Such an attack calls for absolute physical quiet and as much tranquillit
as you can muster. The victim should lie flat with coverings above an
underneath him if he is outdoors. Leave him on the floor instead of movin
him to a bed if the attack strikes him indoors. A doctor should be called t
the scene to give pain-relieving injections. An oxygen-equipped ambulanc
or rescue squad can help, too, but by giving oxygen at the scene, not b
moving the patient. Adequate pain relief and complete control of shock ar
much more important than getting the patient to a hospital. In fact, th
prevailing medical view is that the patient should not be moved under an
circumstances until his pain is completely relieved and shock has been con
trolled—usually two to four hours after the onset of the attack.

THE OUTLOOK IN HEART DISEASE

In one center recently established to help heart patients get back to work
almost half of the patients were found to have just one disability: misap
prehension about their disease. The idea that the least overexertion woul
kill them instantly was very common. An unnecessarily discouraging view o
their future also ran rife. "Once you've had heart trouble, you're finished,"
one patient remarked.

The actual facts are much more hopeful. If a person with a bad hear
overworks, he gets shortness of breath or swelling of the ankles or discom
fort. He does himself no permanent harm so long as he heeds these warn
ings. He doesn't suddenly drop dead. Moreover, work actually helps hi

ondition. Heart victims recover more quickly and more completely if they lo as much as they can without developing symptoms, once the healing rom their initial attack is complete (usually six to eight weeks). The vast najority of heart attack victims get back to full time work, and many others ecome useful to some lesser degree. Heart disease may impose limitaions on its victims, but those limitations should be based on either doctor's rders or definite symptoms revealing overindulgence, not upon undue fears nd old wives' tales.

CHAPTER 22

How To Avoid or Contro Other Common Chronic Diseases

CHRONIC DISEASES ARE DISEASES WHICH SMOLDER ALONG FOR MONTHS OR YEARS often for a lifetime. Their accumulated burdens and residuals involve almos everyone by age sixty-five.[1] Yet it is a mistake to think of chronic illness as problem mainly of old age. You can fight disease much more effectivel before it appears or at its onset than after it has wreaked its ravages. Olde people may bear most of the burdens of chronic disease, but its conques calls for action throughout your earlier years. You cannot take steps too earl against the common chronic illnesses considered in this chapter.

CANCER

At this moment, millions of cells within your body are in the process o growing or reproducing themselves. This process will continue as long a you live. Cells grow in well-disciplined order to replace normal wear an tear, to heal injury, and to meet special body needs.

Occasionally, a clump of body cells grows without detectable purpose resulting in a tumor. The undisciplined growth may continue without invad ing normal surrounding tissues: then a so-called *benign* tumor results Such growth may continue for a time and cease without interfering in any way with the body's biological efficiency. It may continue until the mass i unwieldy, until it causes disfigurement or disability, or until it causes bodily disorder by pressing on neighboring parts, but it does not spread to distan body organs.

The undisciplined tumor growth may invade and destroy surrounding tissue and spread through body fluids to distant sites, where it sets up new focuses of purely parasitic growth. Any tumor capable of such growth i

[1] Twenty out of 22 old people surveyed had one or more chronic illness which eithe interfered with daily activity, limited daily activity, or required continual care accordin to Statistical Bulletin, March 1959.

alled a cancer. However, there is a stage in the existence of almost every ancer when its cells are 100 per cent localized to a body part which can be emoved or within which cancer-destroying radiation can be concentrated. cancer is not a tumor which has spread beyond the range of cure: it is a umor which has that potential if its progress is not arrested.

Irritation and Cancer

Take a group of body cells which are growing only enough for self-eplacement. Submit them to some form of injury which kills out many of eir number each day without impairing the capacity of the others to grow. he remaining, live cells then multiply rapidly in the normal process of ssue repair. Now continue this growth-spurring process over a period of any years. Isn't it reasonable to expect that the process of cellular growth ill ultimately overstep the bounds of useful self-repair?

Such cancer-spurring irritation seems to be a definite factor in bringing n certain cancers. Various substances, irradiations and conditions play their arts. For example:

1. Farmers, sailors, and other workers who are exposed constantly to the un have many times as many cancers of the skin as office workers.
2. Physicians specializing in x-ray suffer substantial extra risk from leu-emia (cancer of blood-forming cells).
3. Most cancers of the mouth of the womb apparently occur in conse-uence of smoldering, untreated infection.
4. Cancer of the lip and tongue usually occurs in pipe smokers, and most always springs from the site where the stem or smoke stream strikes.
5. Cancer of the mouth usually starts in the exact spot where jagged teeth : ill-fitting dentures rub and press.
6. Cancer of the penis is very common among uncircumcised desert ibesmen who lack water for body cleanliness.
7. Workers who come in contact with certain chemicals in the course of eir daily work suffer cancer of the skin, nose, bladder (from chemicals assing through into the urine), or other organs depending on the nature of eir exposure.
8. Several pieces of strong evidence point toward a true cause-and-effect elationship between cigarette smoking and lung cancer (see Chapter 7).

How to Avoid Cancer-Spurring Irritation

Most people readily agree that these steps for avoiding cancer-spurring ritation, which do not conflict with prevailing attitudes and practices, are efinitely worthwhile:

1. Prompt repair of jagged teeth and ill-fitting dentures.
2. Cleansing beneath the foreskin in uncircumcised males.
3. Biannual pelvic examination with prompt care of any infection found at the mouth of the uterus.
4. Proper protective measures against excessive radiation or dangerous chemical exposures at work.

Two further means of avoiding irritation of types clearly associated with increased occurrence of cancer also deserve your attention:

1. Shielding your skin from prolonged, intensive sun exposure either with a hat, a thin layer of yellow vaseline, or a suntan lotion should substantially reduce your chance of suffering cancer of the skin.
2. Shielding your lungs from tobacco smoke, and especially from frequently-inhaled cigarette smoke (whether filtered or not).

Cancer Vanguards and Early Growths

The transition from normal cellular growth to the wildly undisciplined growth of a cancer sometimes occurs in stages. A cluster of pigment cells on the foot grows until it constitutes an ordinary mole. After years of irritation by the pressure and rubbing of a shoe, this cluster of cells might begin to grow more wildly and to cast living sprouts into nearby body fluids, thus becoming malignant. A patch of cheek lining rubbed by a rough tooth responds for a time by white, leathery thickening before its cells become cancerous. The cancer vanguard phase of tissue growth often permits treatment before cancer has even begun, totally preventing a hazardous malignancy.

Even if cancer starts without a vanguard phase or has already become malignant, prompt treatment cures more than half the victims. As long as the abnormally growing cells remain in nearby tissues, doctors can usually remove or destroy them totally. The result is permanent cure, not for five years or ten years but for life. Doctors commonly report results in terms of "five-year cures" to permit prompt comparison of results with various treatment measures, not (as many people seem to believe) because a five year interruption in the course of the disease is all they hope to achieve. Actually, the percentage of five-year cures and the percentage of lifelong cures are almost identical, because the occasional case in which cancer reappears after five or more years is balanced statistically by other cases in which death from noncancer causes occurs within the first five years.

How to Detect Possible Cancer Vanguards and Early Growths

Periodic medical examination frequently detects cancer vanguards or early cancers in time for complete, lifelong cure. Your personal physician can detect the vast majority of cancer vanguards and early growths in his own office. A cancer detection clinic can find a few vanguards and curable cancers which an individual physician would miss, but not enough to justify any considerable delay in seeking attention. Most people do better to use the facilities readily available to them than to let things slide in hopes of later arranging slightly more thorough care.

Between medical examinations, a monthly self-inspection often proves helpful. During the reproductive years, a woman should perform this self-examination the day after the cessation of menstrual flow, when new breast lumps can be most readily detected. Postmenopausal women and men of all ages find the first day of each month easiest to remember. Self-inspection is best performed in the nude, in a well-lit room, and with the aid of both a full length and a shaving mirror. Area by area, here are the findings which should send you to your doctor:

Skin. Horn-like, heaped up piles of dry skin cells or rough, dry plaques often prove to be cancer vanguards. These occur chiefly on the face and backs of the hands. Hard little bumps with a shiny surface, scab-covered depressions which have persisted for more than two weeks, and pits eaten into the skin often prove to be early cancers.

Lips, tongue, and mouth. You can see best if you remove all dental appliances and use a magnifying mirror. Leathery white patches, hard lumps or pits eaten into the underlying tissue call for prompt care.

Breast. A woman can examine her own breast quite effectively in search of lumps. Key points are systematic examination of each breast quadrant, use of the palm surfaces of joined fingers instead of the fingertips, and rolling the breast tissue against the underlying chest wall. Examination is best performed in the reclining position, and shortly after menstruation ceases.

Genitalia. An inspection of the readily accessible folds of tissue at the opening of the female organ for white patches, pits and lumps occasionally proves fruitful. Lumps in the testicles and scab-covered or open sores of the penis can also be readily noted on self-examination.

General. Any lump, bump, or bulge under the skin or elsewhere deserves evaluation.

In addition to these relatively urgent conditions, you can note several other conditions on self-inspection in order to ask your doctor about them on your next visit. Moles of the feet or shaving area and raised moles subject to irritating pressure or friction (such as at the beltline) and bony irregularities in the vicinity of your joints fall into this category. Any noticeable change from month to month puts these conditions in the urgent category.

The vast majority of conditions you find by self-inspection will prove noncancerous upon medical examination, especially in your early adult years. However, if during your whole lifetime you get attention for one tumor several months earlier by this program than you would by waiting until its progress or your annual examination makes it manifest, your efforts will have added substantially to your life span.

Alertness for Complaints Possibly Signifying Cancer

In addition to lumps or sores within range of self-inspection, several other evidences of possible cancer merit prompt attention. To be specific:

1. *Unusual bleeding from any body cavity.* Bleeding from the nose or mouth, coughed-up blood, bleeding from the nipple or rectal bleeding usually occurs in readily recognized form. Vomited blood may look like coffee grounds, due to the action of stomach acids. Intestinal bleeding may reveal itself as soft, bulky, pitch-black stools. Bleeding between menstrual periods always deserves attention, even if it only amounts to a few spots on the panties or occurs only after sexual relations. Menstrual bleeding which becomes unusually heavy [2] or causes passage of large clots also deserves evaluation.

2. *Unexplained weight loss.* Ten pounds loss within six months always deserves full evaluation.

3. *Watery or irritating vaginal discharge.* Although commonly due to noncancerous conditions, a watery discharge which burns, stings, or itches deserves a doctor's attention.

4. *Persistent indigestion or difficulty swallowing.*

5. *Change in bowel habit.* Abrupt onset of constipation, of alternate periods of constipation and diarrhea, or of frequent false alarms from the rectum may signify tumor.

6. *Persistent hoarseness.*

[2] A woman of average fastidiousness generally uses ten napkins or less during each menstrual period. If she soaks up twelve or more, medical examination is wise.

7. *Cough or change in the character of cough.* Enough mucus runs down from the back of the nose into the throat to give most people a slight persistent cough, which is usually unimportant. Any increased brassiness, depth, discomfort or frequency of cough deserves prompt medical evaluation.

How to Muster Cancer-fighting Courage

If you have yourself checked every year, inspect your body surface every month and remain constantly alert for possibly cancer-caused complaints, you should become suspicious of the presence of cancer very promptly if it should attack your body. However, the idea that cancer might be present is such a profound threat to your peace of mind that you can rarely face facts immediately. At some subconscious level, your mind usually argues:

"If it is cancer, I don't want to know. I'll have to change all my plans, my way of thinking, everything. I just can't face it right now."

Against this perfectly natural human tendency, you can muster three facts:

First, the complaints or findings may not signify cancer at all. The signs listed above are sufficiently suggestive to deserve attention, but will usually prove to be due to something other than a cancer. Prompt medical evaluation will probably set your mind at rest, not confirm your fears.

Second, the disruption of your living pattern involved in treatment of early cancer probably will be quite brief. Most people have a discouraging picture of cancer care, since the only cases they know about are those in which the disease progresses inevitably and painfully for months. In the early case (which even the victim usually does not know to be cancer), operation or x-ray therapy often involve no more than two to four weeks disability.

Third, cancer care is exceedingly hopeful. Permanent, lifelong cure seems possible in at least half the cases with prompt attention. Cancers commonly detected through a preventive program, such as cancer of the skin and breast, have a much higher rate of permanent cure.

Scientific Cancer Care

The primary aim of cancer treatment at present is destruction of the abnormal cancer cells. The most efficient way to do this is often to remove those cells along with a margin of normal neighbors. In some instances, the rapidly growing cancer cells can be selectively destroyed by radiation with x-ray or radioactive substances. These methods often prove curative.

If total destruction of the cancer cells is impractical, their rate of growth

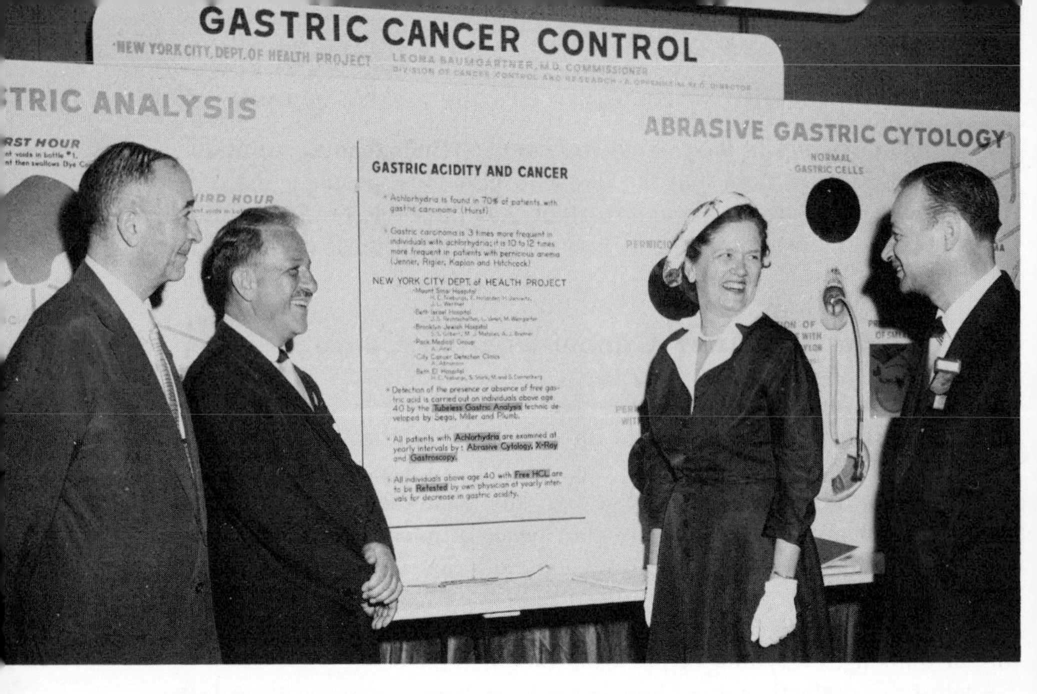

Figure 86. Cancer detection exhibit at medical convention. *Courtesy New York City Department of Health.*

can sometimes be slowed or temporarily halted by the use of hormones or other chemicals. Thus cancer of the prostate gland in men often melts away and remains apparently cured for months or years in response to injections or tablets of female sex hormone. To date, however, no methods other than surgery or radiation have produced lifelong cures. If your doctor advises surgery or radiation, a search for alternative means of treatment is usually worse than futile: the attendant delay wastes a substantial portion of your chance for cure.

COMMUNITY ATTACKS ON THE CANCER PROBLEM

Government agencies and voluntary health organizations attack the cancer problem in many ways. Probably the most effective in the past has been *public education.* Thanks to community efforts, a great many people know today that cancer can be cured and that the danger signs listed on pp. 278–9 might point to its presence. This knowledge makes for earlier care, which increases the rate of cure.

Cancer detection clinics also aim at earlier identification and cure of cancer victims. The detection clinic approach works less effectively for cancer than for such diseases as tuberculosis because of the lack of a single, quick and easy screening test. A complete physical examination and several special procedures are required to detect a fair proportion of early, curable malignancies. Moreover, the detection and care of one cancer does not make further malignancy among the remaining population less, as is the case with tuberculosis. However, cancer detection clinics have undoubtedly saved many lives and advanced medical knowledge of cancer in many ways.

Community sponsored research affords the great hope of the future in the cancer field. In separate units like the National Institutes of Health and in universities and hospitals throughout the land, scientific inquiry moves forward on many fronts. While no one expects a great breakthrough which will suddenly solve the cancer problem, new and effective measures for prevention, detection, cure and alleviation have been and will continue to be devised.

CHRONIC DISEASES OTHER THAN TUMORS OR INFECTIONS

Early and persistent care is the keynote for holding down damage from most chronic diseases. In general, one can say that:

1. Chronic diseases deserve attention according to their potential long-range effects, even if they cause little discomfort or inconvenience at the moment. Every substantial unexplained change in any body function or contour deserves a physician's evaluation. Every continuing, active disease deserves continuing, active care. For instance, an abrupt and substantial decrease in the volume of urine you pass deserves prompt and probably heroic medical care even though your comfort and capacities seem unimpaired. If tests prove that nephritis is present, continued careful adherence to a prescribed program may be wise for ten years or more, even though you feel perfectly well. This is true because nephritis usually leads to disabling or deadly effects over a period of years if it remains unchecked, not because immediate complaints will punish you for its neglect.

2. Chronic disease victims must rate the value of medical and other measures by comparing their condition at any one time with the state to which their disease would presumably have reduced them by that time, instead of comparing their state of health at the beginning and end of a treatment period. Almost all victims of chronic disease become slipshod in the management of their conditions at one time or another on the basis of one of two problems: undue discouragement or undue optimism. "My joints hurt just as much now as they did when we started this treatment," says the arthritic

who would almost certainly have sustained permanent crippling and felt much worse without care. "I didn't think I really needed shots any more, I felt so well," says the pernicious anemia victim who neglected his disease until he got a recurrence even though he had been repeatedly warned that his problems would come back as soon as he discontinued his injections.

3. Chronic disease sufferers must sometimes work for worthwhile improvement in ability to enjoy life or perform useful service instead of pursuing cure. They must often aim for restoration of over-all personal efficiency, not freedom from a diagnostic label or restoration of exactly the same capacities previously enjoyed. For example, one young lady was unable to work or to manage her own affairs because poliomyelitis had left her unable to get up and down stairways and curbs. A rehabilitation center fitted her with braces and taught her how to manage this task. She took secretarial training and became entirely self-sufficient. Her impaired muscular function remains unchanged, but her total functioning as an individual is tremendously improved. Like many other victims of chronic disease, she did not arrange this rehabilitation promptly, however: seven years of discouragement with the unavailability of cure preceded her first effort to seek such help.

Preventing Allergic Disease

Allergic diseases such as asthma and hay fever spring from abnormal sensitivity to certain ordinarily harmless substances or conditions. This sensitivity is usually based upon formation of chemical neutralizing bodies of the same sort your body uses very effectively in combating infection. When an antibody meets the substance it was formed to neutralize, known as its antigen, the ensuing reaction liberates a group of chemicals with strong effect upon nearby blood vessels and smooth muscle. These chemicals are histamine and several similar compounds. Their effect is usually desirable: it helps to open tiny blood vessels and bring extra blood supply to the scene of incipient infection. However, the effect can be very undesirable indeed when antibodies have formed against some ordinarily harmless substance such as ragweed pollen. Compared with the minute quantities of chemical associated with bacteria, the amount of pollen in each breath may be tremendous. The histamine and histamine-like substances liberated in your nasal lining or bronchial tree causes distressing swelling, irritation and muscle spasm. If the nasal lining is affected, the sneezing and congestion of hay fever result. If allergic effects strike mainly in the bronchial tree, the wheezing, cough and breathing difficulty of asthma follow.

Three different methods have proved highly efficient in preventing serious allergic disease:

1. *Decreased allergic exposure.* Since allergies usually develop quite early in life, measures for their complete prevention work best if applied from early childhood. If a child's family history suggests unusual liability to allergic disease (see Chapter 8) he should be shielded from common allergy-causing substances. Sample precautions: special techniques for infant feeding, no house pets or stuffed animals, scratch tests for grass and ragweed pollens before choosing the appropriate season for summer camp, special house-cleaning methods to cut dust exposure, avoidance of raw egg or other raw foods. Your physician can give detailed guidance, of course.

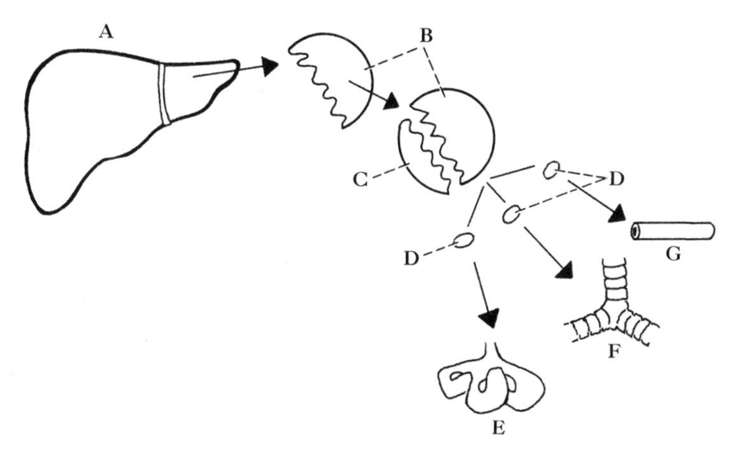

Figure 87. Reticulo-endothelial cells in the liver and spleen (A) make anti-bodies (B) which combine with antigen (C) in the tissues. Histamine-like compounds (D) liberated during the antibody-antigen reaction act on nasal lining tissue (E), bronchial tubes (F), or tiny blood vessels (G) to cause allergic disorders.

2. *Prompt identification and avoidance of allergens.* The body reacts to any occasion for antibody formation by speeding its production of all antibodies, so that any allergic exposure (and any infectious illness) increases all allergies. Moreover, the lining layers of the nose, lungs, and intestinal tract offer less barrier to penetration of substances capable of generating further allergies when their functioning is impaired by any disease, including allergic disorders themselves. One allergy thus predisposes to further allergies and contributes to its own further development.

Infants and small children commonly start their progress toward serious allergic disease with apparently mild food allergy or eczema. Introduction of one food at a time with alertness for possible allergies often pays off in long-term allergy control. Prompt consultation with a physician and thorough allergy testing when eczema, hay fever or recurrent bronchitis occur may allow avoidance of allergy-generated substances and complete control of allergies before they become multiple and severe.

3. *Desensitization.* Other than avoidance, desensitization is the only method of allergy control which substantially alters development of further allergies. Desensitization involves injections of gradually increasing amounts of purified antigen. This combines with harmful antibodies faster than the body can form new ones, and effectively reduces the concentration of antibodies in the blood stream and tissue fluids. The decision as to whether to use this method of allergy control must be left to your physician, of course. Its efficiency in preventing further allergies frequently makes desensitization worthwhile even when your complaints are not so severe as to demand it. Certainly, any trace of asthma calls for discussion of desensitization with your physician well in advance of your usual season, leaving plenty of time for possibly necessary tests and graduated injections.

ARTHRITIS

Probably the commonest form of joint disorder is osteoarthritis, which stems mainly from wear and tear. This disorder almost never leads to severe crippling or deformity, but causes considerable discomfort and disability. You can hold down joint damage through the years and decrease the onslaught of osteoarthritis by measures aimed at decreasing joint strain such as:

1. *Weight control.* Excess weight affects ankles, knees, hips and backs far out of proportion to the percentage of overload. Shedding extra pounds saves considerable wear and tear.

2. *Lifting technique.* A lifting position with the back upright and legs bent throws most of the load on the thigh muscles instead of the small spinal joints, and helps cut down arthritic change.

3. *Decreased mechanical vibration and jolting.* When you ride a truck or operate a heavy machine, vibration and jolting create considerable joint strain. Farmers often get back pain from rough-riding equipment. Proper springing, hydraulic cushioning or other means of smoothing the ride offer real joint-preserving benefits.

The other exceedingly common form of joint disease is *rheumatoid arthritis.* Before modern treatment made control of this smoldering, jointreezing inflammation possible, rheumatoid arthritis frequently led to crippling and deformity. Modern care of the active phase of the disease, combined with modern measures for preserving or restoring joint motion, almost always allow victims of rheumatoid arthritis to avoid marked bodily distortion or loss of function. The very long duration and commonness of the disease still makes it a major health problem, however.

DIABETES

Early detection is the keynote in preventing lasting damage from diabetes. Diabetes impedes the use as internal fuel of sugars and starches. The victim's body soaks up normal amounts of sugar from his food, but does not burn it normally. Sugar accumulates in the blood, and ultimately flows through into the urine. Sugar passing through the kidneys pulls extra water with it, thus increasing the volume of urine passed. Meanwhile, body parts which normally would operate with sugar as their main fuel begin to burn other compounds instead. The body burns some of these other compounds, particularly fats, in ways which lead to accumulation of harmful acid bodies in the blood and to accelerated hardening of the arteries.

Early Detection of Diabetes

In its earliest stages, diabetes can be identified only by laboratory tests of the victim's urine or blood. The period when diabetes remains undiscovered, with its deteriorative effects therefore unchecked, averages at least as long as the period of known disease. The potential damage which diabetes can do to your body if you wait until disease-caused complaints drive you to a doctor is thus very much greater than that you might suffer if you detect the disease promptly by laboratory means and bring it under control.

During diabetes detection week (the third week in November), most communities arrange free urine tests either by laboratory technicians or through self-performed home procedures. A urinalysis in your own doctor's office during a routine annual examination also accomplishes this end.

When to Suspect the Presence of Diabetes

The early manifestations of diabetes relate mainly to poor fuel use and increased volume of urine. Victims complain of fatigue. They lose weight in spite of good appetite. They often suffer intense and frequent thirst. They urinate frequently and voluminously. Poor resistance to infection often reveals itself through sieges of boils, poor healing of minor cuts, and prolonged illness with every cold.

Without adequate treatment, further difficulties develop. The accumulated poisons derived from faulty use of fats lead to episodes of unconsciousness. Accelerated hardening of the arteries leads to visual difficulties, to problems in circulation (sometimes even to gangrene) in the legs, and to a general speeding up of physical decline.

Insulin and Diabetes

Insulin is a substance poured into your blood stream by certain cells in your pancreas. It has an indispensable function in facilitating your body's use of sugars as fuel, and usually overcomes completely the diabetic's deficiency in sugar use. This does not mean that diabetes is caused by an insulin deficiency—faulty tissue response to normal insulin levels is undoubtedly at fault in some cases. The dosage of insulin required to control cases of diabetes is often much more than that required to correct sugar use after complete removal of the pancreas, for instance. However, insulin injections usually permit substantial control of the disease without undue dietary restrictions.

Several compounds have also been discovered which aid sugar metabolism in certain types of diabetes when taken in tablet form. These have not replaced insulin, but offer your doctor an additional, often-useful weapon against certain diabetic states.

CONVULSIVE SEIZURES

Convulsive seizures are fits of unconsciousness, usually accompanied by jerking muscular movements, which occur when certain brain cells are submitted to abnormal stimulation. Anyone will get a convulsive seizure from certain stimulating drugs or from the sharp drop in blood sugar after an overdose of insulin. Some people get convulsive seizures under unusual physical stress such as abrupt, high fever, lack of oxygen to the brain during a severe fainting spell, or upset in the body's chemical balance during an attack of diarrhea. Some other people get convulsive seizures without obvious precipitating stress. Such proneness to spontaneous seizures is known as epilepsy.

Certain laws, customs and common attitudes tend unjustly to set epileptics aside as second class citizens. Several states still have laws on the books forbidding epileptics to marry. In many states, a history of epilepsy suffices to keep a person from getting a driving license, even if proper care has kept him free of seizures for many years and attacks have always been preceded by preliminary warning symptoms. Employment opportunities and advancement often are denied because of the widespread notion that epilepsy leads to steady and inevitable mental decline.

The actual facts are much more hopeful. The probability of an epileptic's children suffering from spontaneous seizures is only slightly above the general average—certainly not sufficient to restrain his marriage and reproduction. Treatment controls epilepsy to the point where it usually becomes no substantial handicap. Virtually all epileptics can keep their disease under sufficient control to permit gainful employment. The mental deterioration which was once thought part of the disease virtually never occurs with proper treatment, and is now recognized to have resulted mainly from chemical and physical damage to the brain during uncontrolled seizures. Misinformation about epilepsy probably does much more harm than the disease itself, and certainly deserves whatever efforts you can devote to its correction.

NERVE CELL LOSS

Unlike other body tissues, nerve cells in your brain and spinal cord never replace themselves. Your original crop has to last for life. Any physical or chemical injury which kills these cells therefore leaves a lifelong defect.

Neurological defects often involve very specific areas, and interfere in no way with uninvolved functions. The polio victim who cannot raise his foot may still be able to straighten his knee. Similarly, the channels through which people communicate and relate to one another, including voice, facial expression, bodily posture and deliberate or unintentional gesture, frequently become impaired in neurological disease. Unless you recognize the fact that you constantly view the victim's mind and personality through a smoke-screen, you may not give him his due as a possible friend, student, or business associate. The grimacing, inco-ordinated victim of cerebral palsy usually has perfectly normal mental and emotional patterns, and deserves opportunities to exercise them.

Different neurological disorders cause different types of nerve cell damage and follow different courses, many permitting a normal life span while others lead rapidly downhill. In some, like cerebral palsy and poliomyelitis, skilled assistance allows the victim to make the most of the capacities which remain unimpaired and permit a full and useful life. In others, such as muscular dystrophy and multiple sclerosis, the outlook at this time seems rather bleak. Prevention, rehabilitation and research all offer hope in these disorders, however, and deserve your full support.

CHAPTER 23

Preventing or Managing the Problems of Old Age

WHEN A GROUP OF COLLEGE STUDENTS STATE THEIR MAIN HEALTH PROBLEMS, difficulties with aging relatives always rank quite high on the list. Of course, life can continue to be satisfying and pleasant right up until its termination, and some old people in their eighties and nineties create no problems whatever for their relatives and associates. However, each year on earth takes an almost inevitable toll. Injury or disease, including such almost universal disorders as arteriosclerosis, smolders along and leaves impairment in its wake. Age itself imposes burdens of wear and tear, even in the absence of any detectable disease or injury. A great many people live on beyond the point of total self-sufficiency, requiring everything from mild concern to constant attention or help during their period of decline. This problem-generating phase of old age involves decrease in protective or adaptive responses to extra stress. It involves changes in appetite, energy and environment which predispose toward malnutrition. It involves gradual erosion of sustaining personal and community relationships, with distinct threats to living satisfaction and to feeling of worth. It involves memory loss, emotional instability, and other undesirable mental changes. Although you might hope to see the oldsters in whom you have personal interest live out their lives happily and contentedly, you should prepare to watch for and control such difficulties as frequently arise.

Sluggish Protective and Adaptive Response

Old people respond less vigorously and less specifically to physical disorders, physical dangers and situational threats than young ones do. This sluggishness and vagueness of response creates many practical problems.

Difficulty deciding when a doctor's care is needed

Old people may have little or no fever in response to infection. They may have poorly localized and ill defined pain in conjunction with disease. They may have no distinct complaints with disorders which in younger persons would cause considerable discomfort or loss of function. To cite actual cases:

••• Seventy-two year old Mrs. B. fainted at the dinner table, and awoke complaining of vague, generalized discomfort. Laboratory tests led to an abdominal operation, which revealed that her illness was due to a ruptured appendix. She apparently had no symptoms whatever until the appendix actually burst, and only vague, atypical difficulties thereafter.

••• Eighty-one year old Mr. P. put off visiting his doctor for several days in spite of almost overwhelming fatigue, because he had no fever or other complaints to show that he was ill. When he finally got around to medical examination, he proved to have pneumonia.

This tendency toward obscure onset of illness makes it logical to call a physician for any suspicious alteration in a senior citizen's state of health. All too commonly, serious disease gets an almost insurmountable foothold through the regrettable tendency to shrug one's shoulders at vague complaints in the aged. While old people often have to bear up under some physical discomforts which are not sufficiently specific to permit medical relief, new complaints can only be evaluated by skilled medical examination. Periodic examinations are of increased value, also, both because complaints are a poor guide to need for medical care in the aged and because serious chronic diseases grow more common as the years go by.

Extra accident hazards

An old person's slowed muscular responses may let him suffer falls, sustain burns and otherwise receive injuries which a younger person's prompt responses would prevent. Older industrial workers do not have a markedly high rate of injury, presumably because of highly developed work skills. However, an old person's more brittle bones, slower healing, and tendency toward complicating disorders make home and other injuries quite common and hazardous. Thus home safety is especially important where senior citizens are concerned. Nonskid floor wax, rubber bathtub mats, and sturdy hand grips beside the tub; well-lit, uncluttered stairways; sturdy, stable household ladders and various household safety precautions save many an old person's life.

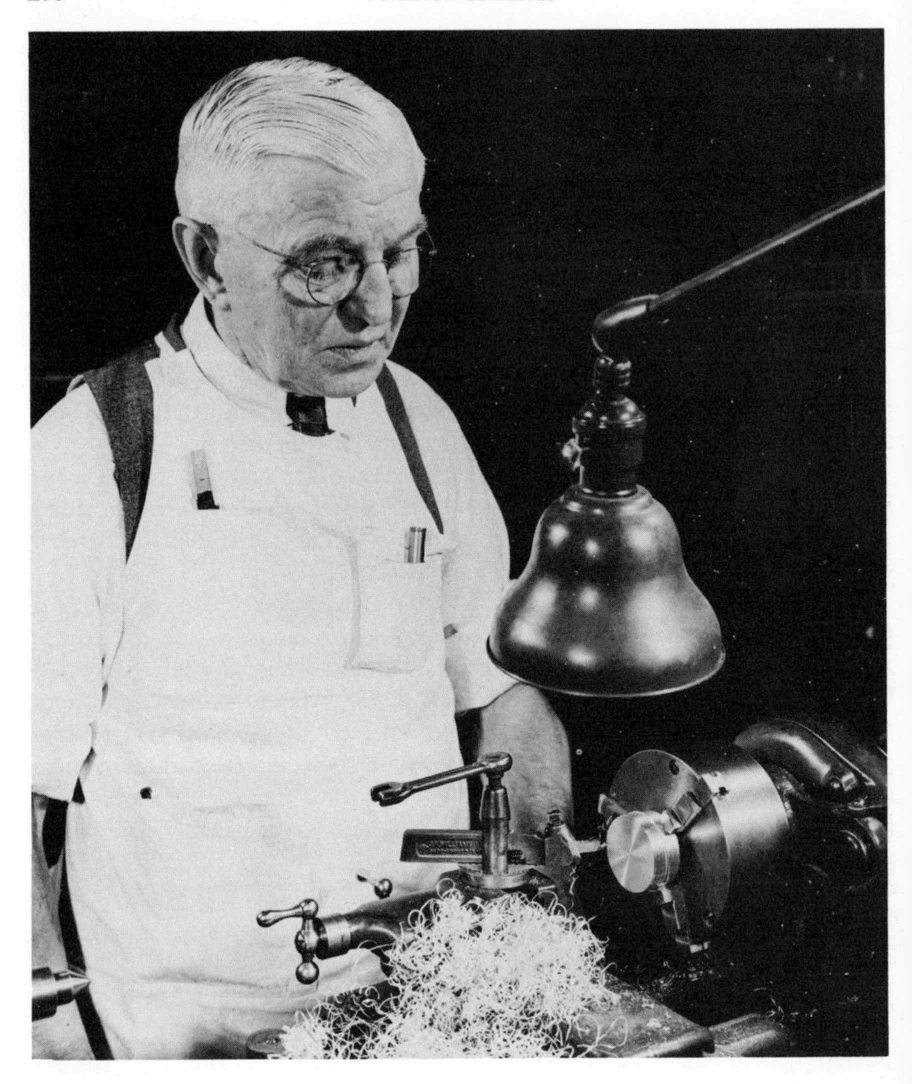

Figure 88. Skills built through a lifetime more than make up for lack of adaptiveness in this precision worker. *Ewing Galloway.*

Decreased adaptiveness

The response of the whole individual as well as the response of his various organs and parts slows somewhat in old age. Slow or inadequate response to new threats or demands often impedes an old person's adaptation to new circumstances. Old people often have thoroughly tested and refined skills with which to meet both vocational and personal needs but they do not have much capacity for quickly revamping their approach to meet altered circumstances.

This decreased adaptiveness makes at least a partially self-determined schedule almost essential for older people. Institutions for the aged must provide relative privacy and a flexible schedule. If you keep an older relative in your home, a separate exit and partial cooking facilities often let him continue his own living pattern with less friction than complete absorption into your household.

Nutrition in Old Age

Even if your activity level remains the same, your body's need for fuel falls by seven to eight per cent every ten years after full maturity. Decreased physical activity cuts your fuel needs further. Yet your need for vitamins, minerals, varied protein sources and so on remains virtually unchanged. You tend to eat much less, but require almost as much assortment of foods as ever.

At the same time, various pressures tend to decrease your food selection. Most old people suffer some budgetary restrictions which they meet by limiting meat, eggs and fruit. Poor teeth impose further limitations in selection of foods. Many old people live alone, and find it difficult to fix complete and varied meals for themselves. A can of peas lasts four or five meals, for instance. Its proprietor is fed up with both the cooking effort and the peas before it is gone. Prepared food mixtures like TV dinners and frozen meat pies afford some relief, but impose still another burden of expense.

If you have an older relative who lives alone, his grocery purchases give a better clue to his diet than his answers to inquiry. You can often arrange to drive him to and from the store without offending him, while he will treat questions as busybodyness. Sometimes you can arrange gifts of casseroles and other nutritious food combinations prepared as small-sized duplicates of your own family meals. Proper use of a freezing chest or compartment to permit preparation of larger quantities of food and spacing out in consumption of foods often proves very helpful to aged householders.

Sustaining Relationships

The web of affection and respect which everyone needs to sustain his ego gradually weakens with the advancing years. Old people inevitably lose friends and loved ones through death. They generally occupy a shrinking part in the lives of their children. They lose the feeling of worth that comes with useful employment, and often find their participation in church and community affairs curtailed.

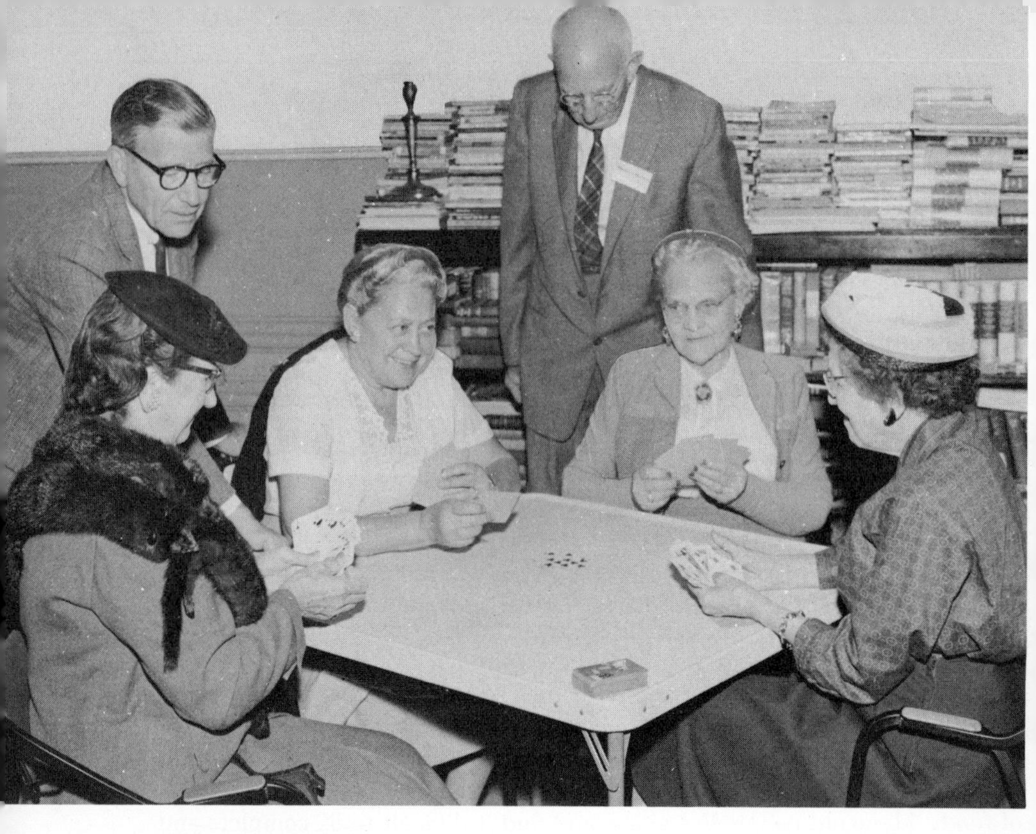

Figure 89. Fun in a Senior Citizens' Center. *Courtesy Senior Citizens Center of Schenectady County, Inc.*

Regular family activity and participation in community affairs help to ward off these difficulties. In some cases, a shift to an old people's home, active membership in a community recreation program for senior citizens, or work with religious organizations proves helpful.

Mental Changes

Changes in intellectual capacities and emotional stability almost always occur in old age, although these changes usually do not greatly impede active people with sound personality structure. Two fundamental alterations are quite common: memory change and emotional instability.

Memory change

Three separate functions seem to be involved in memory:

1. Immediate recollection, typified by your ability to dial a telephone number which you have just looked up.

2. Recent memory, typified by your ability to remember what you had for breakfast this morning.

3. Distant memory, typified by ability to recollect experiences from childhood and the past in general.

When old age leads to memory loss, ability to form permanent, new mnemonic impressions suffers first. Recent memory becomes inaccurate, even though immediate recollections are sound and distant memory may actually be heightened—a flood of new memories apparently obscures old ones to some extent. The lost memories do not necessarily stand out as blank places in the recent past, though. Your mind tends to fill in the gaps with logical but inaccurate subconscious fabrications. If you are concerned with the welfare of an older relative, this fact often creates many problems. You ask him what he had for breakfast and he answers: "Two eggs, bacon, toast and coffee." Then you find that he has not bought an egg for two months. Disagreements with the bank and with creditors also are frequent: the old person distinctly recalls paying all his bills or swears that he never made a certain purchase, and there is no way you can convince him that he is wrong.

One good protection against these difficulties is patterned or structured living. This case is an extreme example:

• • • Seventy-six-year-old Mrs. D. had virtually no memory for recent events, but she managed to live alone with very little help from her relatives. System was the keynote of her survival. She checked off each day on her calendar when she got up in the morning and consulted her reminder lists repeatedly. She had adopted a uniform weekly menu when her husband died some years before, and bought the same groceries every Tuesday and every Saturday. She paid for everything she bought in cash, put utility bills and such into a separate pigeonhole of her desk until they were paid, then filed them in her bottom drawer. Every Saturday she wrote checks, often carrying them downtown with her. The only time Mrs. D. got into trouble was when Tuesday or Saturday proved to be a holiday. On several such occasions, she went to do her shopping and found the stores closed, then became very confused and upset. Her relatives finally discovered the nature of her problem, and arranged to take her for a drive and supply her groceries for her when Tuesday or Saturday was a holiday, solving even that difficulty.

After recent memory has faded, immediate recollection and distant memory may gradually become inaccurate, too. This usually causes episodes of confusion and mismanagement of personal affairs.

Emotional instability

Many old people have abrupt mood swings. They sometimes move from tears to laughter and back to tears again in a matter of seconds. The proper approach to gloom in old age must be based upon this fact: where you need to show sympathy before you can give much comfort to a younger person, a bright greeting, pleasant remark, or quick switch to a pleasant (even if well-worn) topic works well with old people. Typical dialogue between a very old patient and a favored (for obvious reasons) nephew:

Old man (in tears): Nobody gives a hang about me.

Nephew: Say, why don't you tell me about the time Teddy Roosevelt shook hands with you. I certainly like that story.

Old man (brightening almost instantly): Well, like I've always told you, Teddy was nobody's fool——.

Old man (becoming aggrieved again): I haven't heard from your mother in months.

Nephew: She is quite well. Look here, I've got my picture album along. Want to see how the family's grown?

Old man: You bet I do! (Adjusts his glasses.) Say, look here at little Tib! Isn't he something!

A number of mementos, souvenir books, and other reminders of past pleasures may help an old person to remain content, even though these things seem useless to younger eyes.

LIVING ARRANGEMENTS FOR OLD AGE

The old person of today belongs to a lost generation. When he was young, old folks got family aid as their just reward for having reared, educated and given opportunity to children. Now that he is old, young people have different views. They hold that each person deserves as a sacred right all the education and opportunity which his gifts permit him to utilize, and should look to the government or to insurance rather than to the family for security. This leaves little room for profound feelings of family obligation to their own parents and old relatives.

Few people arrive at age sixty-five with enough money to manage their full support during the average of fourteen years which remain to them, few can support themselves entirely by working, and relatively few can count on extensive family aid. Most must depend mainly upon public assistance, social security, pensions, or investments.

Public assistance

Funds administered by the welfare departments of state, county and municipal governments help to sustain old people who have no other means. In most cases, assistance granted becomes a lien against any property the old person possesses. This policy is intended to keep people who accept no obligation toward their older relations from later profiting from their relationship through inheritance, not to keep down utilization of funds by the needy who still own property or a home. Such assistance usually maintains no more than a minimal standard of living, however, and is difficult for people with strong feelings of pride to accept.

Social security

Social security is a compulsory program for financial protection against dependency, paying benefits to the worker in case of permanent disability or retirement and to his family in case he dies leaving dependent children or an aged widow. The reserves accumulated by the social security administration are nowhere near sufficient to pay benefits to all the people who have contributed, so that the present arrangement imposes the burdens of retirement for each generation upon the next. However, the enormous reserves necessary to make each generation truly self-sufficient would alter the entire capital structure of our economy. The program is secure, since receipts from future subscribers undoubtedly will provide adequate cash to pay benefits when present subscribers die or retire, and discontinuance of the program is politically impossible. Benefits received by each group since the inception of the program have generally matched or exceeded in value the benefits purchasable from private insurance companies for similar premium outlay. The only trouble with social security as an income supplement in old age is that benefits are not paid until age seventy-two if the old person continues to work, so that the person who wants to remain productive sacrifices his social security benefits for several years. People in their sixties are thus discouraged from continuing to work, with harm both to themselves and to the economy.

Pensions

Industrial and union pensions increasingly assist with the financing of retirement. Funds vary in extent and administration, but deserve close attention in arranging employment and establishing a retirement plan.

Annuities and investments

Only about one person in eleven in the general population supports himself by income from investments today, partly because of the extensive wartime and post-war inflation. Insurance and other fixed-return investments enjoyed high favor for building retirement funds in the thirties and forties. Such investments give no protection against inflation, and many people who retired on what they thought was an adequate income found themselves in dire straits when their dollars shrank in purchasing power.

Investment counselors today advise accumulating retirement funds partly in fixed-dollar form (insurance policies, bonds, savings accounts) and partly in inflation-riding form (real estate, stocks, mutual fund shares). An early start means a smaller annual burden in accumulating retirement funds, of course.

Retirement

Although they do not realize it, most people gain from their work several important forms of satisfaction and psychologic support in addition to the recognized material rewards. When they retire, they often miss these non-material compensations very much, even if they do not miss their wages. That is why many people want to keep working, even if they can afford to retire. For instance, one man who depended heavily on his continued employment to justify his self-respect complained: "I'm worth just as much this month as I was last. Why do they have to cast me aside like an old shoe?"

The other side of this question might be termed the boss's dilemma. "How in the world can you decide when a man has lost his sharpness?" one employer remarked. "And if you do decide, how do you tell him so without *really* bruising his ego?"

Since this latter problem proves almost insurmountable, most organizations have a definite retirement age. After age sixty-five or so, the chances are that you will have some degree of difficulty finding further opportunities for gainful or even useful activity. Only four channels are frequently open: irregular, not too challenging work such as odd jobs, piecework or commission selling; operation of a small business which is primarily an investment, and therefore involves some risk if your estimate of your capacities is in error; useful activity in conjunction with church or some other organization; and useful activity within your own family group.

Hobbies sometimes serve to fill the gap, especially if they have been developed during earlier, more active years. An old person can achieve the feeling of worth which he needs so desperately by winning a game of checkers or carving a soap statue even if he does not earn a dime in the process.

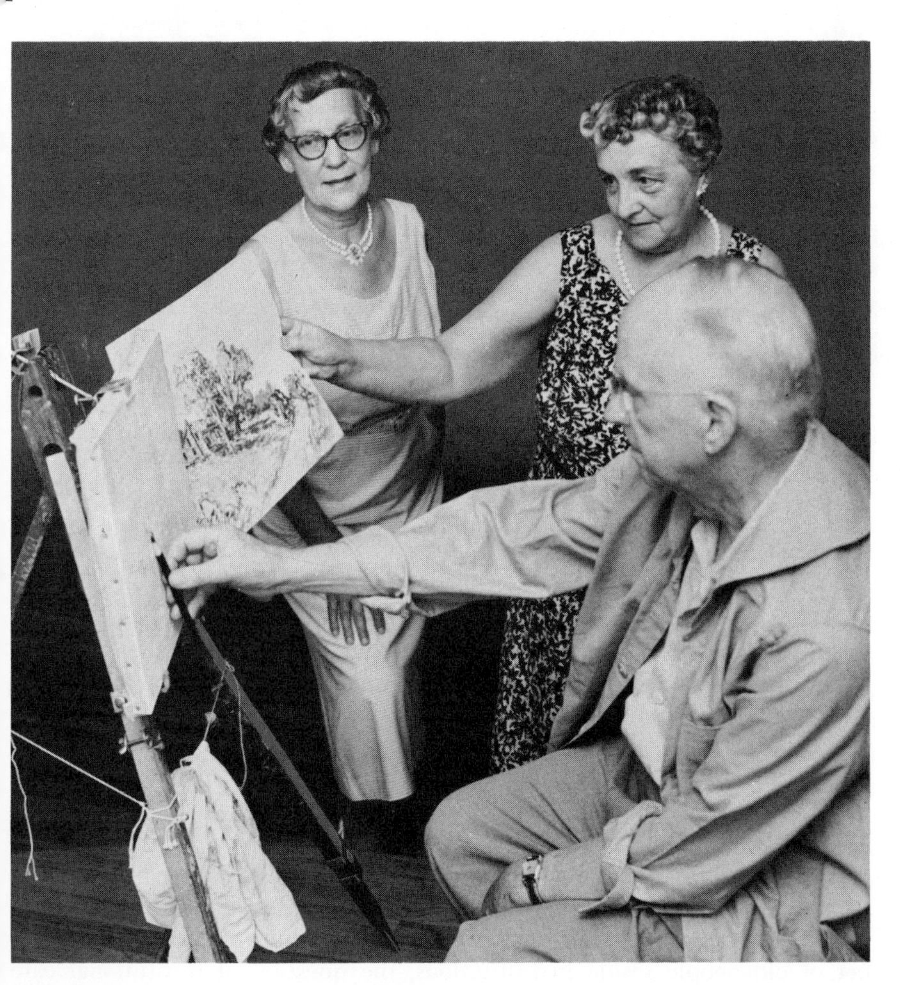

Figure 90. Absorbed in a hobby. *Courtesy Senior Citizens Center of Schenectady County, Inc.*

Most people do best if they plan the way of life they will pursue after retirement, test it out in small doses over the years, and edge into it gradually. Remembering the limited adaptability of the aged and the relative paucity of emotional supports available to them, doesn't it make sense to spend several vacations down in Florida instead of moving there from a midwest farm without any preliminary trial? Doesn't it make sense to get a

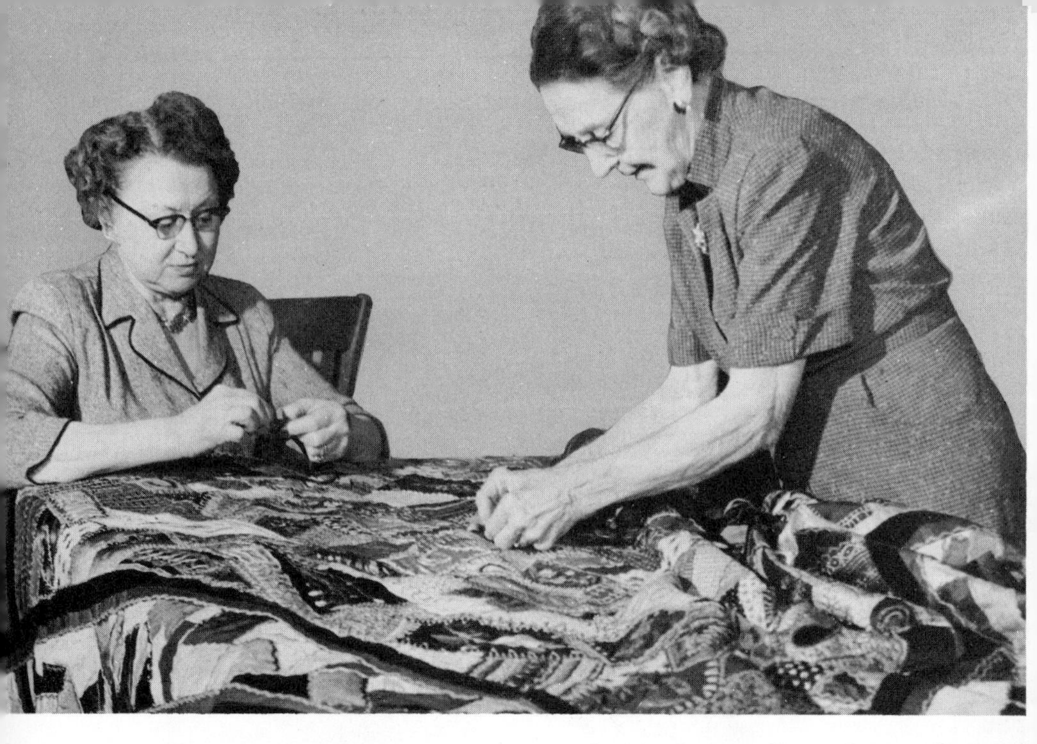

Figure 91. Organization projects give satisfaction. *Courtesy Senior Citizens Center of Schenectady County, Inc.*

job relieving a hotel's night clerk two or three evenings a week instead of spending your life savings on a motel without ever trying the business? Unfortunately, people do not always take time for such testing until retirement is already upon them and abrupt action seems required.

Special Facilities for the Aged

Institutions aimed at providing comfortable and pleasant living facilities for older people can be found in every part of the country, although most of the better ones have long waiting lists. Although a relatively small number of old people reside in institutions, the question of institutional care often comes up. Some homes for the aged make special financial arrangements whereby a person can sign over a certain amount of property and be assured of a home for the rest of his life: if he dies in a week, the institution makes a profit with which to offset the losses they might suffer on clients who live to age one hundred. Other institutions operate on a weekly or monthly charge like any boarding house.

Facilities or areas in several states, especially Florida, California and Arizona, are oriented toward the needs of older people who maintain independent households. Certain trailer courts and rental units cater to retired people, often providing social centers where they can congregate, shuffleboard courts, and other suitable recreations. Individual units are generally compact and easy to maintain, providing welcome relief from heavy household chores.

An increasing number of municipal recreation agencies now operate senior citizens' clubs or other programs providing recreation, crafts, and social exchange for older people. These clubs promote better physical and mental health to a measurable degree: one Brooklyn district found that decrease in the welfare department's medical expenses after institution of an active recreation program for old people actually paid the entire cost of the recreation program twice over.

All of these facilities blend privacy and independence with social opportunity and personalized care in a way which exactly suits the needs of many old people. Although each individual's interests and needs must be evaluated in deciding what type of living arrangement will suit him best, it is no longer true today (as it may have been a generation ago) that families place their old folks in an institution or send them to a distant retirement center only out of disinterest and neglect. Very often, they encourage such arrangements wisely for the good of the individuals concerned.

Hospital or Nursing-Home Care

You may well have to decide some day at what point an aging relative needs constant supervision and care. These points may help you:

1. Inability to recognize familiar people and locations, or to know the date (month, day and year) within two or three days, usually goes along with dangerous loss of memory and judgment.
2. The feeling that others are taking advantage of him or cheating him may make minor degrees of memory loss cause serious friction for an old person. For example, the man who simply does not remember whether he got his pension check yesterday or not may be able to make out well outside an institution, while the one who automatically accuses his wife of stealing it usually requires institutional care.
3. Periods of confusion, dizziness or unconsciousness usually call for continual supervision.

CHAPTER 24

Safety

IT TAKES COURAGE TO PLAY SAFE, AND BEFORE YOU CAN EVEN START YOU MUST get past the fear-dictated "personal immunity factor." Most people think "It can't happen to me," and proceed blithely, completely neglecting ordinary precautions. Ironically, their associates often credit them with intestinal fortitude instead of recognizing the fact that they simply haven't enough courage to face the facts.

Before you can deal with a hazard effectively, you have to acknowledge it deliberately. You never feel that your own chance of falling down stairs or being caught in a fire justifies the effort of a home safety inspection, or that your own chance of being killed in an automobile accident really justifies the "chicken" tactics of defensive driving. It's emotionally disturbing (and therefore very difficult) to face the extent of your own liability to accidental injury or death. Most people have to drive themselves to this unpleasant task by a very definite periodic exercise of will rather than depend on regular, everyday thinking processes.

HOW TO DISCOVER HAZARDS

At least once a year, perhaps as part of your New Year's observance, a brief hazard hunt usually proves worthwhile. Walk through your home from attic to cellar with safety uppermost in your mind. You'll often find accumulated paper and oily or waxy rags in which fire can start, cluttered stairways or broken stair treads, wiring defects, and a dozen other risky states you can easily set straight. A similar tour of work and play areas may pay big dividends.

Mental review of planned activities may help, too. Will your vacation involve boating where life belts should be routine? Do you change your storm windows without benefit of a sturdy ladder? Do you tackle household repairs in a harum-scarum way instead of setting up a safe and efficient work bench?

As a running check on safety hazards, you can also organize a record for close calls and minor injuries. Such incidents often reveal potentially serious risks. If you have a definite safety notebook and encourage every member of the family to write down each injury or close call along with the exact particulars, you will often discover and correct substantial risks.

Injury	Place	What happened	How further trouble might be avoided	Family counsel's actions
Potential Burn	Kitchen stove. Baby at right side.	Baby climbed on stool and tried to cook in pot—tipped it toward him. Fortunately, I caught him up out of the way.	Rearrange furniture with work table to block off area beside stove. Keep pot handles turned in—get rid of stool.	First two suggestions adopted. Mom needs the stool to reach shelves safely.

Figure 92. A safety notebook makes minor incidents into major warnings and often prevents later accidents. Last two columns discussed thoroughly in family group.

Important hazards

Perhaps comparisons with problems whose magnitude you already recognize may lead you to appreciate the importance of the commoner accident risks. As a whole, accidents cause more death and disability before retirement age than heart disease, cancer or any other type of health threat. Automobile accidents are so common that you have a better-than-even chance of being killed or seriously injured in one during your remaining years of life. Many other types of accident kill or disable far more people every day than poliomyelitis, which most people acknowledge as a risk worth attacking. Falls, drowning, fires, burns and scalds, poisoning, electrical hazards, accidents involving machinery and livestock, and accidental shooting all deserve preventive action.

Dealing with Hazards

Once you recognize a hazard, you can lessen it in several ways.

Elimination

If a given piece of equipment creates more hazards than it is worth, you can eliminate it. You can discord left-over medicines which have no foreseeable future use, for instance. You can disconnect unused electrical outlets within the reach of small children. Clutter from stairways, throw rugs and ragged carpetings require attention, especially if you have fall-prone old people in the house.

Guards on the article

You can often eliminate most risks without impairing utility by fitting a misuse-preventing guard. Iron grillwork or security screens on second-story windows let in light and air while still preventing falls, for instance. Non-skid rug pads prevent many falls. A kitchen arrangement which keeps toddlers away from the sides of the stove may prevent fatal scalding.

Guards available for users

Sometimes the person using equipment can increase its safety by taking steps which you can make more convenient. Hot pads stored within reach of the stove are one example. Calked boots for old people to wear during icy winter also help.

Consolidate the hazards

Often if several risky items are put in one place, protective measures or safety rules are easier to enforce. You might collect household poisons into a single box which can be locked or made definitely off bounds for children, for instance. Similar treatment works well for firearms and for sharp or dangerous tools. Stacking stored materials in one area and covering them with canvas helps keep youngsters from climbing on them, experimenting with risky materials, and so on.

Safe and effective habits

If you devise and establish a new, less hazardous but equally efficient way of accomplishing a given purpose, you serve the cause of safety. Learning to lift with leg power and an upright back is one example. You might have to concentrate on it for a few weeks, but after that you automatically continue the habit.

Learn safety-promoting skills

Behind-the-wheel driver training measurably decreases highway risks.

The heavy drowning toll among children is a potent argument for swimming instruction, not against it. Wading, boating, and falls into the water and through thin ice account for most of the casualties. Swimming at unguarded beaches and foolhardy overconfidence account for most of the rest. Proper instruction could prevent many of these tragedies.

Follow a blazed trail

In many instances, experts have studied the facts and made rules or suggestions which outline safe ways of achieving your end. When you drive a strange road, for instance, the speed limit signs are a better index to probable traffic conditions and hazards than any other means of instantaneous appraisal. Even if you travel a road every day, you do not have the facts and knowledge about accident frequency, cross traffic and the many other factors a traffic expert applies in setting a speed limit. Why not use his considered opinion of proper speeds, at least as a general guide?

COLLEGE SAFETY

You will avoid considerable burdens of misery and disability if you can decrease your chance of suffering laboratory, sports, and traffic accidents during your college years. These three types of accident account for most collegians' injuries. You can prevent many adversities with practical, simple measures.

Laboratory safety

You can prevent many accidents by developing safe and effective work habits in laboratories. For instance glass tubing goes through a cork readily if you roll the cork thoroughly, bore a proper size hole, always use water or glycerin, use a towel to protect both of your hands, and feed through the tubing a little at a time. Always study the manual or check with an instructor to learn safe techniques before trying new tasks with glass, strong acids or alkalis, electricity, etc. Try to work out uniform work habits, too. A single area designated as "hot spot" for recently bent tubing, etc., saves you many minor burns through the years. A standard approach to routine chores, from assembling apparatus to cleaning equipment, helps you work faster as well as stay safer.

Many laboratory accidents can be kept from doing serious harm by prompt use of emergency equipment. A water bath or shower should always be nearby when you are working with acids. The habit of setting out water for use as an eye bath if necessary may be worth forming. You should check where fire extinguishers are located and which one to use for each kind of fire.

One approach to laboratory safety is to ask each instructor during your first or second session with him to discuss the accidents or close calls he has seen during his teaching career and how each might have been prevented or kept from doing as much harm.

Sports safety

The vast majority of college sports injuries occur during unorganized or intramural rather than varsity participation. In these situations, and to some extent in understaffed physical education courses, your safety rests largely in your own hands. You have to rate your own condition and skill, arrange for proper equipment, and see that everybody sticks fairly close to the rules.

Condition and skill

Conditioning definitely helps to prevent injury. One of the best ways to keep from becoming a sports casualty is to anticipate active sports seasons with some conditioning activity. Some athletes do this by arranging some kind of sports or physical activity throughout the year, others start a calisthenic program a few weeks before their most active season. Either way, you'll avoid many injuries by getting into condition before you compete.

Skill enters the injury picture whether you compete against the elements or against other players. Most skiing accidents, many drownings, and quite a few gymnastic injuries stem from overconfidence. Difficulties sufficient to give you a thrill of accomplishment when you overcome them always involve some hazard, and deserve full respect. Perhaps someone else's estimation of your readiness for a certain feat might be more accurate than your own, or at least prove worthy of consideration.

Unequal competition between players leads to frequent injuries. Without in any way meaning to do so, an experienced two-hundred-pound football player is likely to mangle a lightly built novice. Such encounters never happen in varsity ball, but frequently occur in unorganized touch games.

Equipment and grounds

If varsity football matches were played on bumpy fields in deficient or misfitted pads, few coaches would be able to field a team two weeks in a row. Many of the injuries from unorganized and intramural games stem directly from such poor grounds and equipment. If better equipment is available at reasonable cost, the decrease in ijuries may make it worthwhile. An alternative approach is to modify the rules of the game to suit your facilities. Football players without pads and helmets should set up special rules to eliminate all kick plays, for instance: downfield blocking without pads is foolhardy. If a softball catcher has no mask, best eliminate base stealing so that he can back up to a safe distance behind the plate. If the playing field has certain rough areas, see whether you can rearrange boundaries to eliminate them (e.g., a hit into the hummocks is an automatic double).

Officiating

In some colleges, injuries during unorganized and unofficiated games were once so frequent that recreational workers were assigned to the available

Figure 93. Regular practice makes a difference—to skill *and* safety. *Gary K. Cowell.*

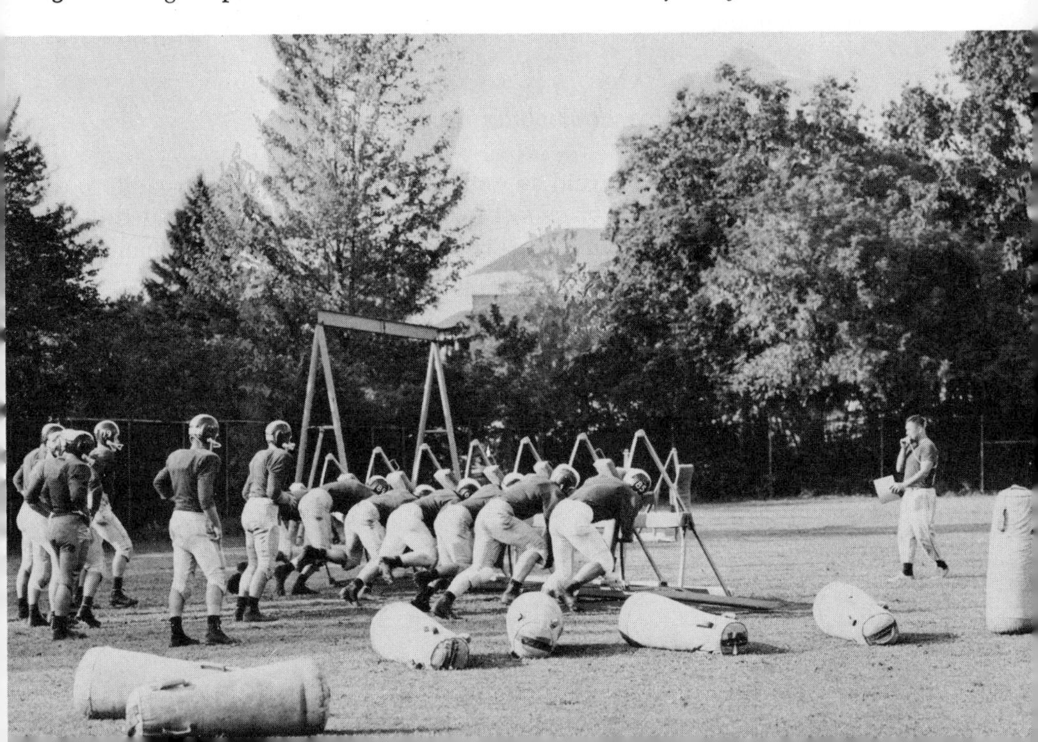

playing fields. The decreased cost of friendly mayhem has generally proved sufficient to pay their salaries with interest.

Reasonably tight officiating helps to keep down injuries in most games. You can rotate the officiating chore among players in an unorganized game or ask your physical education department to provide officials (since many would-be physical educators are as interested in officiating as in playing the game). If no official is available, scrupulous calling of fouls even on your own team makes for a cleaner, better, and infinitely safer game.

Traffic

It's human nature to make the chore of getting from place to place into a game. Children do it by skipping, doing cartwheels, and walking along the tops of walls; teenagers do it with drag races; and somewhat juvenile adults do it by racing at stoplights, weaving through traffic, and ignoring speed limits. The speed laws are one of the few sets of authoritarian regulations you can break without marked social disapproval.[1] Discourtesy is much more socially acceptable behind the wheel, too: many drivers find horn-blasting, crowding and cutting-in effective outlets for their hostilities, although most would admit that many less hazardous outlets are available.

The actual time gained through frantic driving seldom merits the nervous strain and effort, much less the risk: a top-notch driver racing through city traffic (with police permission) saved less than two minutes on a twenty-minute run when he ignored traffic regulations instead of obeying them. Complete obedience to traffic laws and bland unconcern with whether others are getting ahead of you or violating your rights cost you surprisingly little time, if you can only adopt a viewpoint which keeps them from rending your emotions.

Injury-reducing automobiles

Even if you cannot avoid an automobile accident, you can quite possibly avoid or decrease your chance of injury in it. Safety belts, padded dash and visors, remodeled steering wheels and collision-cushioning bumpers are a few of the measures which have proved helpful. The collision crouch, in which you hug your chest to the steering wheel or brace your body against

[1] If you doubt this statement, compare the reception your friends give you if you get tagged for reckless driving with their attitude toward any other crime of comparable magnitude under the law such as drunk and disorderly conduct or shoplifting, and their attitude toward valid measures of law enforcement which make unmarked cars for speed control "sneaky" while viewing plainclothes detectives as perfectly proper protection for property.

he dash, definitely keeps down injury if you have the presence of mind to ssume it. Riding small children in the back seat or in a seat attached backvard to the back of the front seat helps keep them free of injury.

Pedestrian accidents

A surprising number of college students hurt themselves while walking rom place to place. Icy steps and walks certainly deserve attention. Fads in ootwear have some effect: from slick sneakers to spike heels, all extremes eem to increase injuries. Haste and inattentiveness create further problems.

CHAPTER 25

Meeting Health Emergencies

YOU NEED A GREAT DEAL OF FIRST AID TRAINING TO HANDLE INJURIES ON THE battlefield, in an atomic air raid, or out in the wilderness. Much simpler techniques suffice (and often are much better) in the ordinary civilian situation where you can reach a doctor or nurse by telephone in a few minutes and transport a casualty to the hospital rapidly. Everyone—even people already accomplished in more elaborate, special-situation first aid methods—should learn the fundamentals presented in this chapter.

INSTANT EMERGENCIES

A few accidents and illnesses call for such prompt action that you have no time to call a doctor for help or advice. You should strive to get medical aid to the victim as quickly as possible in all such cases, even while you are doing what you can for him yourself. However, you will have to proceed with certain procedures in the meanwhile.

Poisoning

When you suspect that a person has recently swallowed some poisonous substance, look into his mouth. Unless you see considerable evidence of chemical burns—and unless the patient is unconscious or the poison is a petroleum product—you should induce vomiting. Turn the victim on his stomach and keep his hips higher than his head to keep him from sucking vomited material into his lungs. If the victim is a small child, you will usually find it best to hold him across your knees. Tickle the back of his throat with your finger, until the stomach has been thoroughly emptied. A small volume of water or milk followed by immediate induction of vomiting may wash some further poison out.

If mouth burns show that the substance was caustic, vomiting may tear the damaged tissues of the gullet. Probably the commonest serious caustic poisoning occurs when young children eat drain-clearing preparations containing lye. Vinegar contains enough acid to neutralize such alkaline poisons. Dilute half a glass of vinegar with a glassful of water. Acid poisons, such as glacial acetic acid from a photographic darkroom, can be neutralized with a solution of baking soda. Milk works fairly well in neutralizing both acids and bases, and should be administered if caustic poisons of unknown nature have been swallowed.

Always save the container from which the suspected poison came, and take it along to the hospital or doctor's office. An exact knowledge of the ingredients in the poison often proves very helpful to the victim's physician. Immediate medical care is always wise, even if you think you have recovered all of the poison.

Blocked Breathing

Sucked-in food chunks or pieces of plastic toy sometimes lodge in the throat to block breathing. The nature of the problem is often confused by the victim's violent attempts to breathe. Close observation will show that as the diaphragm pushes the abdomen out it sucks the lower part of the chest in. The apparent breathing motions are see-saw in character instead of being properly coordinated. When this happens, you have only five minutes or less in which to reestablish flow of air into the lungs before the victim expires. Attempts to remove the offending object with your finger only pack it down harder and cause more object-retaining swelling. Your best bet is to keep hands off, place the victim in a slightly slanted, face down, hips high posture which encourages the object to fall away from its blocking position when unconsciousness relaxes the surrounding muscles, and simultaneously make arrangements to get skilled help. The postural program works well in an automobile, so the ideal course in most circumstances is to rush the victim to a car, place him stomach down and partly on his side, and head for the hospital or for a doctor's office by a predetermined route. Someone else can call the doctor meanwhile and ask him to meet you halfway. Both you and the doctor should blow your horns constantly and keep your headlights on so that you will recognize each other instantly.[1]

[1] You have read about heroic first aiders who cut into the windpipe and inserted part of a fountain pen cap into the wound to provide a breathing passage. In an isolated spot, such measures might be truly heroic. When they are done within a block of the nearest medical building (as was the case in one recent episode), you can't help but wonder whether instant mobilization from one or both ends would not have solved the problem more satisfactorily.

Respiratory Arrest

Victims of drowning, electric shock, and brain injury or disease often cease breathing when otherwise capable of recovery. In such instances, you should start artificial respiration immediately and continue it indefinitely until medical aid appears. In electrical accidents, you must be careful to interrupt the flow of current before touching the victim, of course.

The mouth-to-mouth method of artificial respiration seems simple, safe, and effective. Its principal plus points are that it leaves your hands free to deal with any blockage in the breathing passage, makes you continually aware of how much or how little air you are getting through into the victim's lungs, and is much less fatiguing than methods calling for use of the victim's chest as a bellows. Clear the breathing passage by removing loose dentures or other objects from the mouth if necessary. Place the victim on his back. In this position, the muscular relaxation of unconsciousness usually lets the jaw bone drop straight back, permitting the back of the tongue to block the breathing passage. Pull the jaw straight forward so that the chin juts well in front of the upper lip to keep the passage clear. Encompass the victim's mouth with your own and close off his nose with your fingers. If the victim is an infant or small child, you may need to encompass both his mouth and his nose with your lips to get a tight seal. Press upon his abdomen with your free hand if any air is passing into the stomach. Blow into his mouth until you see or feel a definite rise in his upper abdomen. Remove your mouth and take a breath while his lungs deflate naturally. Blow into his mouth at brief intervals, aiming for about twenty breaths per minute.

Heavy Bleeding

Occasionally, an accident involves such heavy bleeding as to create an immediate threat to the victim's life. Bleeding must be exceedingly heavy to create immediate danger: totally uncontrolled bleeding from the largest wrist artery generally takes about twenty minutes to cause fatal changes. Even heavy bleeding usually slows sufficiently when you place direct pressure on the wound to permit a doctor to reach the scene before serious harm results. The best method of controlling bleeding in civilian accidents is therefore direct, firm pressure through several layers of cloth, continued without interruption for at least four minutes or until professional help arrives. In the excitement that follows an accident, most people give direct pressure much too little time to do the job. One minute seems an eternity, so they interrupt pressure every few seconds to see if bleeding is still active and never allow a hemorrhage-stopping clot to form. The intense color of blood lets a few tablespoonsful soak through a coarse towel or undershirt in a frightening fashion, often making the excited first aider quit direct pressure and try a tourniquet. In my years of practice, I have never seen a wound short of amputation in which bleeding could not be controlled by direct pressure. I have seen a great many patients with heavy bleeding while a tourniquet is in place who stopped bleeding as soon as the tourniquet was removed,[2] and at least one patient who lost an arm due to arterial injury resulting from application of a poorly padded tourniquet. As long as medical aid is fairly readily available, you virtually never should apply a tourniquet.

Shock

Severe injury, hemorrhage or overwhelming pain cause a harmful bodily response known as shock, which disturbs the nervous system's regulation of circulation and other automatic body processes. The most critical problem in shock is effective decrease in the volume of blood available to the brain and other organs because of pooling in engorged abdominal veins. Lack of blood supply to the brain leads to dizziness or unconsciousness, lack of circulation to the muscle makes for overwhelming weakness, and lack of blood in the skin makes for extreme pallor. The pulse becomes weak and rapid, the blood pressure very low. Shock also causes profuse perspiration, making for a cold, clammy skin. When these evidences suggest shock either after an injury or in the course of an illness, the victim should be laid out flat or with his feet a few inches higher than his head, which promotes return of venous blood to his heart. He should be kept warm to prevent shivering, which would otherwise demand extra blood flow through muscles and leave that much less for the vital organs. He should be protected from further painful or emotionally disturbing experiences (e.g., transportation with an unsplinted fracture or a chance to look at any severe wound). Most of the circumstances in which shock occurs involve possible abdominal injury, emergency surgery, or tendency toward vomiting, so you should not ordinarily let the victim drink water until the doctor comes.

Unconsciousness

Whether unconsciousness results from injury or illness, you can apply certain emergency measures while awaiting medical aid. Lay the victim flat

[2] Even a well-padded tourniquet is downright painful when tight enough to stop all flow of blood through the arteries in an extremity. Consequently, most tourniquets are applied tight enough to stop flow in the veins, but not tight enough to dry up the arteries. The blood moves almost unimpeded into the extremity, and then has no place to go but out on the floor.

on his back, especially if injury, stroke, or circulatory disturbances (such as fainting) seem at fault. Remove chewing gum, loose dentures, and other objects which might drop back into the victim's throat. Pull his jaw forward into the jutting position described in conjunction with artificial respiration above. This step is especially important if breathing is noisy or snoring in quality: noisy breathing is partially obstructed breathing. If the victim starts to vomit or regurgitate, you must generally roll him quickly to the side so that his face points at least partially toward the ground. Then gravity will carry the vomitus away from the breathing passage. Sometimes you must mop out mucus or secretions from the mouth and throat, too.

Victims of convulsive seizures require some further assistance to keep down bodily injury during attacks. A convulsive seizure is an attack of unconsciousness accompanied by violent twitchings or rhythmic movements. A sucked in moan or involuntary cry often heralds the seizure, giving bystanders an opportunity to help the victim avoid injury during the fall which usually occurs immediately thereafter. Seizure victims frequently bite themselves on the tongue or bruise themselves against nearby furniture during their violent muscular twitchings. A few layers of cloth (e.g., a folded handkerchief) or of felt (e.g., a hat or blackboard eraser) between the teeth helps to prevent tongue injuries. You must be careful not to push the lip or cheek between the teeth while inserting such a gag, and not to use any object which might break or might injure the teeth. It is better to let the victim bite his tongue than to break off three of his teeth by shoving a knife handle into his mouth, as an ardent first aider did for one of my patients.

People frequently make the mistake of trying to force some "stimulant" such as brandy (which is not a stimulant anyway) or coffee down an unconscious person's throat. The victim often sucks said substance into his lungs, with resulting blocked breathing or later pneumonia. Your best bet is to leave stimulants to the physician.

Community Emergency Facilities

Most communities provide aid for instant health emergencies in addition to and in conjunction with the normal hospital and medical installations. You can get help from the rescue squad, whose members have training in all types of emergency care, by calling the fire department. Most hospitals provide emergency care and advice around the clock. Some communities maintain a Poisoning Control Center in one of the major hospitals, providing doctors and first aid workers with an immediately available source of information on what products contain which poisons, appropriate antidotes, and so on. The Red Cross, Civilian Defense agencies, Boy Scouts, and other agencies provide instruction in first aid and emergency care to interested parties.

CONJOINTLY HANDLED EMERGENCIES

You can get medical aid and advice before you have to take any particular action in handling most injuries and illnesses. When an emergency does not involve an instant emergency, you should usually do as little as possible until you have discussed the situation with a doctor. If a man's leg is bent double at a fracture site, leave it bent double until the doctor comes. Protect an accident victim from the elements instead of moving him out of the cold or rain. If he is lying in the middle of the street, leave him in the middle of the street and stop traffic to help protect him. The only exception to this rule occurs when further injury is imminent: when fire might soon reach the gas tank, or fast-moving traffic comes zooming over a hill toward the original accident's scene.

A great many injuries and illnesses involve possible need for urgent care. Here is a brief consideration of the commoner injuries in the order of their actual urgency, followed by common illnesses in the same order.

Fractures and dislocations

Shock accompanying fractures and dislocations often requires urgent care. Otherwise, fractures and dislocations can be handled in a deliberate, unhurried fashion. Proper splinting generally controls pain, and precise replacement of parts knocked out of place can wait.

Figure 94. Poison control in New York. *Courtesy New York City Department of Health.*

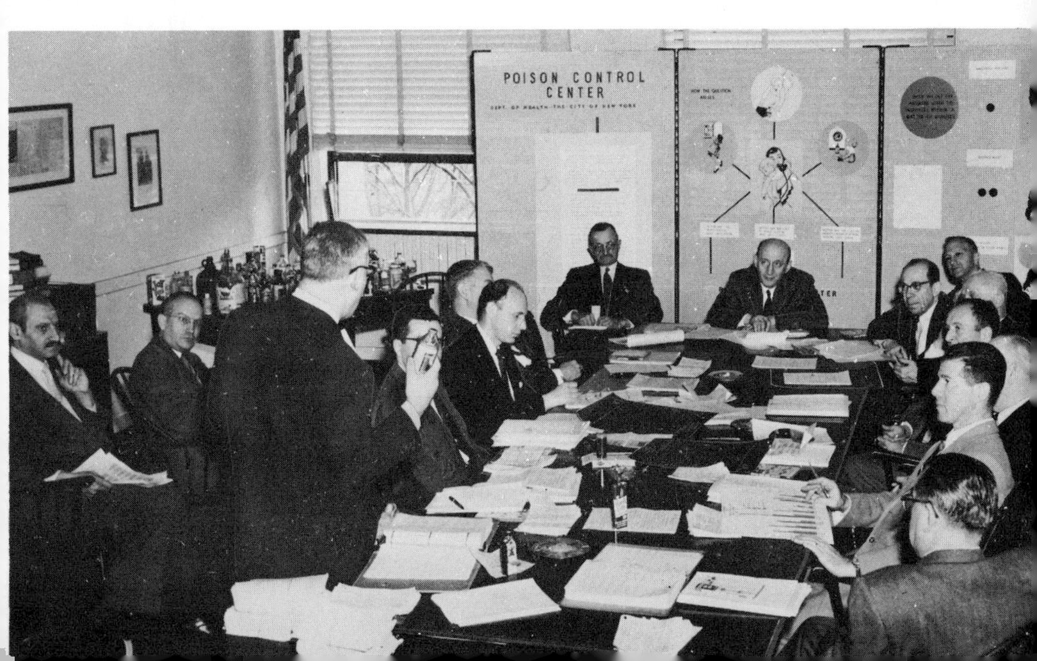

If you face a situation in which a fracture or dislocation may be present but there is no heavy bleeding or shock, the key problem is prevention of further damage by the displaced bony fragments. Certain corollaries of this statement help a lot in practical emergency management of fractures and dislocations:

1. *Possible fractures of small extremity bones need not have immediate professional care unless there is gross deformity.* Small bone fractures with-

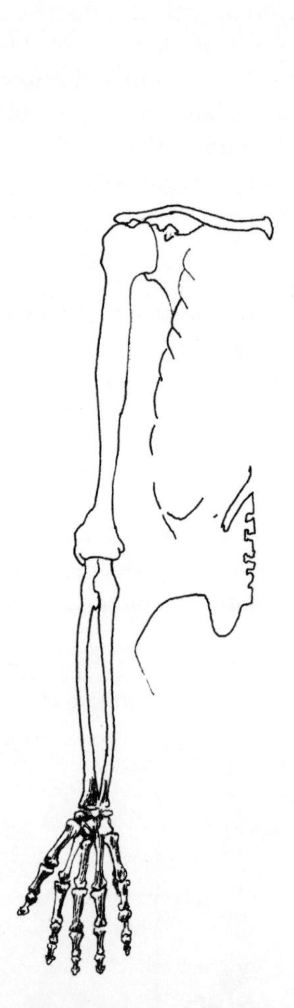

Figure 95. Arm bones. Fractures of bone shafts and elbow (unshaded) must be splinted before the victim can be moved. Fractures of wrist and hand (shaded) need not.

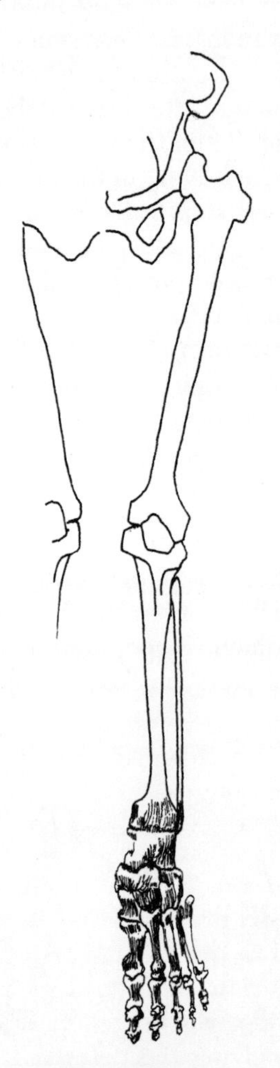

Figure 96. Leg bones. Fractures of bone shafts and knee (unshaded) must be splinted before the victim can be moved. Fractures of the ankle and foot (shaded) need not.

out gross deformity can generally be handled with simple splints or bracing bandages and non-use of the affected part until your doctor's next scheduled office hours. Thus a possibly broken finger can be protected from motion by bandaging it to a stiff wood or cardboard support. A possibly broken ankle can be wrapped with an elastic bandage and protected from the strains of walking through the use of crutches or by other improvised means until your doctor's regular office hours. An ice bag and rest in an elevated position (e.g., propped on two pillows) may help to keep down swelling in the meanwhile. Face bones require somewhat more urgent care. Nasal bones begin to heal within a few hours and become hard to put back in place. Other facial fractures frequently extend into the sinuses or the brain cage, making prompt medical treatment worthwhile.

2. *Possible fractures of large, long bones should be splinted before the patient moves.* Even if normal conformation suggests that any broken bones are not grossly out of place, bone shaft fragments may slip apart during slight body movement. Proper splinting should be used to prevent further damage whenever bony tenderness indicates possible fracture of any long bone. In most such cases, you will find it easier to summon a rescue crew, ambulance, or physician than to carry out the necessary procedures yourself.

3. *Back pain or bony tenderness after an accident always calls for on-the-spot medical care.* Displacement of vertebra fractures, which may cause only slight discomfort and little or no tenderness, may allow adjacent vertebrae to slip out of proper alignment and shear off or injure the spinal cord. Since the nerve fibers of the spinal cord perform vital functions (such as control of muscular movement) and never heal once destroyed, serious and permanent damage may result. Any back or neck injury of consequence thus calls for special care in lifting the patient or allowing him to move. Full precautions should be observed until the presence or absence of fracture has been proved by adequate x-ray evaluation. On-the-spot supervision by a physician usually proves best, with rescue squad or trained first aid workers the only acceptable second best.

4. *Markedly displaced fractures and dislocations.* Generally speaking, a markedly displaced fracture cannot be splinted satisfactorily without at least partial replacement. Any deliberate replacement of bone fragments calls for a physician's skill (and for pain relieving agents only accessible to a physician). You should generally send for a physician and attempt to relieve pain by steadying the deformed part rather than try to improve the fracture's position yourself. This is especially true if a bone fragment has pierced the skin and protrudes into the open air.

In dislocations, the problem is a little different. Here the displaced bones have smooth edges, the intact muscular attachments virtually eliminate movement of the fragments, and the big problem is that pressure against blood vessels and nerves might do damage. After careful all-over evaluation to make sure that no other injuries are present, you can usually transport a person with a part out of joint to the nearest physician or hospital for further care.

Burns, scrapes, and cuts

Unless extensive involvement or heavy bleeding makes shock a danger, preventing infection is the key problem with surface injuries. Germs invade your body surfaces fairly slowly, taking several hours to spread beyond the range of ready removal. Surface wounds therefore call for prompt but not instantaneous medical treatment. Thorough washing with soap and water helps remove germs which might be present. Application of a sterile bandage or clean cloth cover (e.g., an ironed handkerchief or sheet) prevents other germs from getting into the wound. Doctors like to sew up any gaping wound within six or less hours after injury. Painful wounds and burns call for prompt attention in order to restore comfort. Other surface wounds usually deserve attention within a few hours, but not immediately.

Bruises, strains, and sprains

With bruising or rending injuries, emergency measures are mainly aimed at stopping leakage of blood and fluid into the tissues. Cold applications help: either cold cloths or padded ice bags make torn blood vessels in the area shrink and decrease seepage. Smooth pressure such as that obtained from an elastic bandage may help, too. If the affected part can be held above the level of your heart so that blood flows downhill through the veins, part of the pressure which otherwise pushes blood and fluid out through leaky vessels is relieved. You can achieve such downhill drainage by lying flat with an injured leg propped up on two pillows (but level with the floor so that muscles are relaxed and do not press on veins at the back of the knee) or with an injured arm supported across your chest. Do not continue cold applications too long: your doctor will probably advise you to use heat instead after a day or two, when torn blood vessels have sealed and extra circulation will help carry leaked-out fluid away.

You usually cannot distinguish a strain or sprain reliably from a fracture. Patients can often move a fractured part or even walk a few steps on it without much pain. You should usually brace any severely injured part and protect it from the strains of use until your doctor's regular office hours, then let him decide whether it is broken.

Heart attacks

Smothering-type heart attacks, which show up mainly as shortness of breath out of proportion to exertion, call for prompt transportation to a hospital or other oxygen source. Heart attacks with chest pain and shock-like collapse deserve care on the spot by a physician. The patient should be kept flat on his back until a doctor arrives. A wild ambulance ride has distinct disadvantages in such a situation. For further details see Chapter 21.

Abdominal pain

You should regard abdominal pain as possibly serious until proven otherwise. Even if diarrhea, onset of menstruation, or the fact that "stomach flu" is going around suggest an innocent cause, you must base your actions on the possibility that you might have appendicitis, intestinal obstruction, or other critical disease. You should avoid laxatives and hot water bottles. You should call your doctor promptly and see him within a few hours of onset if even mild cramps persist.

Abdominal pain following an accident always calls for prompt action. Even mild discomfort may signify disruption of intestine, liver, kidney, or spleen. Dizziness or pallor in association with discomfort might stem from internal hemorrhage calling for very urgent care (although it might also stem from emotional reaction or other innocent causes, of course).

Severe abdominal pain in an individual who has recently suffered daily or almost daily indigestion quite frequently stems from a perforated ulcer. In such cases, even a few minutes makes a big difference. Shock often follows soon after the onset of the pain, so transportation in an ambulance to permit the reclining posture may be worthwhile.

Infection-generated complaints

In evaluating the urgency of an infection, the organ involved usually deserves more emphasis than the height of the fever or the extent of discomfort. Earache, deep cough or spitting of blood, rapidly spreading, red swelling somewhere on the body surface or red streaks running up the involved extremity from an infection, a burstingly intense headache with poker-stiff neck and back (generally signs of meningitis) or abdominal pain make even mild fever reason enough for urgent care.

Infants and children lose considerable fluid through perspiration, vomiting, diarrhea or other processes connected with infection. This often makes dehydration a fairly immediate threat. Fluid loss occurs in proportion to body surface, and infants have much more body surface per pound (inside and out) than adults. One way to evaluate fluid loss is to weigh the patient accurately as soon as any sign of illness appears, and figure that replacement of lost fluid becomes urgent when the weight has dropped by about 3 per cent. Doctors usually suggest hospital care with replacement of fluid by injection if loss seems likely to reach 5 per cent.

Until you get in touch with your doctor, you can take several helpful steps to combat infections. Rest in bed always seems worthwhile. Unless nausea or vomiting interfere, or abdominal pain makes emergency surgery a possibility, you get help in combating infection-spurred dehydration from extra juice, clear broth, or carbonated beverages other than cola drinks (which contain enough caffeine to add at times to the patient's restlessness).

CHAPTER 26

How To Choose a Health Adviser

MOST PEOPLE PLAN TO GET TOPNOTCH MEDICAL CARE WHENEVER THEY GET ANY serious disease, but relatively few realize how much hangs in the balance in their choice of an adviser for ordinary care. Even the best doctors often have trouble in promptly identifying the serious conditions which sometimes underlie mild difficulties. Moreover, a doctor who takes the time to be thorough can make lifesaving discoveries while giving care for the simplest ailments by detecting unrelated but serious conditions.

The only way to get prompt and adequate care for serious illness is to consult a well-trained, thorough physician every time you get sick.

Even when complaints stem from minor illness, good medical advice has much to offer. Simply avoiding serious errors and abuses is crucially important. Medical errors contribute considerably to human miseries, from disabling penicillin reactions when proper study would have proved that the original infection was with organisms for which penicillin would give no help to appendectomies erroneously done for green-apple stomachaches. Unprincipled callowness in the healing professions (fortunately rare among medically trained doctors) can lead to expensive courses of treatment, manipulations, or operations recommended for no reason other than the healer's own benefit. Both honest errors and deliberate deception can cost you dear in health affairs. Best keep them to a minimum by careful selection of a health adviser.

Nonmedical Sources of Advice

As a college student, you probably come from a family which handles its health problems by going to a physician for advice whenever substantial signs of illness are present, and sometimes even for preventive care, too. However, this policy prevails only among the better educated, more intellectually oriented social groups. Unskilled and semiskilled workers and their families ask for advice first from members of other health professions more often than from physicians.[1] The pharmacist in the corner drug store, the osteopath or chiropractor, and the registered nurse down at the industrial plant are favorites.

Pharmacists

While nobody can argue with the pharmacist's skill in compounding medicines or his knowledge of their effects, the popular custom of using him as a medical adviser has several glaring faults. Pharmacists receive no training in distinguishing mild from serious disease, identifying disease entities, or selecting the proper medications for a given illness. Many of the most important elements in care of disease (e.g., rest, diet, control of communicability,

[1] See *The Health of Regionville* by Earl Lomon Koos, Columbia University Press, New York, 1954, which elucidates the health practices and attitudes of people at various social strata in a typical New York town.

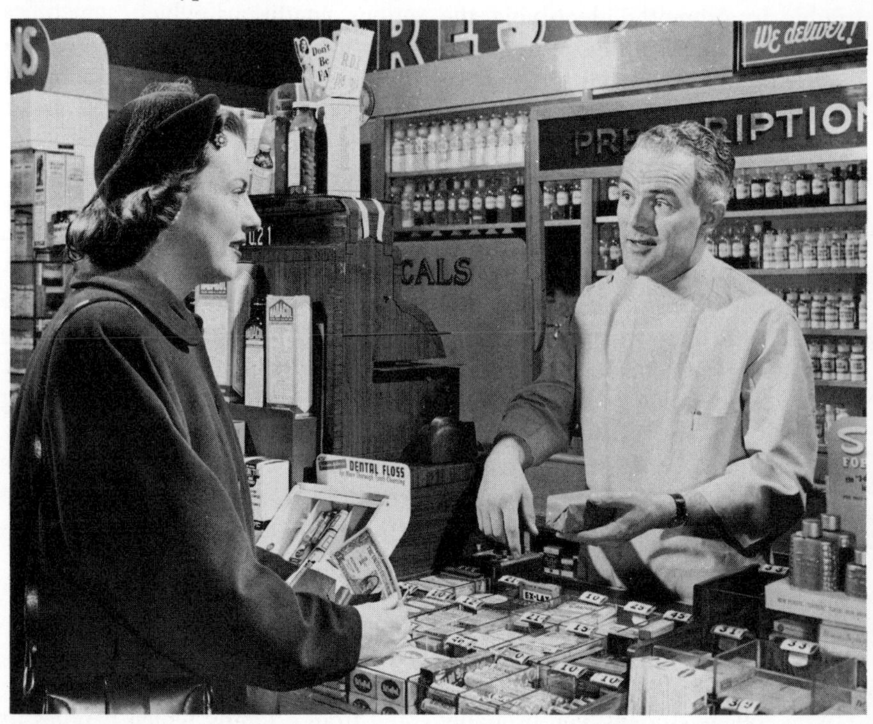

Figure 97. A good place to get your medicines, a poor place to ask which ones to use. *Ewing Galloway.*

use of physical agents such as heat and cold, enemas, and similar procedures) involve no medications and are completely outside the pharmacist's scope. Even if pharmacists knew everything necessary to prescribe for illness, complaints alone constitute a poor basis for selecting ideal measures. Most physicians require a detailed history, a physical examination and sometimes several laboratory tests to make that choice, but these procedures are never done at a prescription counter.

Osteopaths

The osteopath today occupies a changing place among the health professions. A generation ago, osteopathy was a clearly nonmedical cult whose practitioners applied only manipulative means to the care of disease. Training for an osteopathic career omitted many elements essential for broad scientific practice, and often included material sharply conflicting with generally held scientific views. Today, the curriculum in a college of osteopathy closely parallels that of a medical college. Osteopaths prescribe medicines and nonmanipulative treatments quite freely in many states. At the same time, M.D.'s have adopted some elements of manipulative therapy (used in combination with, rather than as replacement for, other available methods of treatment). The theoretical differences between the two professions seem almost resolved. However, three practical problems remain:

1. Many practicing osteopaths received their training in the old days when the manipulative approach disproportionately dominated instruction.
2. With virtually no M.D.'s on their faculties,[2] osteopathic training in some fields has had to get off the ground by pulling on its own bootstraps. The situation is not quite one of the blind leading the blind, but osteopathic instructors are frequently hampered by lack of direct association with medical authorities.
3. A good many people get into the osteopathic profession who have failed to make the grade in medicine. If the admissions committees and faculties of our various medical schools know what they are doing, a profession made up to any major degree of their rejects presumably carries some degree of comparative stigma. This does not mean that every osteopath is a frustrated M.D. or that every osteopath has less ability or character than his physician counterpart, but it strongly suggests that the osteopathic profession may include a higher proportion of poorly qualified individuals than the medical profession.

[2] After extensive study of the question, a committee of A.M.A. doctors recently recommended that M.D.'s be allowed to teach in colleges of osteopathy, but the organization's governing body did not pass the enabling resolution. With osteopathy still officially regarded as a cult, medical ethics thus prohibit physicians from teaching in its schools.

Chiropractors and other cultists

A number of healing cults base their approach to illness on theories at distinct variance with generally accepted scientific views. Chiropractors attribute virtually all illness to displacement of bones in the spine, for instance. A variety of quasi-scientific theories have provided a basis for other healing cults.

I have no doubt that chiropractors and other cultists superintend the recovery, relieve and even cure a considerable number of their patients. Any convincing attack upon disease (even one deliberately designed to be futile) will accomplish these objectives at times. Doctors who have done research on new medicines for arthritis, for instance, find that sugar pills or shots of plain water give considerable help to more than half the sufferers as long as they think a new medicine is being tried. With a piece of red string and a convincing line of chatter, one of my doctor friends cured almost two-thirds of the patients who came to him with warts. However, the wisdom of replacing prompt, scientifically oriented investigation and care with less orthodox forms of treatment seems very questionable. Even assuming that all cultists have the moral restraint to send you away instead of mulct you out of as many fees as possible if they recognize a serious disease (which sometimes seems a false assumption), many of them have no suitable training or equipment with which to identify such disorders.

Registered nurses and other subsidiary health professions

Nurses in industry, schools, and summer camps often give sound help and advice for minor illnesses and injuries, but cannot replace thorough medical evaluation and care in any disorder of consequence. Their training (and that of laboratory technicians and so forth) embraces very little specific skill in identifying ailments and selecting apt treatment measures.

A PERSONAL PHYSICIAN

The personal-physician approach to obtaining medical service consists of selecting one medical adviser whom you consult for virtually all of your medical problems whether you expect him to handle them himself or not. In this way, you can obtain medical service for most illnesses from a doctor who is familiar with your total health and situation, plus skilled guidance in deciding upon the need for specialized services, selecting proper specialists, and arranging well-coordinated, effective specialized care. Your personal physician under this system acts as a case manager rather than a jack-of-all-trades: he does not attempt to treat all of your illnesses himself, but brings all the resources of the medical community to bear upon your problems. In fact, some of the best personal physicians are not general practitioners at all. Specialists in internal medicine frequently fulfil the personal physician's role. Pediatricians and geriatricians often act as personal physicians for very young and very old people. While general practitioners probably render more service as personal physicians than any other medical group, they have no monopoly.

The personal-physician approach usually proves highly efficient for several reasons. The doctor's interest in your total health often leads him to detect and arrange care for crucially important conditions not yet causing substantial complaints. His long-term acquaintance with your condition and situation saves a great deal of otherwise duplicated effort, thus permitting quicker visits and lower fees. His capacity to handle minor or incidental problems simultaneously with care for your major complaints improves care without extra expense, too. His guidance helps you find the right man when you need specialized care. Last but not least, emotional support plays a big role both in your comfortable adaptation to disease and in your recovery from it. The long-term association of a personal physician relationship often proves more helpful than the briefer, more complaint-centered attention of various specialists.

Different doctors for different problems

Many people do not always go to a certain physician or group with each medical problem. Some consider one doctor or group as their primary

Figure 98. Situation well in hand—and the patient's confidence helps to keep it that way. *Gary K. Crowell.*

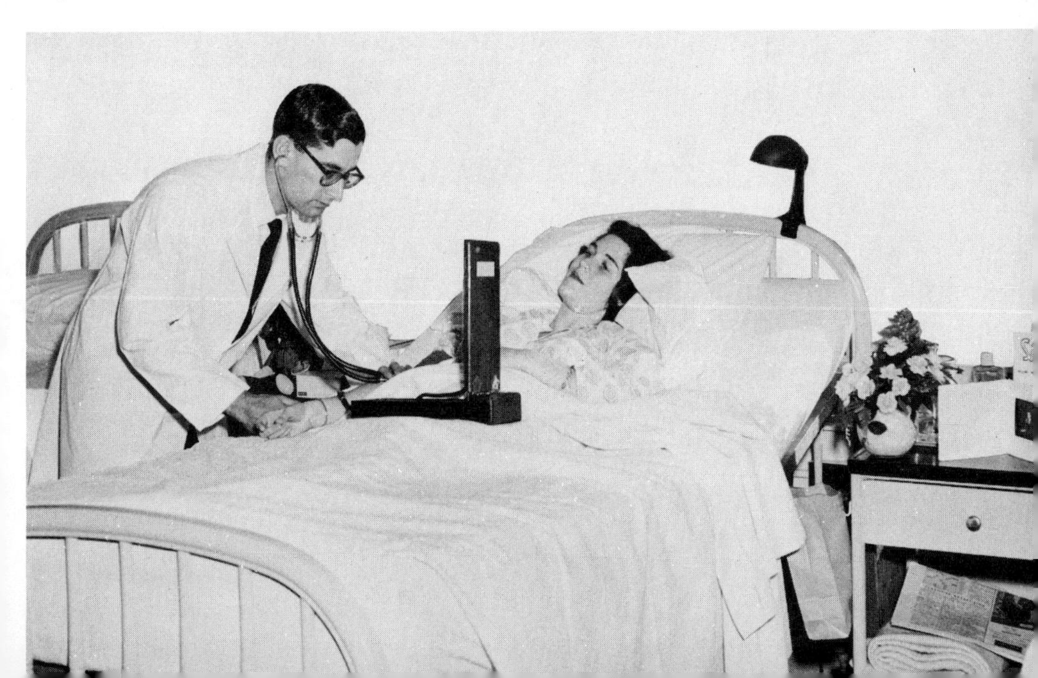

medical adviser, but handle problems in certain fields such as eye trouble and skin disease by going straight to a specialist. Others do not have any one doctor to whom they take their health problems regularly, but attempt to pick the right doctor for each individual medical service they require: usually the cheapest and most conveniently available for apparently minor conditions and a highly touted specialist or clinic for complaints which arouse any deep concern.

This approach at best saves one office call fee per illness in exchange for the effort and risk involved in selecting an apt adviser for each new difficulty. At worst, it involves either considerable waste of costly services or misdirected, incomplete care. To cite two typical examples:

••• A young man with pain in his left chest went to a heart specialist, who performed almost a hundred dollars worth of studies before concluding that the difficulty was out of his field, probably being indigestion.[3] A general practitioner could almost certainly have identified the difficulty in one visit, or at least directed the patient to a member of the correct specialty.

••• A young lady with bunions went directly to an orthopedic specialist to arrange care. Since his concern was with her feet only, she did not mention the thickening in her left breast. Three months later, after the bunion problem was solved, she finally consulted her physician about the breast tumor, which proved at that time to be incurable. Had she visited a good general physician to start with, he would have almost certainly done a complete examination, put first things first, arranged treatment for the tumor rather than the bunion, and quite possibly saved the lady's life.

You will almost certainly get better care for less money in the long run by sticking to the personal physician pattern. While you might make an occasional exception for a clearly defined specialized problem (e.g., need for new glasses), a personal physician's evaluation of your complaints, over-all view of your health problems, and guidance on the specialists who can give you the most help usually prove well worth a visit in any illness.

SELECTING A PERSONAL PHYSICIAN

You will have a hard time selecting a doctor (specialist or general practitioner) on the basis of what people ordinarily tell you about him. Satisfied patients mean little or nothing: the lady who raves about the terrific job her

[3] The doctor's behavior was perfectly proper in this case, since a practitioner in a narrow specialty has to perform complete study even if he is almost sure that the problem lies outside of his field from the start. His reputation hangs in the balance, and his work habits and routines are established to fit difficult, life-and-death problems irrespective of cost.

doctor did in removing her appendix was actually asleep when he was doing the work, wouldn't have known if he was doing it right anyway, and has no certain way of telling whether he performed the operation because her appendix was causing trouble or because he needed the surgical fee. A doctor's results are hard to evaluate, too. Unless you know at least as much as he does, how can you say whether some other measures might have been more effective than the ones he used?

You need to investigate several specific points to get a real picture of a doctor's competence. While none of these points directly measures the doctor's professional skill, they have considerable bearing on his effectiveness as a personal physician.

Thoroughness

Thoroughness means more than any other quality you can evaluate in judging a physician's worth. The world's most brilliant man cannot interpret and use observations he does not bother to make. Besides, thoroughness correlates very well with professional skill in studies made of doctors in action, yet is easy for you to appraise.

Ideally, your personal physician should do a complete physical examination early in the course of your association with him, at least annually thereafter, and whenever required for evaluation of obscure or generalized complaints such as weakness, fatigue, or unexplained fever. He should at least examine all body parts concerned with disordered bodily functions (e.g., the nose, throat and lungs with cough, the entire abdomen with indigestion) for illnesses that arise between complete examinations. A complete examination should include a searching review of health background and a head-to-toe examination with clothing completely removed. Careful thumping and listening to all areas of the chest, thorough exploration of the breast for lumps, and feeling all areas of the abdomen are always part of a thorough examination. Investigation of the rectum with the examining finger should ideally be part of a complete examination, being especially important in patients over forty. The female generative organs deserve evaluation even in somewhat younger individuals, since cancer and other serious disorders of this area become fairly common in the late twenties and thirties.

You can also judge a doctor's thoroughness from frequency of hospital visits, completeness of instructions, and so on.

Availability

If you plan to call a certain physician every time you get sick or need advice, you want to choose one who is reasonably available to you. A number of points affect availability. Is he in individual practice, taking care of his own emergency work at nights and on weekends, or is he a member of a medical group which rotates off-hour responsibility among all its members? Will he come out to your home in case of need? Can you get to his office easily (considering distance, parking difficulties, public transportation if necessary and so on)? Are his fees within your proper range so that you can call upon him fairly freely? Will he be able to take care of you in the hospital which you prefer if you become seriously ill?

Observance of limitations

When a general practitioner sends a patient elsewhere for surgery or asks for a consultation, some people seem to feel that he is admitting a degree of incompetence. Perhaps he was, under the old jack-of-all-trades theory. In the modern medical framework, though, he is showing commendable restraint. You want a doctor who provides you with the best available care for every illness, not one who does everything he thinks he can get away with. When a practitioner calls upon his colleagues frequently, the chances are that he considers himself one of a medical team rendering service rather than a totally independent, monolithic source of all your care. A specialist or a member of a large medical group almost always thinks of himself as a member of a medical team, which gives him some advantage in this regard. However, many general practitioners also qualify.

Staff memberships and credentials

You can get some idea of a doctor's reliability and skill by investigating his staff memberships and credentials. If a group of physicians have checked upon a doctor's skill and found him a suitable associate, that fact deserves some weight in your considerations. How much weight depends on the group of physicians and the circumstances: a teaching appointment in a medical school or visiting staff membership at a large and reputable hospital usually shows a high level of professional skill, while staff membership in a private or in an open staffed hospital (i.e., one to which any physician in good standing can take patients) may mean absolutely nothing. Clinic membership also varies in significance: the top consulting clinics have to maintain their reputation under the constant scrutiny of the hundreds of physicians who supply them with patients, and generally select well-qualified medical scientists for their staff. Total-care clinics vary in nature from groups of highly qualified specialists in well-coordinated practice to doctors of quite ordinary ability, banded together for the sake of convenient working conditions as much as for complementary scientific skills. The clinic label itself means nothing, and doctors practicing a given specialty in a clinic are not necessarily well qualified in that specialty.[4]

You should check on the credentials of any individual doctor you plan to visit, and confirm the qualifications of several members of any medical group you plan to patronize. Meaningful credentials, which you will find listed in the A.M.A. Directory at the nearest library, include membership in the local medical society, in the American Medical Association, in the American Academy of General Practice, certification by the appropriate specialty boards, and fellowship in the American College of Surgeons or the American College of Physicians.

Personal compatibility

When you pick your personal physician, remember that one of his most important functions is to give you emotional support. The man you see for a cold today may act as your main source of counseling in emotional upheaval tomorrow. You cannot usually tell how you will get along with a doctor beforehand, but you should reconsider your choice if you find that you do not like, trust, and respect the physician you have been seeing.

MEDICAL SPECIALTIES

Since medical knowledge and techniques have far outdistanced any one person's capacity for mastering them, you will almost certainly need to consult medical specialists on occasion over the years. A knowledge of the recognized specialties and subspecialties may prove quite helpful.

Internal medicine

A specialist in internal medicine, or internist, provides all varieties of nonsurgical medical and diagnostic service for adults. Internists act as personal physicians for some of their patients, and have specialized training and experience in the care of such disorders as heart disease, diabetes, and

[4] For example, three brothers who had been in general practice recently decided to band together in a clinic, each confining his attentions thereafter to his field of special interest (surgery, medicine, or obstetrics). While this was perfectly legal, none of these men would have represented himself as a specialist in individual practice. A similar tendency to specialize according to interest pattern rather than extra training frequently reveals itself in the clinic framework.

ulcers. Internists also serve as diagnostic consultants, identifying and evaluating the various disease states which afflict a patient with puzzling or extraordinary complaints.

Pediatrics

A pediatrician provides medical and preventive service for growing children, either as a personal physician or as a consultant.

Other non-surgical specialties

The box below shows other specialties in which surgery plays no major part. The first group are considered completely independent specialties, while the second are subspecialties within the field of internal medicine—that is, doctors in these fields usually qualify in internal medicine before concentrating their energies upon the smaller area within that field. Bracketed fields are frequently combined.

Specialty	*Concerned with*
{Dermatology	Diseases of skin
{Syphilology	Syphilis
{Neurology	Diseases of the nervous system
{Psychiatry	Mental disorders
Anesthesiology	Anethesia and pain relief
Physical medicine	Use of heat, massage, exercise, and so on in treatment of disease or in rehabilitation
Radiology	Use of x-rays and radioactive materials in identifying and treating bodily disorders
Pathology	Study of disease processes, especially cellular and chemical changes associated therewith
Public health	Community health promotion and preservation
Cardiology	Heart and blood vessel disorders
Gastro-enterology	Digestive problems
Allergy	Allergic disorders
Endocrinology	Diseases of growth and metabolism
Phthisiology	Diseases of the lungs (especially tuberculosis)
Geriatrics	Disorders of old age

General surgery

A general surgeon determines the need for surgical attentions, performs such surgery as is necessary, and supervises or assists the patient's recovery.

Most general surgeons emphasize abdominal surgery, but also handle breast surgery, female organ disorders and so on.

Surgical specialties

Although the distinguishing skills in surgical specialties are dexterous operative technique and ability to decide on the spot which procedure to perform, each of the surgical fields also includes skill in determining need for operation and in supportive care. The surgical specialties in the second group below also embrace medical and other measures required to give complete care for all the difficulties with which they concern themselves rather than confining themselves to surgery alone. Bracketed fields are often combined.

Specialty	*Concerned with*
Thoracic surgery	Surgery within the chest
Plastic surgery	Restoration and repair of externally apparent defects
Neurosurgery	Surgery of the brain and nervous system
Vascular surgery	Correction of varicose veins and other circulatory disorders amenable to surgery
Orthopedic surgery	Surgery of bones, muscles, tendons, and joints
Urology	The urinary and the male generative systems
{Otorhinolaryngology (ENT)	Diseases of the ear, nose, and throat
{Ophthalmology	Eye disorders
{Obstetrics	Pregnancy, labor, and postparturient rehabilitation
{Gynecology	Female organ disorders

Nonmedical practitioners often confused with medical specialists

A doctor cannot become a specialist in any of the fields discussed above until after he has completed his general medical training. Specialists therefore have acquired considerable knowledge of the whole field of medicine, usually sufficient to warrant their licensure as general practitioners. Then they have had further training and concentrated their energies in the specialized field. None of the titles listed below indicate medical school training, and practitioners in these groups should not be confused with medical specialists.

Osteopath	Chiropractor	Chiropodist
Naturopath	Optometrist	Podiatrist

Dental specialties

In dentistry as in medicine, several fields of practice require special training, skill, experience, or equipment. These specialties are listed in the box below.

Specialty	*Concerned with*
Oral pathology	Study of disease processes within the mouth
Public Health Dentistry	Education and other means of promoting the public's dental health
Pediatric dentistry	Children's teeth
Orthodontia	Prevention and cure of irregularities, malalignments and malocclusions
Prosthodontia	Artificial teeth and appliances including bridges, partial, and full dentures
Periodontia	Health of gums, tooth sockets, and tooth-supporting structures
Oral surgery	Surgical measures for relief of disease, injury, or malformation

CHAPTER 27

Hospitals and Other Health Facilities

THE PROVISION OF FOOD AND ACCOMMODATIONS FOR THE ILL CONSUMES A RELAtively small proportion of your hospital dollar. Around-the-clock nursing, special services in identification and relief of illness, a broad array of scientific equipment, and a selected, supervised staff of physicians and surgeons are the key elements in hospital care. A good hospital provides all of these, usually on a distinctly nonprofit basis.

Hospital management and control

Few people realize that doctors have no financial stake or administrative control in most hospitals. The hospital administrator works directly under a governing board which usually includes no physicians. Ownership of nongovernment units is usually by a nonprofit or religious organization. The medical staff is set up mainly to determine each doctor's qualifications and to supervise his work, and has no direct power over other hospital policies. Your doctor gets absolutely no portion of your hospital dollar and has no responsibility for the hospital's financial affairs.

This arrangement actually works to your advantage as a rule: your doctor decides all questions on the basis of your need for care rather than the hospital's need for customers,[1] and the hospital provides new facilities according to your health needs instead of potential profit.

[1] By contrast, I have observed at least one private hospital in which the doctor-owner's view of his patients' need for hospital care fluctuated sharply with the number of empty beds he was supporting out of his own pocket. In slack seasons, a bad cold became "beginning pneumonia" and became plenty of reason for hospital care, x-rays, and so on. The profits were high, but the net effect on total cost would make such an approach disastrous if widely adopted.

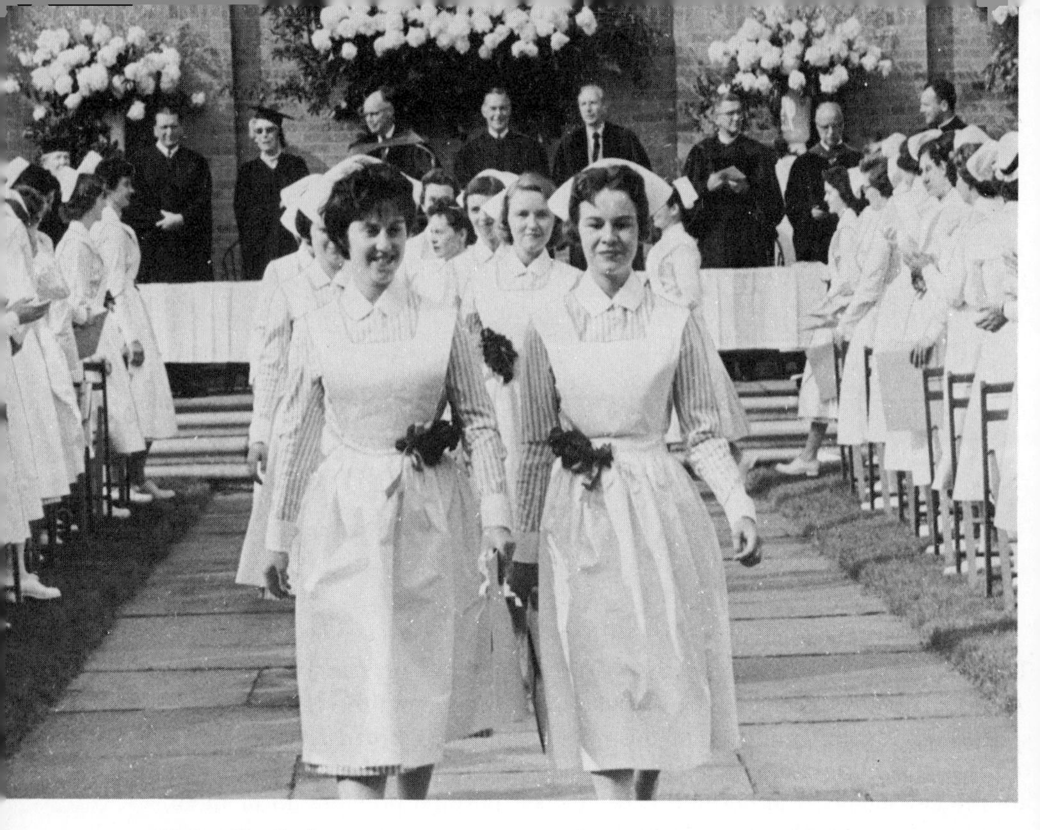

Figure 99. Graduating nurse—an asset to the community, whose training deserves community support. *Courtesy Columbia-Presbyterian Medical Center.*

Hospital services to the community

Early hospitals were devoted to management of illness among people who otherwise had no one to care for them. Most governments have nominally taken over this responsibility as part of their welfare program. However, church-sponsored, nonprofit, and teaching hospitals provide care for welfare patients in many areas without being fully compensated out of welfare funds. In a sense, hospitals thus meet some welfare responsibilities in behalf of the community.

The community has a special stake in proper hospital care for certain illnesses. For example, tuberculosis hospitals help limit the spread of infection besides healing the present victims of disease. Mental hospitals keep patients from harming other people as well as contributing to their cure.

Stand-by service is also a community function in a sense. A substantial part of hospital costs consists of maintaining more beds and more facilities than it usually can utilize, so that adequate facilities will be available during periods of special need. This stand-by service for epidemics and catastrophes is similar in all respects to other stand-by services maintained by the community—firefighting equipment, military establishments, and so forth—and deserves general support.

Education and research are valid community aims served by hospitals, which frequently provide training for student nurses, medical students, interns, and residents at a cost which generally exceeds the value of their services. Research also serves the entire community rather than the patients ill at the moment, and deserves some public support.

Perhaps the most valid protest over the cost of hospital services is that sick people should not have to bear the cost of the hospital's community services. In a sense, this is what happens in nongovernmental hospitals today. The hospital includes all its expenses in determining what it costs to operate beds, including operating expenses of welfare, stand-by, educational, and research programs. Contributions generally come in only for construction of new facilities or for meeting deficits in an emergency: few communities offer sustaining funds for normal nongovernmental hospital operation. Hospitals extend services which they do not feel can be retrenched, and have no recourse except to pass the cost along to patients in the form of higher fees.

Hospital costs

In spite of the sometimes considerable overload attributable to community services, you get a lot for your hospital dollar. If you went to a decent hotel, ordered three meals a day sent to you in bed, and compared your total cost with the nearest hospital's daily rate, you would probably find very little difference. Yet meals and maintenance amount to less than a third of most hospitals' costs, with the remainder going for nursing service, drugs, specialized equipment, and so on. Your hospital bed represents a considerable investment because of all the behind-the-scenes equipment: it costs more to build and equip each bed-unit of a hospital than it does to erect a completely furnished family home. Hospital costs usually prove quite burdensome to people already suffering disability and other high expense, but they generally allow no profit even in efficiently administered units. In fact, the vast majority of hospitals operate at a deficit in spite of their seemingly high charges.

Choosing a Hospital

If you want to choose your hospital on the basis of its most essential assets, you must delve beneath appraisals of its atmosphere and food to get some facts about its nursing staff, medical staff, and equipment. These points deserve your attention:

An adequate nursing staff

While the exact number of nurses required in a hospital varies greatly with the variety of cases treated, the presence of a registered nurse on each ward at all times seems an irreducible minimum requirement. A sufficient staff of fully qualified nurses to supervise all medications and treatments during busy hours seems a fair requirement, too. If former patients in a hospital tell you of practical nurses or aides being in charge during the night, changing sterile dressings or administering intravenous infusions, you should question the adequacy of the staff.

Accreditation

You can easily check to see whether a hospital carries current approval by the Joint Commission on Accreditation of Hospitals. An accreditation certificate should be plainly displayed in the waiting room or admissions office, or your county or state medical association will gladly give you the information. Accreditation covers many points from fireproof structure to proper kitchen technique, plus such professional matters as the adequacy of care and supervision. In an accredited hospital, proper records of your illness and care are thoroughly reviewed by a well-organized medical staff to be sure that no doctor performs unnecessary operations or does slipshod work.

Hospital equipment

Equipment for emergency and technically difficult diagnostic, medical and surgical procedures deserves (and usually gets) priority over attractive furniture and decoration in hospital management. Machines worth thousands of dollars may sit in a cupboard somewhere for months on end, but still save lives by being instantly available when needed. If you have a choice between hospitals, best ask your doctor whether he thinks all are equally well equipped instead of going on impressions or reports based entirely on the appearance of the rooms and building.

Varieties of Hospital Accommodations

Most hospitals other than government-operated welfare units offer several grades of accommodation. You must usually choose between three common varieties:

Ward

Ward accommodations generally are provided at less than actual cost as a means of simultaneously serving the sick person's needs and providing training for medical students, interns, and residents. Most ward service is provided in large rooms with several or many beds. The hospital's charges include all expense as a rule, including physician's services. The interns and residents, who are graduate physicians but generally not very experienced ones, perform most or all of the required medical and surgical services. Good-quality care is assured by the supervision and assistance of experienced physicians on the hospital's visiting staff. Medical students serve mainly as observers, clerks and minor participants or assistants. Although some hospitals perform considerable research, any deviation from standard treatment measures can only be undertaken with the patient's specific written consent. You can accept ward accommodations with confidence that you will receive standard rather than experimental treatment unless you specifically consent to the latter. However, you have no choice of physician under the plan.

Semi-private

Semi-private arrangements permit you to choose your own physician or surgeon and receive care primarily from him rather than from interns and residents. You can get semi-private service in multibed accommodations also known as "wards." Thus a ward patient is one under the house staff's care without the services of a private physician, while a four-bed ward, eight-bed ward or open ward is a multibed accommodation in which patients often receive care from their own physicians under the semi-private plan. Semi-private accommodations generally are priced to be self-sustaining, and

Figure 100. Ward for postoperative patients. *Courtesy Columbia-Presbyterian Medical Center.*

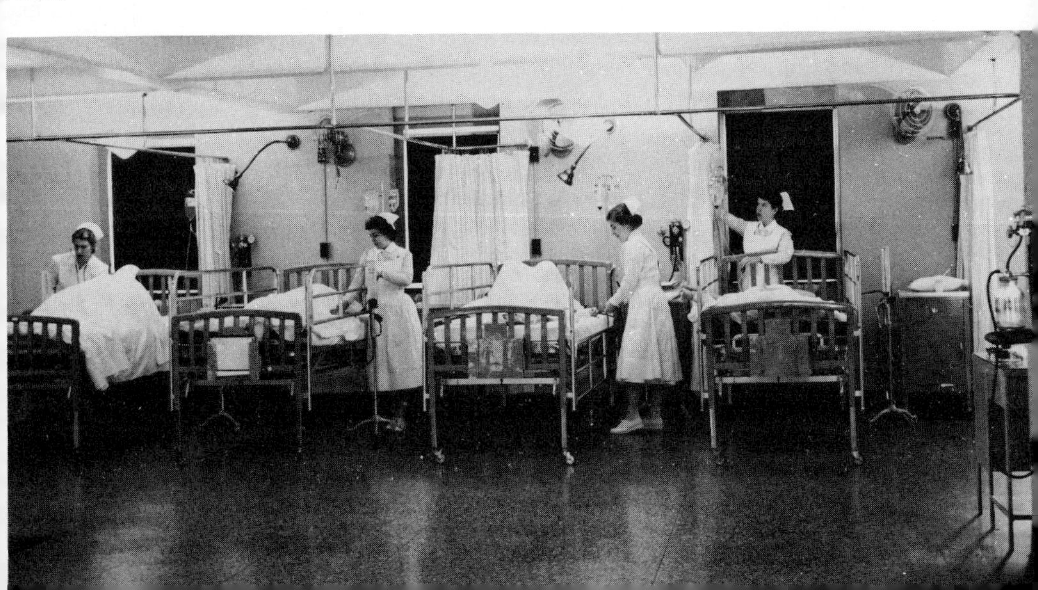

patients usually receive nursing care, food and other services similar or identical with that given to private patients. Hospital charges do not include the cost of physicians' or surgeons' services, which you must pay separately.

Private

When you get a room by yourself in the hospital, you consume a somewhat larger amount of nursing time and other services than you would in semi-private accommodations. Moreover, many hospitals operate somewhat on the soak-the-rich-and-spare-the-poor principle. Private accommodations therefore often cost considerably more than semi-private without actually giving any essential additional benefit.[2]

Help and Advice with Choice of Hospital Accommodations

People frequently choose hospital facilities on purely emotional grounds. Everybody is worried about Mama when she has a heart attack. The best is none too good, so she sits in a private room with bath for the first, bedridden week, has to move out into the open ward for lack of funds by the time the bathroom would do her any good, and winds up so far in debt for the unused luxury accommodations that she has to scrub her own floors for months instead of hiring needed help after she goes home.

A more rational approach to selection of hospital accommodations could prevent many such tragedies. In larger hospitals, you can plan a sound long-range program easily by discussing the situation with a social worker before arranging accommodations. Most social workers feel that they can accomplish more by counseling people with moderate means in ways of remaining self-sufficient than by aiding the destitute. A trained social worker knows what a patient with a certain diagnosis can expect in the way of expense and disability both in the hospital and out. He knows how to appraise a family's financial picture, and where they can best cut down expenditures. He knows what other facilities—child care, home nursing for follow-up attention, vocational rehabilitation centers, and so forth—might prove useful. And he knows where loan or welfare funds can be obtained if necessary.

If the hospital you enter has no social worker available, perhaps you can get similar counseling from a family service agency in your community. Otherwise your doctor probably is the best source of such aid.

[2] In cases where privacy is actually necessary to the patient's recovery, as in the critical stages of a heart attack, most hospitals have arrangements whereby even a ward patient gets a room to himself or its equivalent.

OTHER USEFUL COMMUNITY HEALTH FACILITIES

Some community health facilities come into play primarily when you have reached or seem likely to reach the end of your resources. Others constitute joint attacks on common problems, and carry no such implication.

Welfare Agencies

You can get complete medical care for any substantial illness or injury any place in the United States regardless of your ability to pay. Most stories about people suffering for lack of money with which to buy medicines or to obtain medical care are completely groundless.[3] Although a few people may choose to suffer rather than accept either public or private charity (whether for reasons of pride, ignorance, or fear), the facilities are available, and generally are provided in a way which is as dignified and pleasant as is consistent with efficient administration.

If you want to arrange care for someone who cannot pay the entire cost of an illness or who seems likely to exhaust his resources before the illness is at an end, your first contact should be with the city or county welfare department. Social workers in this agency can direct you to the other community resources, and simultaneously make such arrangements for government assistance as may be required.

Social Services

In most urban and suburban communities, one or more social agencies affords each of the services listed below.[4] Patients who are able to pay as well as indigent or part-pay clients frequently utilize these facilities, since many specialized services can be obtained more easily through social agencies than from other sources.

Adoptions: Children studied and selectively placed in homes for adoption.

Aged: Nursing homes; recreation centers; low-cost housing; old-age assistance.

[3] On several occasions, county medical societies have conducted intensive advertising campaigns offering to arrange medical care for any such people. Such campaigns have generally failed to produce a single complaint which could not have been managed through ordinary channels, and often produce no complaints at all.

[4] From Agatha Hopkins, M. S. W., "What Social Workers Can Do For You," *Medical Economics,* November 10, 1958, pp. 237–53.

Blind: Home instruction; talking-book machines; financial assistance; job placement.

Budgeting: Advice and assistance; consultation on food and nutrition.

Camps: Resident and day camps for healthy youngsters; camps for the handicapped, retarded, and underprivileged.

Children's Services: Residential treatment of the disturbed; classes for the retarded; aid to the dependent; help with personality disorders.

Chronically Ill and Handicapped: Homes; nursing care; homemaker service; educational training; special workshops; rehabilitation.

Citizenship: Special services to foreign born; financial assistance; housing; health care; immigration help; education and Americanization.

Day Nurseries: Daytime group care for children of working mothers.

Employment Agencies: Vocational guidance; counseling in regard to employment; selective job placement of physically and emotionally handicapped; help in processing claims for unemployment and disability insurance.

Family Services: Help with personal relationship problems, with economic and environmental difficulties, and with emotional disorders.

Financial Assistance: Public assistance for living expenses; medical services and supplies; aid to dependent children; Federal disability assistance; aid to needy blind.

Foster Homes: Where children may live healthy, normal lives.

Homemaker Services: Specially trained women whose job it is to provide continuity to family life during periods of a parent's acute illness or absence from home.

Housing: Processing of applications for Federally subsidized housing for low-income families.

Legal Aid: Advice and legal services to those who cannot afford an attorney.

Mental Health: Agencies for education, research, use and development of psychiatric facilities.

Neighborhood Centers: Educational and leisure-time activities for different age groups.

Nursing Services: Beside care in the home, regardless of ability to pay; education in disease prevention.

Prosthetic Appliances: Help in renting, purchasing, or learning to use prosthetic appliances.

Psychiatric Clinics: Help in getting diagnosis and treatment of personality disorders of children and adults.

Rehabilitation: Physical restoration; vocational retraining; job placement for physically and mentally incapacitated.

Special Schools: Classes for retarded, blind, deaf, physically or emotionally impaired.

Transients: Temporary shelter, food, clothing for homeless; work program.

Travelers' Aid: Information regarding housing; travel service for children and the handicapped.

Unmarried Mothers: Help in getting maternity care, financial assistance, temporary boarding of babies, adoption.

Widows: Help in obtaining survivors' insurance, employment; counseling to ease problems of adjustment.

Control of Disease Spread and Nuisances

Most health department efforts to control diseases and nuisances continue automatically whether you request them or not. Control of communicable disease, community water and sewage systems, laboratory services, and so on give you substantial protection against disease even though you take no initiative. You can also call upon health department workers for aid in any situation involving threats or potential threats to your health and comfort. A few common examples:

1. *Nuisances.* Health department responsibility comes into play whenever your health, comfort or safety are impaired by actions of your neighbors. Everything from noisy parties to unleashed dogs may legitimately send you to your health department, which often has greater authority than the local policeman to deal with nuisances.

2. *Independent sanitary provisions.* If you must get your water from an individual well or dispose of your sewage with a septic tank and cesspool, your health department can often offer guidance.

3. *Infant care.* Well-baby clinics provide advice and help with the hazards of early infancy, including formulas for infant feeding, necessary inoculations, instructions in skin care, and general child-rearing suggestions.

4. *Pollution problems.* If an individual or firm dumps chemicals into water, ground or air in a way that impedes your use of public grounds or waterways, you can often get help from your health department.

Educational Materials

You can get a great deal of educational material and assistance from various health agencies, both official and voluntary. Your state health department probably can send you considerable pamphlet material regarding any health problem with which you are concerned, from ordinary infant care to problems of the aged. If you ever assume responsibility for obtaining programs for P.T.A. or other organizations, you will find the health agencies a splendid source of speakers, movies, and other materials. Public health departments, voluntary agencies (e.g., American Heart Association, National Association for Mental Health), and local medical or dental associations frequently provide adult education service.

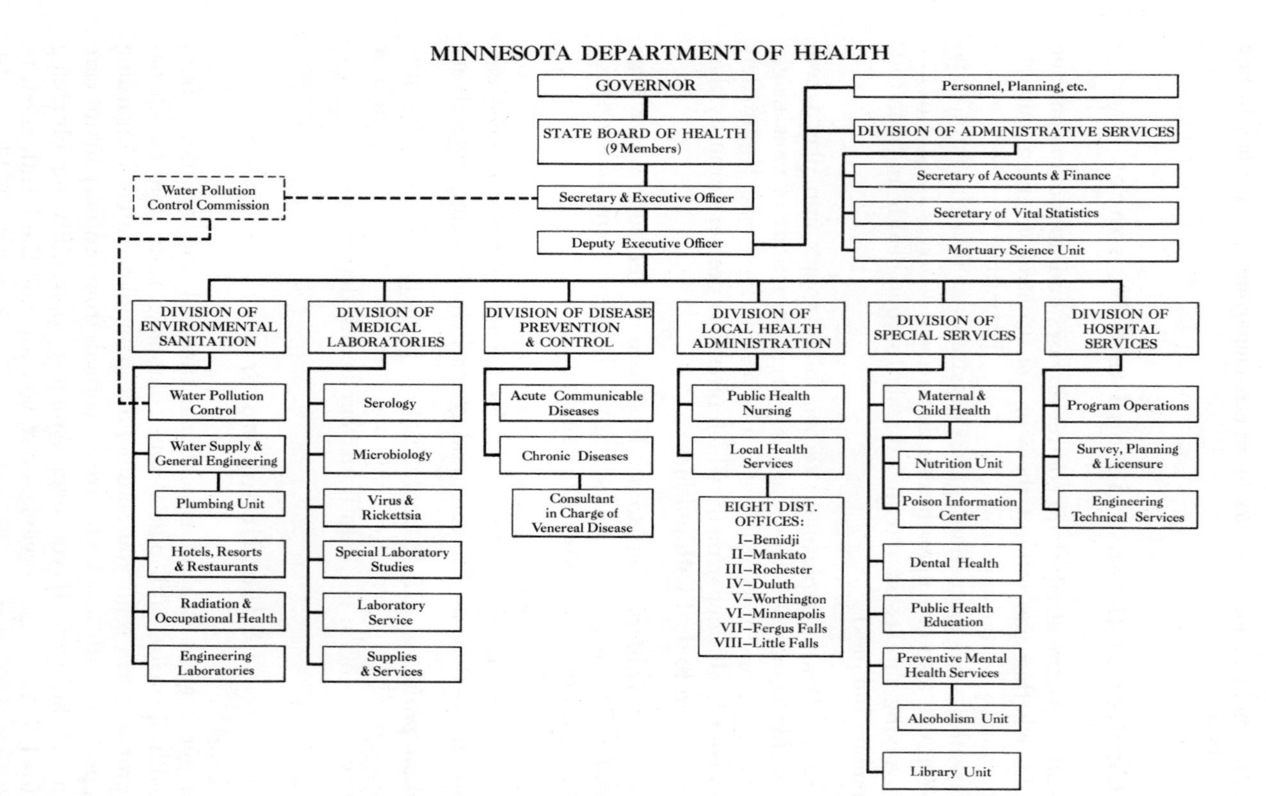

Figure 101. Administrative structure of the Minnesota Department of Health. Each box represents specialized functions requiring a trained staff and supervisors.

Research

Research into the causes, prevention, and cure of disease obviously serves the entire community or the whole world. The wonderful tools of space-age science promise great new discoveries when applied to the field of health. Such application costs large sums of money, though. Most modern medical research is carried out by teams of specialists. The unsolved prob-

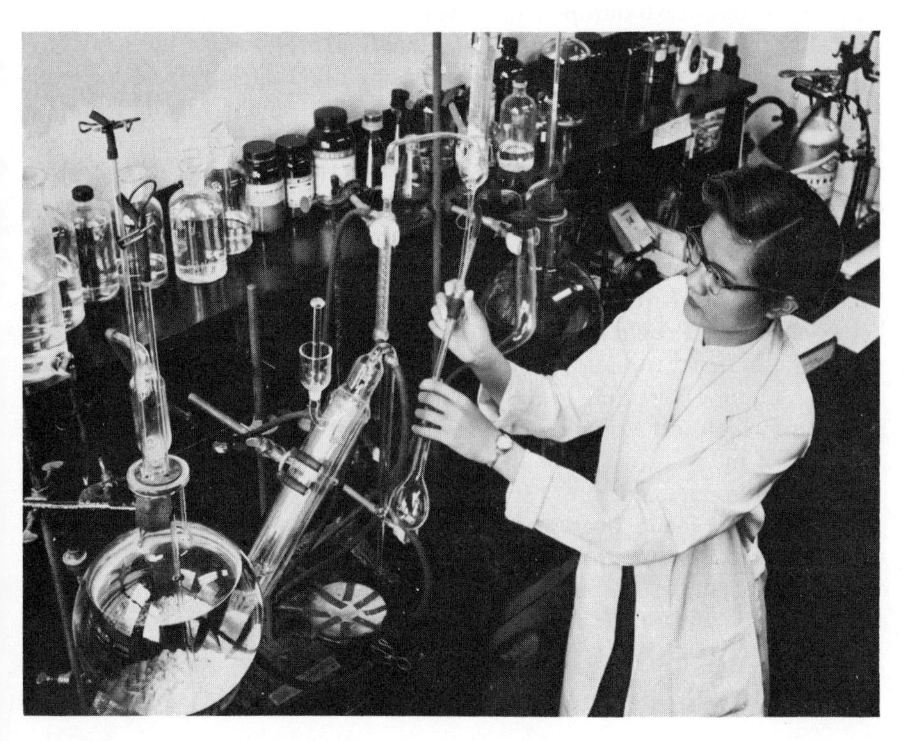

Figure 102. Research in action. *Courtesy Columbia-Presbyterian Medical Center.*

lems of today involve such complex phenomena as cellular growth and the bodily controls which keep cellular growth from becoming cancerous, body use of fuels and the bodily processes which keep down hardening of the arteries, and immunology (emphasizing body processes through which people might avoid such plagues as the common cold). These problems seem better suited to all-out, well-equipped, full-time researchers' attack than to armchair thinking or individual inquiry. Both government and voluntary agencies have tremendously increased their research expenditures to aid the attack.

Generally speaking, government agencies contribute rationally planned balance to our research program, while voluntary agencies contribute flexibility. Prior to the government's post-World War II expansion of its research program, several major problems were left almost unattacked, simply because they had not caught the public's fancy. Research funds were available for almost any project related to poliomyelitis, but were almost totally unavailable for the mental illnesses which cause hundreds of times as much disability and death, for example. Today, government funds help fill such gaps, and substantial research funds are devoted to every major cause of death or disability. The National Institutes of Health in Bethesda, Maryland have brought together teams of leading scientists to attack each of these big problems, and government grants support a great deal of the research done in private institutions. On the other hand, government research projects usually must be justified by some promise of concrete and immediate application, and often must be authorized through slow and cumbersome channels. A crash program like the National Foundation's all-out effort to develop, try, and encourage production of Salk polio vaccine would be almost impossible to achieve through official channels. This whole program was completed before a proposal could have been prepared and funds authorized through normal legislative processes. An arrangement like the American Heart Association's lifetime research grants would also be impossible, because this program (which sets a number of research leaders free to pursue any matter they find of interest) would be difficult to pigeonhole as "heart" or "cancer" or other authorized pursuit. Yet many crucial scientific discoveries in the past have been made by researchers who started out in pursuit of some entirely different goal and presumably would have had to stick to their original quest under the standard government contract. Thus government and voluntary research fit well into a complementary overall program.

CHAPTER 28

The Financial Aspects of Illness

YOU WOULD RATHER NOT BE SICK AT ALL. YOU WOULD RATHER NOT ACKNOWLEDGE that you might some day have mental illness, tuberculosis, or some other major, long-drawn-out disorder. So you have a natural human tendency to put off concrete planning for illness and its consequent expense. However, the financial burdens of illness usually can be met much more easily if you have made suitable provisions in advance.

YOUR HEALTH INSURANCE OR PREPAYMENT PROGRAM

You can meet burdensome medical expense most easily through health insurance or other forms of prepayment. You have to pay something extra for the privilege: a dollar's prepayment will not bring you a dollar's worth of insurance-compensated service because of administrative and other expense.[1] However, prepayment provides immediate protection and spreads extremely heavy medical expense from a few people's shoulders to a larger group, while other programs for developing emergency resources (such as savings or investments) do not.

The average expenditure for medical and hospital care in America is not very burdensome. You will pay many times as much during your lifetime for pleasure driving, tobacco products, and alcoholic beverages as for physicians, hospitals, and drugs. But the man about to drown in a river takes little comfort from the fact that its average depth is only two feet, and the

[1] Nonprofit health plans currently pay out 90 cents for each premium dollar collected, commerical group plans 77 cents, individual commercial insurance only 53 cents, according to the Health Insurance Newsletter. Cooperative, student health, labor union, and other prepayment programs are harder to appraise because of varying accounting procedures.

person whose medical bills exceed his total income for a given year feels much the same way. Very few people have sufficient reserves to handle some of the financial burdens illness can impose. Almost everyone needs some form of insurance or prepayment in his personal program of health finance.

What Should You Prepay?

Your prepayment plan should cover medical expenses which you will feel individually obliged to pay and which you will be unable to meet out of reserves, out of current income, or through incurrence of readily manageable debt. You are underinsured if any predictable hazard will force you and your family to sharply curtail their living standard. You are overinsured if you pay an administrative overload to spread costs you could easily manage out of reserves and current income, if you place yourself under financial strain to pay in advance for varieties of care for which you would not otherwise feel individually obligated (e.g., if you pay heavy premiums to provide protection against the expense of prolonged hospital care for tuberculosis when your financial position is such that you would otherwise depend on state-provided facilities), or if your premiums leave you unable to build reserves with which to meet generally uninsurable hazards like the mounting disabilities of old age.

As you can see, your prepayment program should vary with your income and financial position. Let's examine the various means of prepayment to see how each might fit your needs as the years go by.

Closed panel, limited service groups

Many student health services provide for medical care on a closed panel, limited service plan. The physicians working in the student health facility are available to you at certain hours and for certain services. Care you receive from other doctors or care beyond the specified limits of coverage must be paid for separately (although insurance-type benefits are often also available either as part of the standard plan or as a supplement to it). Other closed panel plans operate as cooperatives or under sponsorship of union and other groups. They often place special emphasis on preventive care and management of early or mild illness, since these are important elements of care which are difficult to provide efficiently under a straight insurance program.

The closed panel plan works very well in meeting the needs of students, who need prepayment on this basis mainly for minor illnesses and who can easily utilize one centralized facility. However, this approach has certain drawbacks in more general application. The services best rendered through this plan (namely preventive care and care of everyday illness) are not those which most people find very burdensome. Overuse or abuse of certain services increases cost and impairs the doctor-patient relationship at times. Limited choice of physician may create problems, especially if the patient feels that more competent doctors are available elsewhere.

Hospital insurance

Most of the illnesses which impose heavy financial burdens on you involve hospital care. The expense of hospitalization in these cases amounts to a substantial part of the total, and usually must be paid in cash. Hospital insurance has therefore become the most popular form of protection against burdensome medical expense.

Most hospital insurance contracts do not pay the entire hospital bill, mainly because total coverage encourages overuse. Some pay a stated daily rate plus specific sums for extra hospital services. Others pay a certain percentage of the total hospital bill. Almost all hospital insurance contracts cut off after a certain period, and most exclude certain long-lasting diseases (especially nervous and mental diseases). However, people who can pay for mild illness and must resign themselves to taking state aid with catastrophic difficulties can get an excellent cushion against the financial burdens of severe-but-not-overwhelming disease or injury at reasonable cost through a well chosen hospital insurance contract. Your Blue Cross organization offers such contracts on a nonprofit basis. Many commercial insurance companies offer well-designed hospital contracts, too.

Medical and surgical policies

Hospital illnesses generally involve considerable medical and surgical expense in addition to hospital costs. Insurance against these expenses helps to make these bills less burdensome. The Blue Shield plans generally offer a true service contract to people of moderate means: doctor-members, who usually include almost all the local physicians, have agreed to accept the payment made under the policy as their total fee unless the patient has an income above a certain level. Other contracts offer straight cash payments which may or may not meet the whole bill.

Major medical and semicomprehensive insurance

Major medical and semicomprehensive coverages pay a certain percentage of medical expenses above a certain minimum due to a given illness or during a single calendar year. Hospital bills, medical expense including office care and home visits; and in some instances drugs, nursing in the home and other incidentals are all covered. In a major medical contract, you might pay the first $250 in any illness and 10 per cent of the remainder. In a semi-comprehensive contract, you might pay the first $50 of expense attributable to illness during any one calendar year and 20 per cent of the remainder. Everything except completely optional services (preventive examinations, cosmetic surgery, and the like) is usually covered.

These policies offer reasonably complete coverage after the initial, patient-borne deduction, yet avoid the excessive administrative expense of numerous small claims. A small proportion of expense is always left uninsured on the assumption that patients will not call for truly unnecessary services if they have to pay a portion of the fee, and that doctors and hospitals who might raise their fees or multiply their services if nobody would be hurt but the insurance company will hesitate to do so if part of the cost comes out of the patient's own pocket. Unfortunately, this assumption has not always proved entirely valid, and abuses have added somewhat to the predicted cost of the policies. However, they still offer a very logical attack on the problem of burdensome medical expense, and measures to curb abuse may well keep them reasonable in cost.

Income replacement and overhead insurance

As soon as you assume responsibility for your own support or for support of a household, you need protection against lost earnings during any prolonged disability. A good income protection policy certainly is worthwhile until you can build savings and reserves. If you go into an independent profession or business, you can make substantial tax savings by acquiring part of your disability insurance specifically to meet continuing business overhead.

Specific hazard policies

A great many health insurance contracts pay benefits only if certain specific untoward events occur. These offer protection against "Ten Dread Diseases" such as poliomyelitis, scarlet fever, and so forth, against accidents without coverage for illnesses, or against accidents occurring only in one specific place (e.g., school accidents, accidents on the public highway). Such policies actually have no place in a well-rounded health insurance program. Most of them pay out as benefits only a very small percentage of premiums collected: often 10 per cent or less. You cannot fit them into a comprehensive program without duplicating coverage, yet you need just as much protection against multiple sclerosis as against poliomyelitis and against pneumonia as against a broken leg.

Provisions to Look for in Selecting Coverage

No matter what your need for insurance or prepayment might be at any one stage of your career, you should try to fulfil it with policies or contracts with certain provisions:

1. Minimal exclusions

Most health insurance contracts exclude plastic or cosmetic surgery. Many exclude any elective surgery (i.e., surgery which can be done at the patient's convenience) for the first six months. Obstetrical benefits may not commence for ten months or a year, and preexisting illnesses may remain uncovered for a stated number of months or years. These exclusions have proved necessary to avoid abuse (e.g., a person in need of an elective operation might pay one small premium, have his operation, get the insurance company to pay the hospital and the surgeon, then drop the policy). Other exclusions definitely decrease the value of your contract. A clause excluding nervous and mental disease crops up quite commonly. Hospitalization for diagnostic study is excluded in some contracts. Tuberculosis, venereal disease and several other diseases may be specifically excluded. While you will almost certainly have to accept some undesirable exclusions, be sure that you know what they are and take them into account in appraising each contract.

2. Assured maintainability

You will need prepaid coverage especially badly if you get diabetes, heart disease, cancer, or any of a variety of diseases making repeated hospitalizations necessary. Yet many contracts contain loopholes whereby your insurance can be withdrawn at such times. Even policies labeled "noncancellable" in big black letters may contain a clause to the effect that "this policy is renewable at the option of the company only." This means that your insurance can be discontinued at the end of any premium period by the company's refusal to accept another payment. Most group contracts can only be cancelled for the whole group, which gives each individual a degree of protection. Provisions whereby you can keep up your insurance if you change employers or residence are important in these contracts, too.

3. High limits or nonaggregate provisions

One of your main purposes in prepayment is usually protection against big bills, so any provision limiting the insurance company's liability leaves you with the potentiality of losing protection just when you need it the most. Sometimes the policy gives an aggregate total which limits total payments during its entire life to a certain sum (e.g., $10,000 in one major medical contract). Other policies pay for a limited period on any one illness or disability (e.g., up to 30 days' hospitalization, up to 100 months' disability). You should be sure that any such limits imposed are very liberal.

4. Appropriate definitions

Disability insurance is only as good as its definition of the term "disability." If you are only disabled when you are unable to carry out any gainful employment, you might find your benefits shut off as soon as you are capable of selling magazines by telephone. "Partial disability" is another term which often means something different than you expect. Some insurance policies use the term "accidental means," which does not include many mishaps you would ordinarily think of as accidents. You should go over the entire contract word by word whenever you buy any form of health or income protection. If you do not understand certain provisions, ask for a letter of clarification from the company's home office, which you can keep with the contract if you decide to accept it.

Periodic Prepayment Review

At least every three years (and every time you change employment, residence or family situation), you should review your health and disability insurance coverage. Write down first the facts determining what coverage you need: how big a bill you could stand out of reserves and current income, whether you can afford coverage against catastrophic illness or must plan on state facilities in such event (possibly best determined by evaluating the premium cost each way), what responsibilities demand income protection. Next, write down the coverage you have, including coverage through your employer (especially sick leave or disability arrangements). Last, investigate the means by which discrepancies can best be eliminated and take appropriate action.

THE SHIFTING ECONOMY OF MEDICAL SERVICE

As a future leader in your community, you should have a sound viewpoint toward the economic framework through which you receive medical services. The prevailing fee-for-service system of private medical practice is under heavy pressure to be revamped in certain respects or be replaced. Your position will carry considerable weight in this period of possible change.

HOW DOCTORS RECEIVE PAYMENT

Although other factors also influence choice of profession and professional behavior, economic factors have definite effects. Each of the common modes of payment rewards or discourages certain professional acts. The quest of success coincides somewhat with the quest of goods, so that even relatively altruistic doctors are not entirely unaffected by economic motivation.

Fee-for-Service

Fee-for-service compensation awards the physician a certain amount for each procedure he carries out. An office call, a complete examination or an operation each rates a certain fee. A physician increases his earnings by performing more services or by performing more difficult, and therefore more expensive, services.

Advantages

The outstanding advantage of fee-for-service care is that it maintains or even concentrates care upon stubborn or incurable conditions. The system encourages general practitioners and specialists in the broader fields to spend a great deal of time and effort on patients with difficult or insoluble problems and permits doctors with special interest in certain such problems to concentrate their entire professional energies upon them. This orientation dominates the whole profession through its effect on prevailing norms and attitudes. Medical talent concentrates itself upon presently incurable illness, making progress almost inevitable and service for major difficulties superb.

The fee-for-service system also encourages amelioration of disease, which is second only in importance to cure (or possibly even exceeds cure in importance, if you consider the help doctors give for conditions they cannot eradicate such as diabetes, psoriasis and the common cold). And it encourages doctors to go out of their way to satisfy patients: to treat them considerately, to be pleasant to them as people, and make their care convenient.

Fee-for-service encourages each physician toward constant improvement of his professional skills. He increases his earnings largely through improving his capacity for service as a doctor rather than through seniority or shift to administration. He continually scans the medical literature for new and better treatments with which to help patients unresponsive to standard methods and thus retain their loyalty.

These advantages of fee-for-service operate mainly through broadly disseminated professional norms. They remain effective as long as fee-motivated physicians constitute the professions peer group, even when programs aimed at meeting the deficiencies of the system coexist with this basic plan.

Disadvantages

Although the outstanding disadvantages of fee-for-service (without prepayment) lie on the consumer side, it also has some adverse effects on the service provided. Attempts to satisfy misinformed patients sometimes leads to ill-considered overtreatment. For example, a great many patients receiving antibiotics today have no antibiotic-sensitive infection of consequence. Certain doctors give in to the patient's manifest desire for "something to really knock these germs" in spite of their own knowledge that antibiotics are worthless in such cases. Fee-for-service encourages a problem-centered approach which fits poorly with the people's expanding need for preventive services. When a patient comes in with a common cold, for example, his doctor does not usually urge him to take a complete examination for cancer detection. Many patients would regard such urging as an attempt to force unwanted services upon them and stick them with a higher bill. While preventive services can be rendered under fee-for-service, they cannot be vigorously pushed.

Fee-for-service occasionally encourages doctors to overreach their limitations, too. While we try to check this tendency through medical staff supervision in hospitals, medical society activities, and tightly interpreted malpractice laws, the fact remains that physicians without special training often perform technically difficult operations or continue to muddle along with medical problems beyond their true range. Desire for the fees involved presumably provides at least part of their motivation.

Capitation

Under capitation, each doctor receives a certain amount of money annually for each patient who has selected him as his source of personal-physician type services. Capitation applies mainly to personal physician services, with specialized care compensated in some other way.

Advantages

Capitation preserves or even exaggerates the doctor's desire to please his patients. It eliminates most paper work necessary to collect for services. Capitation certainly encourages a personal physician to observe his limitations and utilize (or overutilize) specialist colleagues.

Disadvantages

As an economic motivator, capitation encourages the physician to do as little for his patients as he can without losing their allegiance. It encourages him to send work along to specialists which he might adequately provide himself if he had any incentive to do so, increasing time spent by patients in getting care and multiplying medical costs. Capitation especially restricts the personal physician in care of chronic illness and incurable disease—fields where he works most actively under fee-for-service. Diabetics who need frequent attention or arthritics who want weekly treatments actually cost the doctor money under capitation, so he shifts them off to the specialists. While exponents of capitation rightly point out that most progress anticipated today is more likely to stem from organized research than from general practitioner's observations and treatment trials, capitation certainly discourages interest in any disorder not readily remediable and militates against any progress which might occur at the practitioner level. The path of self-improvement beckons less cordially under capitation, too: unless a doctor goes all out for specialized training, he cannot increase his earnings by learning new techniques or expanding his professional horizons.

Salary

A salaried physician is paid by the hour, day, or year instead of according to services rendered or patients seen. Salaried compensation presupposes an administrative structure within which the doctor can be assigned certain responsibilities rather than a direct doctor-patient relationship.

Advantages

You can presumably induce a physician to fulfil any community or individual need through payment of a salary, including many needs not readily met under the other frameworks. You can make physicians available in isolated areas, where fees or capitation would not produce a living income. You can encourage teaching, research, public health and other services rendered to the community instead of to individuals.

The fact that a knowledgeable administrator rather than a less well-informed patient acts as the arbiter of adequacy may allow the salary system to improve care in some respects, especially in encouraging uniform application of unpopular but scientifically desirable procedures. For example, an examination in an administratively supervised cancer detection clinic virtually always includes careful examination of the breasts, rectum, and genitalia while only a few, superior practitioners perform all of these procedures on private patients who request an annual checkup.

Disadvantages

The doctor's attitude generally tends to be somewhat different when he is responsible to an administrator rather than the patient. Salaried practice tends to become unsympathetic, impersonal, or even downright inconsiderate unless the administrators make a constant and vigorous effort to combat such orientation. The emphasis is usually on correctly identifying the patient's disease processes and prescribing the correct curative medicines or treatments. Relief-giving measures, attempts to set the patient's mind at ease, and other measures concerned with comfort rather than cure (but often contributing considerably to cure as well, since morale certainly affects your recuperative powers) often suffer substantial neglect.

When salaried practice prevails throughout the medical community, treatment tends to become rigidly fixed. A salaried physician has done his job if he identifies your illness and applies standard remedies to it. He does not need to shift his program to keep you satisfied if the usual prescription doesn't work. The constant adaptation of treatment to disease, treatment to individual response, and treatment to situational demand which prevails in patient-centered systems tends to disappear in administration-centered ones. So does progress, outside of that made by full time research.

Advancement in salaried practice occurs mainly through development of administrative rather than professional skills. The keenly developed capacities of a top surgeon or diagnostician are unavailable when advancement rapidly carries able men off to executive posts.

Mode of Payment in Private and Governmental Programs

A fee-for-service system operates efficiently in private practice. Fee-for-service has been used in conjunction with government programs, too, especially as a small direct payment by each patient for services rendered by a physician whose basic income is provided by salary. This approach retains many of the advantages of fee-for-service, while still providing means of encouraging doctors to practice in isolated rural areas, etc. Part-time and occasional services performed for the government can be compensated by fee. However, fee-for-service has generally proved unsuitable for governmental or institutive plans providing total care and employing physicians full-time. Administrative expenses become prohibitive when a claim, processed at substantial cost, results from each minor illness. A few doctors multiply expense by overtreatment (e.g., treating a minor illness as virus pneumonia with frequent visits and laboratory studies, or prescribing a prolonged series of heat treatments for backaches better handled with aspirin), especially when unsupervised office care is covered. A few patients make many extra demands which fee-compensated doctors have no reason whatever to discourage. These abuses can only be controlled by further administrative expense, which can ultimately triple or quadruple the total cost of the program.

Capitation gets away from this administrative problem. However, capitation applies only to personal physician services. Specialists treat almost all serious and chronic illness under capitation, and specialists must be compensated in some other way, usually by salary. Capitation helps to keep people happy with a medical care plan by encouraging patient-pleasing efforts at the grass roots level, but in matters of consequence the system depends on salaried physicians to get the job done. It must be rated in conjunction with salaried practice, then, rather than independently.

Salaried practice as a basic pattern has many undesirable and irremediable features. However, it is almost inescapable in any plan attempting to render total care to the entire population.

HOW PATIENTS PAY

Your mode of payment influences both your behavior, your doctor's behavior, and the distribution of medical expense.

How Direct Cost Influences Your Actions

Pressures toward immediate care such as pain or disability, anxiety about your disorder and hope for substantial aid, may closely match pressures against immediate care, such as fear of finding out something unpleasant, fear of pain and disability during treatment, and time consumed in getting medical service. Cost sometimes tips the balance toward "wait and see" with resulting hazardous delay. However, this effect has probably been greatly exaggerated. When the British health plan went into effect, for instance, many people expected that the absence of any cost barrier would lead to much more prompt detection and care for cancer with a resulting rise in the rate of cure. The opposite actually happened, suggesting that the cost barrier is less important than prejudices, fears, and misconceptions which can best be attacked by educational rather than economic means.

To a certain extent, direct payment on a fee basis may incline patients toward minimizing problems other than the one for which they are specifically seeking help, while total prepayment encourages them to raise every possible issue. This effect is counterbalanced by an opposite pressure on the physician. Direct payment also discourages overuse of house calls or emergency services, which has proved a difficult problem in totally prepaid plans.[1]

How Direct Payment Influences Physicians

When your doctor knows that his services cost you money, he can work on the assumption that all of your complaints and demands have some substantial basis. A complaint might be neurotic or an emergency call the result of undue alarm, but some uncontrollable, psychological or physical difficulty exists. Not so under prepayment, where the reason for complaints may be a desire to get off work (e.g., goldbricking in the Army) and a house call may be requested in place of an office visit merely for the patient's convenience. The viewpoint and manner of a physician approaching a problem which he knows has real grounds is sympathetic and inquiring, while total prepayment encourages skepticism and quick dismissal for people with obscure difficulties.

Your doctor tends to order less expensive laboratory tests, less prolonged

[1] The extent of this problem can be judged from the drastic remedies applied or proposed for it, which range from a stiff, government collected house call fee (under the former French plan) to a procedure requiring successive approval from a social worker and a public health nurse before a physician's visit would be authorized (under the LaGuardia proposal).

hospital stay, and less expensive drugs when he knows that you must personally pay for them.[2] Although many of these eliminated services are luxury items or unnecessary refinements, objective evaluation shows that a reasonably high proportion would have been worthwhile.

The Problem of Distributing Medical Expense

Without prepayment, medical expenses prove burdensome or catastrophic for some people. The distribution of medical expense strikes old people and chronically ill people very hard: in fact, people least able to pay and most afflicted with other major expenses frequently bear the most burdensome medical costs. Thus some form of indirect payment or prepayment is almost essential in this day of highly developed, and therefore frequently expensive, medical care.

In considering possible approaches to this problem, several points seem worthy of note:

1. *A total care plan would undoubtedly increase total costs.* Although medical care seems very expensive, the costs stem from the need to attract top people, give them strenuous and prolonged training, and draw out extraordinary effort from them. These problems are no easier under an institutive program. Moreover, any system in which patients pay absolutely nothing out of their own pockets is quite subject to abuse. Insurance companies and closed panel plans in this country and governmental programs in other areas and times have uniformly proved that a small to moderate amount of direct payment decreases total costs enormously. Add administrative costs to multiplied services, and total medical expense would undoubtedly increase.

2. *A total care plan means the end of fee-for-service as a factor in establishing professional norms.* Although some fee-for-service practice would undoubtedly continue despite a total care plan, the system's advantages stem mainly from its effects on professional norms. These effects can only be expected to continue as long as fee-for-service physicians constitute the profession's peer group.

3. *Inductive reasoning is almost worthless in considering medical economic issues.* The behavior of patients and physicians in closed-panel plans

[2] The psychologic basis for this difference in behavior is that you can identify with people, but not with institutions. Your doctor knows how you will feel when submitted to a financial squeeze, and sympathy makes him think twice before submitting you to this tension. An institution (whether government, hospital or insurance firm) is not wracked by emotion and evokes no sympathy at all.

and other economic experiments is strongly influenced by community-wide attitudes and professional norms which depend on the basic system. You cannot reason that their success in this framework makes success likely when applied on a national or community-wide basis. Nor can experiments be properly judged in the framework of sharp preliminary selection (either of doctors or patients). The few, highly selected, full-time professors, or a few, highly selected doctors who are dedicated to the cooperative movement might work well on a salary when the less altruistic majority (which must be enlisted to provide total care for the nation) would not. The few prevention-minded patients who sign up for a faculty health plan might come in for regular annual examinations without any educational campaign to encourage this procedure when the average individual certainly will not. Even national programs cannot be quickly judged. Professional norms, attitudes toward physicians (affecting both behavior during illness and attractiveness of health careers), and many other social determinates evolve only gradually from changed position. You cannot pass judgment on the British medical plan today, for instance, without recognizing that many physicians working in the plan chose their profession and developed their work habits before the plan was in operation, that the respectful obedience through which medical recommendations are mainly implemented is to some extent a carry-over from the days when medical practice was not a form of bureaucratic servitude, and so on.

4. The people's true prepayment needs are variable. As we discussed in the previous section, your prepayment needs vary sharply with your situation. A compulsory government program generally must be uniform. If it goes beyond the minimum protection against catastrophic expense which almost everyone needs, it therefore involves costly administrative services which are unnecessary for many of the people covered. Noncompulsory prepayment plans can be adapted much more readily to each individual's needs.

Defining Your Own Ideal

You certainly want an economic system which will provide good medical care for both ordinary and catastrophic illness without excessive total cost (either through fees, prepayment or taxes) and without excessive economic burdens during prolonged or severe disabilities. You probably want to encourage further progress, promote better medical service in isolated areas, and enhance preventive or other unpopular but distinctly valuable programs. Sit down with a pencil and paper to devise a system which will do all this. You will find that if you start with fee-for-service and retain direct payment of at least a portion of expense, you can accomplish virtually all of these objectives without losing the system's fundamental advantages. You can invoke government in place of insurance companies for some prepayment (although that would not be my own preference), you can alter the amount of direct payment or the percentage of doctors' incomes coming from fees, you can devise a dozen workable systems with ease. But unless you have fee-for-service and some increment of direct payment, you will almost inevitably find major defects which cannot be remedied by reasonable supplemental programs. Our present system may look jerry-built and confused, but its fundamental outlines have emerged through a highly selective type of evolution. For all of its deficiencies, it has much which deserves to survive.

GLOSSARY

abortion, expulsion of fetus during first three months of pregnancy (often used as synonym for criminal abortion).
abortion, criminal, deliberately precipitated abortion.
abortion, spontaneous, abortion not precipitated by any deliberate act.
acute disease, a quickly developing and usually promptly resolved illness.
addiction, state of physical drug dependency of such a nature that withdrawal of the drug leads to illness.
agglutinating, causing blood cells to clump.
alleles, genetic determinates competing for the same position in chromosomes.
allergy, a harmful reaction to a normally harmless substance, usually occurring only after previous sensitization.
amniotic fluid, a clear, watery fluid in which the unborn infant floats.
amphetamine, a stimulant drug; one form is marketed as Dexedrine.
anus, opening from rectum to exterior.
appendicitis, infection in the appendix.
arteriosclerosis, a disorder in which firm scales form underneath the artery lining, interfering with the pliability of the vessels and with circulation through them.
association, 1. social contacts and relationships with individuals or groups; 2. a mental connection or linkage by which past intellectual or emotional experience influences behavior, thought, or emotion.
BCG, Abbr. for Bacillus-Calmette-Guérin, a weakened strain of tuberculosis germs used in artificial immunization.
bacteriologic tests, determination of the number and type of bacteria present.
behavior disorder, a failure of social integration, harmful to either the individual concerned or to society at large.
benign tumor, a tumor incapable of spread through body fluids to distant sites.
bronchitis, inflammation of lungs' air-conducting tube.
callus, a hard skin thickening usually on the soles or palms.
calorie, (nutrition) unit of fuel value in food–heat energy required to raise the temperature of one gram of water by one degree C.
cancer, a tumor capable of spread through body fluids to distant sites.
cataract, a vision-impairing opacity in the crystalline lens.
catatonic, variety of schizophrenia characterized by hallucinations and loss of contact with reality.
cerebral palsy, paralysis, incoordination, or other faulty function on the basis of brain damage present from birth or shortly thereafter.
cesspool, a reservoir for refuse and water with walls sufficiently porous to allow seepage into the surrounding ground.

chiropractor, practitioner of healing methods based upon the theory that virtually all human illness results from displacement of bone in and around the spinal column.

chromosome, strand of inheritance-ordaining substance found within each living cell.

chronic disease, a long-lasting or smoldering illness.

colon, portion of large intestine hanging free in abdominal cavity.

commitment, legal process for admission to psychiatric hospital.

community, a body of people joined by some mutual interest or concern, or by frequent association.

conflict, psychologic, a conscious or subconscious struggle between incompatible aims, convictions, plans, etc. generally most stressful when one element seems intellectually more desirable and the other seems emotionally more desirable.

conformity, acting sufficiently like other members of a social group to make yourself acceptable to them.

conscious, (psych.) within your ken or awareness.

corn, a skin thickening, painful on pressure, usually on or between the toes.

cyst, a balloon-like sac without an opening, filled with liquid or semiliquid material.

delirium, a condition in which the victim suffers nightmare visions and sensations which he regards as entirely real, at the same time losing consciousness of the real world around him.

dependency, requiring the actual or emotional support of another.

dermatitis, skin rash or irritation.

desensitization, an allergy-combatting program which neutralizes antibodies by exposure to gradually increasing amounts of antigen.

diabetes, (generally *diabetes mellitus* unless otherwise specified) an abnormality involving passage of large amounts of urine from the body.

diabetes mellitus, an abnormality in the body's use of sugar which allows abnormally large amounts of sugar to pile up in the bloodstream and thence to reach the urine, drawing with it large amounts of fluid.

diarrhea, the discharge of abnormally soft or liquid feces, usually in abnormally frequent movements.

diphtheria, infection with a specific poison-producing family of bacteria.

dissociative disorder, condition characterized by a split between content (what you are thinking about) and affect (your emotional state).

drainage, (purulent infection) creation of an opening through which accumulated pus can escape.

eczema, allergic dermatitis when allergen is unknown.

emotion, feelings which motivate, reward or punish without the intermediacy of intellect.

emotional stability, (*see* stable emotions)

endocrine gland, a gland which secretes into the blood stream rather than into the intestinal tract or to the exterior.

enteritis, inflammation of the intestinal tract, usually characterized by severe diarrhea.

environment, the sum of all elements in your surroundings which affect your health, welfare, or behavior.

epilepsy, a disorder causing attacks of unconsciousness usually associated with jerking motions.

eugenic, for race improvement.

Fallopian tube, narrow muscular tube with a funnel-like end lying near the ovary and a small end communicating with the uterine cavity.

family, (*see* p. 30).

fecal-oral route, (of germ spread) leaving one person's body with the feces and later entering another's through the mouth.

fluoride, the ionized form of fluorine, an elemental gas.

gangrene, death of tissue from inadequate circulation, generally requiring amputation.

genes, units of inheritance arranged in lines along chromosomes.

germ, a microorganism, especially one capable of causing disease.

germ plasm, the portion of the parents from which children take origin, thus giving biological continuity to the family.

gland, a gross or microscopic organ which secretes a substance of physiologic signifiance (a few structures, such as lymphatic glands, retain this designation even although the original presumption that they secreted a substance has since been disproved).

glare, dazzling light, either direct or reflected.

goiter, enlargement of the thyroid gland.

growth, (*see* tumor)

guardianship, legal process whereby another person assumes responsibility for managing an incompetent individual's affairs.

hallucinations, a dream-type experience which the subject cannot distinguish from reality.

hardening of the arteries, (*see* arteriosclerosis)

health, ideal, the state in which one's maximum potentialities in the physical, mental and social spheres are realized.

heartburn, burning and distress in the pit of the stomach or lower breastbone due to digestive malfunctioning (and unrelated to the heart).

hebephrenic, dissociative disorder characterized by childishness and silliness.

heel counters, fitted heel cups attached inside shoes.

hemorrhoids, a swelling or protrusion in the vicinity of the anus, consisting mainly of dilating veins.

hernia, protrusion of an organ or part from the body space which it normally occupies, most commonly the protrusion of abdominal organs through a gap in muscles near the groin.

hormone, a substance which regulates the functioning of body cells without entering into their fuel-burning processes.

humidity, moisture content of air.

identification, a personal relationship so close that the other person's experiences and feelings have the same impact on your emotions and your self-esteem as your own.

indigestion, discomfort of any sort—heartburn, generalized cramps, feeling of fullness—attributable to disorders in the digestive process.

inflammation, bodily response of redness, swelling, and pain frequently associated with infection but also occurring in other varieties of disease.

impetigo, a skin infection characterized by blisters and crusts.

insomnia, difficulty with sleep.

intestine, large, the terminal portion of the intestine which runs in an inverted U shape from the right lower abdomen up across and down to the rectum totalling 4½ to 5 feet in length and 3 or 4 inches in breadth.

intestine, small, portion of digestive tube leading from the stomach to the colon, averaging about 22 feet in length and 1½ to 2 inches in diameter.

isolation, technique of preventing spread of infectious disease by keeping victim alone in a room and preventing his germs from reaching potential victims.

labor, (reproduction) the maternal processes by which a baby is born and the afterbirth extruded.

legumes, seed of pod-bearing plants, such as navy beans and blackeyed peas.

ligament, a strong, pliable, fibrous band which bridges and supports a joint.

liver, large organ in upper right abdomen which functions both as a digestive gland and as a protein-synthesizing center.

malignant, (of tumors) capable of spread through body fluids to distant sites.

malocclusion, a condition in which teeth do not meet in a good bite in part or all of the mouth.

masturbation, stimulation of one's own genitalia, generally to a point of climax.

materialism, a system of values in which goods and the acquisition thereof acquires special significance.

memnonic, of or related to memory.

miscarriage, technically, expulsion of a fetus after three months' gestation and before he reaches viability. Popularly, a synonym for spontaneous abortion.

mood, the emotional substrait or baseline.

mores, customs or conventions enforced by social pressure.

multiple sclerosis, a progressive nervous system disease affecting coordination.

muscular dystrophy, a progressive loss of muscular function, mainly heredofamilial.

narcotic, a pain-relieving drug capable of causing addiction.

nephritis, inflammation of the kidneys.

nutrition, provision of substances needed to maintain your biological processes.

nutrition, state of, condition of health resulting from the adequate or inadequate supply of substances necessary to support your biological processes.

osteoarthritis, a form of joint discomfort unassociated with marked inflammation.

osteopath, member of a healing profession supposedly basing treatment upon manipulative methods, without the use of internal medications (*see* page 321).

pancreas, digestive organ lying below and behind the stomach and pouring protein-digesting juices into the first portion of the small intestine; also contains island cells which function as endocrine glands and aid sugar metabolism.

paranoid, tendency to blame other people or inanimate objects for your own deficiencies or failures; also variety of schizophrenia in which extreme application of this mechanism amounts to mental illness.

peptic ulcer, an ulcer usually located in the lower stomach or first loop of intestine in the formation of which stomach acids and digestive enzymes play an important role.

periodontitis, infection or inflammation of the gums or supporting tissues of the tooth.

pharmacist, a druggist trained to compound and dispense prescription medications.
phobia, an unreasonable and irrational fear.
placenta, a specialized embryonic organ through which interchange of various chemical substances (mainly nutrients and wastes) occurs between an unborn child or animal and his mother.
pneumonia, infection of the lung.
poliomyelitis, acute infectious disease often involving spinal cord cells necessary for the control of muscles.
postparturient, after delivery.
promiscuity, (general) having indiscriminate sexual relationships; (technical) cohabiting with two or more partners.
prostate gland, an accessory sex organ which secretes an important portion of the seminal fluid.
protein, biologically synthesized nitrogenous substances generally having large and complex molecular structure.
psychasthenia, neurosis involving psychologic rather than physical abilities.
psychiatrist, physician specializing in treatment of mental illness.
psychoanalyst, psychiatrist following Freudian theories.
psychopathy, an unusual tendency to rebel against socially exacted standards of behavior.
psychotherapy, treatment via the mind rather than the body, and particularly by planned interaction of personalities or intellects.
purulent, pus-involving.
quarantine, technique for controlling spread of disease by isolating everyone who might possibly have become infected until after illness would have become manifest.
rebellion, renunciation of or opposition to authority, whether governmental, social, familial, or organizational.
rectum, terminal portion of large intestine external to the abdominal cavity.
relationship, an interpersonal bond of interest, concern, or affection.
retina, the sheet of light-sensitive nerve cells at the back of the eyeball.
Rh factor, an agglutinating substance sometimes found in blood and related to a heritable trait.
rheumatoid arthritis, a form of joint disease associated with marked inflammation.
rheumatic fever, a disease characterized by fever, swollen joints, and frequently by heart involvement.
ringworm of scalp, a fungus infection of the scalp, generally confined to the preadolescent age group.
sanitation, practices assuring freedom from agents or substances capable of causing damage to health.
schizoid personality, dissociative disorder which flattens emotional responses but does not interfere with capacity for self-support and independent life.
sedative, drug used to allay nervous excitement and often also to induce sleep.
semen, a thick, whitish fluid produced by the male reproductive glands and discharged at the height of a male sex climax.
sensitization, process by which the skin or other organs become harmfully reactive to a given substance.

septic tank, a reservoir in a sewage disposal system where bacterial digestion liquefies solid wastes.

sinus, paranasal, air-filled hollow in the facial or cranial bones, communicating with the nasal cavity.

slums, crowded and squalid district.

social, pertaining to the relationship and interaction of one person with others, both as individuals and as groups (this term has almost as many meanings as there are social sciences, and is defined here only in the sense usual to health literature).

sprain, a wrenching injury involving the tearing or disruption of visible fibers in a ligament.

stable emotions, controlled and appropriate emotional responses which do not cause disproportionate discomfort or unwise behavior.

sterilization, (in regard to reproduction) procedure rendering one incapable of further reproduction.

stimulant, a substance which speeds or increases physical and psychological response.

stones, kidney, concretions of insoluble material ranging from a fraction of an inch to several inches in diameter which occasionally form in the urinary tract.

strain, a wrenching injury to ligaments supporting a joint, not involving torn tissue fibers (as a sprain does).

stroke, abruptly beginning malfunction of the brain due to either blocked blood supply or a burst blood vessel.

subconscious, (psych.) within your mind but outside your ken or awareness.

sympathetic nervous system, autonomic nervous system in which nervous connection to and from periphery is interrupted outside the spinal column in semi-independent clumps of cell bodies.

symptomatic alcoholism, alcoholic overindulgence due to underlying mental disease other than psychopathy.

tenement, a squalid apartment building, usually defined as one in which several unrelated families must use the same bathroom facilities.

therapeutic, for treatment of a disorder.

tranquilizer, emotion-soothing drug which does not blunt intellectual functioning or induce sleep in ordinary doses.

tuberculosis, an infection with tubercle bacilli usually involving the lungs and persisting for a considerable period of time.

tumor, a swelling; ordinarily the result of undisciplined cellular growth.

typhoid fever, an infection primarily involving the intestinal tract, but often spreading through the blood stream to cause profound illness, usually spread by contaminated water or milk supplies.

ulcer, open sore which has penetrated one or more layers from an external or internal body surface.

umbilical cord, a long, flexible, jelly-like structure containing the blood vessels which link an unborn baby to the placenta.

ventilation, 1. air movement intended to dissipate or replace foul air, gas, etc.; 2. (psych.) airing of grievances and other emotionally significant experiences through any verbal medium of expression.

INDEX